D1614249

MOTOR NEURON DISEASES

CAUSES, CLASSIFICATION AND TREATMENTS

NEUROLOGY - LABORATORY AND CLINICAL RESEARCH DEVELOPMENTS

Additional books in this series can be found on Nova's website
under the Series tab.

Additional E-books in this series can be found on Nova's website
under the E-book tab.

MOTOR NEURON DISEASES

CAUSES, CLASSIFICATION AND TREATMENTS

BRADLEY J. TURNER

AND

JULIE B. ATKIN

EDITORS

Nova Biomedical Books

New York

Library of Congress Cataloging-in-Publication Data

Motor neuron diseases : causes, classification, and treatments / editors, Bradley James Turner, Julie Atkin.
    p. ; cm.
  Includes bibliographical references and index.
  ISBN 978-1-61470-101-9 (hardcover : alk. paper) 1. Amyotrophic lateral sclerosis. 2. Motor neurons--Diseases. I. Turner, Bradley James. II. Atkin, Julie.
  [DNLM: 1. Motor Neuron Disease--etiology. 2. Motor Neuron Disease--classification. 3. Motor Neuron Disease--therapy. WE 550]
  RC406.A24M685 2011
  616.8'39--dc23
                        2011020018

Published by Nova Science Publishers, Inc. † New York

CONTENTS

Contents

PREFACE

Motor neuron disease (MND), also commonly known as amyotrophic lateral sclerosis (ALS), is a chronic neurodegenerative disorder of the motor system in adults, characterized by the loss of motor neurons in the cortex, brain stem and spinal cord. This book presents current research from across the globe in the study of the causes, classification and treatments of MND, including membrane trafficking defects as determinants of motor neuron susceptibility and degeneration in ALS; motorneuron specific calcium dysregulation and perturbed cellular calcium homeostasis in ALS; stem cells and their application in ALS treatment; excitotoxicity and selective motor neuron degeneration and therapeutic invervention and assistive technology treatments.

Chapter I- Motor Neuron Disease (MND) is the most common chronic neurodegenerative disorder of the motor system in adults. It is a relatively rare disease with a reported population incidence of between 1.5 and 2.5 per 100,000 per year worldwide. The only established risk factors are age and family history, with age being the most important factor. The disease occurs throughout adult life, with the peak incidence between 50 to 75 years of age. MND occurs more commonly in men than in women in a ratio of 3:2. MND is characterized by the loss of motor neurons in the cortex, brain stem, and spinal cord, manifested by upper and lower motor neuron signs and symptoms affecting bulbar, limb, and respiratory muscles. Death usually results from respiratory failure and follows on average two to four years after onset, but some may survive for a decade or more.

Whilst the aetiology of MND is unknown, current evidence suggests that multiple interacting factors contribute to motor neuron injury in MND. The working hypothesis is that MND, like many other chronic diseases, is a complex genetic condition and the relative contribution of individual environmental and genetic factors is likely to be small. The three key pathogenetic hypotheses are genetic factors, oxidative stress and glutamatergic toxicity, which result in damage to critical target proteins such as neurofilaments and organelles such as mitochondria.

The symptoms in MND are diverse and challenging and include weakness, spasticity, limitations in mobility and activities of daily living, communication deficits and dysphagia, and in those with bulbar involvement, respiratory compromise, fatigue and sleep disorders, pain and psychosocial distress. Hence, the burden of disease and economic impact of MND upon patients, their caregivers (often family members) and on society is substantial, often beginning long before the actual diagnosis is made, and increasing with increasing disability and the need for medical equipment and assisted care.

At present, the only approved drug treatment for MND in the USA, Australia and in many European countries is riluzole, which is thought to prolong median survival by about two to three months. In the absence of a cure or indeed any medical intervention, which might stop the progression of MND, the management relies mostly on symptomatic, rehabilitative and palliative therapy, which is the focus of this chapter. An update in the symptomatic and disability management of MND is provided, covering the interface between neurology, rehabilitation and palliative care and incorporates issues encountered over the spectrum of disease, including activity and pain related issues, respiratory and dysphagia issues and psychosocial changes. Recent trends, developments and future research in rehabilitation approaches that maintain and restore functional independence and quality of life will be presented.

Chapter II- Amyotrophic lateral sclerosis (ALS) is characterised by motor neuron death and accumulation of ubiquitinated protein inclusions. Motor neurons are large-calibre and long distance projection excitatory cells with unusually high energetic, synthetic and transport demands required for maintenance and survival. These neurons are therefore likely to be uniquely susceptible to intracellular transport abnormalities in cell bodies and distal axons. Here, we review increasing evidence that motor neuron vulnerability in ALS may be conferred by defects in intracellular trafficking pathways specialised for these cells. Firstly, many of the genes implicated in familial forms of ALS encode molecular machinery or enzymes directly mediating intracellular transport. Secondly, these ALS gene products and additional constituents of trafficking pathways form core components of pathology in familial and sporadic disease. Lastly, defective membrane, vesicle, protein and mRNA transport features prominently and early in motor neuron degeneration in ALS models. We provide a systematic summary of ALS-linked proteins including ALS2, CHMP2B, FIG4, FUS, OPTN, p150Glued, SOD1, TDP-43, VAPB and VCP with respect to their localisation, function and dysfunction in intracellular trafficking pathways, such as anterograde and retrograde axonal transport, endoplasmic-Golgi, endosome-lysosome and nuclear transport. The role of molecular motor-linked proteins such as kinesin, dynein and neurofilaments in motor neurodegeneration will also be addressed. We propose that intracellular membrane trafficking defects affecting key neuronal functions, such as neurotransmission, extracellular signalling and synaptic activity, may be an early determinant of motor neuron loss and common denominator of potentially many ALS-linked proteins.

Chapter III- Amyotrophic lateral sclerosis (ALS) is a fatal neurodegenerative disorder characterized by the selective loss of defined subgroups of motoneuorn populations in the brainstem and spinal cord with signature hallmarks of mitochondrial Ca2+ overload, free radical damage, excitotoxicity and impaired axonal transport. Although intracellular disruptions of cytosolic and mitochondrial calcium and in particular low cytosolic calcium ([Ca2+]i) buffering and a strong interaction between metabolic mechanisms and [Ca2+]i have been associated with selective motoneuron degeneration, the underlying mechanisms are not well understood. The present evidence supports a hypothesis that mitochondria are a primary target of mutant superoxide dismutase1 (mtSOD1)-mediated toxicity in ALS and intracellular alterations of cytosolic and mitochondria-ER microdomain calcium accumulation might aggravate the course of this neurodegenerative disease. Furthermore, chronic excitotoxicity mediated by Ca2+- permeable AMPA and NMDA receptors seems to initiate a vicious cycle of intracellular calcium dysregulation which leads to toxic Ca2+ overload and thereby selective neurodegeneration. Recent advancement in the experimental analysis of calcium signals at high spatiotemporal precision has allowed investigations of calcium regulation in different cell types, in particular selectively vulnerable/resistant cell types in different animal models of this motoneuron disease. This chapter provides an overview of recent advances in this field and discusses in detail what has been learned about Ca2+ homeostasis and the role of mitochondria in motoneurons in pathophysiological conditions such as ALS

Chapter IV- Amyotrophic lateral sclerosis is a devastating neurodegenerative disorder that results in motoneuron loss, paralysis and ultimately death due to respiratory failure within 3-5 years after disease onset. Currently, there is no effective treatment that exists despite the substantial numbers of approaches that are under investigation.

The development of the stem cell field brings promise due to the fact that these cells are self-replenishable and either pluripotent or multipotent and give rise to various cell types. This review will focus on the in vivo applications of these stem cells for ALS treatment. The progress, as well as the advantages and limitations of utilizing each variety of stem cell or their derivatives for ALS treatment, is reviewed in this book chapter. Transplantation of these cells may benefit the diseased tissue by cell replacement therapy or by non-cell replacement functions such as delivery of trophic support. The generation of MNs from stem cells in vitro could enable a significant contribution to cell replacement therapy. However, the need to protect grafted cells highlights the importance of developing an effective trophic therapy.

The recent development of induced pluripotent stem cells and the mobilization of endogenous stem cells shed light on the possibility of autologous treatment. However, several challenges need to be overcome to achieve an effective treatment including timing of transplantation, immune system attack, systematic delivery of the cells and their integration, and especially the hostile environment that would exist in a individual with ALS disease.

Chapter V- A proportion of patients with motor neuron disease (MND) exhibit frontotemporal dementia (FTD) and some patients with FTD develop the clinical features of MND. Frontotemporal lobar degeneration (FTLD) is the pathological substrate of FTD and some forms of this disease (referred to as FTLD-U) share with MND the common feature of ubiquitin-immunoreactive, tau-negative cellular inclusions in the cerebral cortex and hippocampus. Recently, the transactive response (TAR) DNA-binding protein of 43 kDa (TDP-43) has been found to be a major protein of the inclusions of FTLD-U with or without MND and these cases are referred to as FTLD with TDP-43 proteinopathy (FTLD-TDP). To clarify the relationship between MND and FTLD-TDP, TDP-43 pathology was studied in nine cases of FTLD-MND and compared with cases of familial and sporadic FTLD–TDP without associated MND. A principal components analysis (PCA) of the nine FTLD-MND cases suggested that variations in the density of surviving neurons in the frontal cortex and neuronal cytoplasmic inclusions (NCI) in the dentate gyrus (DG) were the major histological differences between cases. The density of surviving neurons in FTLD-MND was significantly less than in FTLD-TDP cases without MND, and there were greater densities of NCI but fewer neuronal intranuclear inclusions (NII) in some brain regions in FTLD-MND. A PCA of all FTLD-TDP cases, based on TDP-43 pathology alone, suggested that neuropathological heterogeneity was essentially continuously distributed. The FTLD-MND cases exhibited consistently high loadings on PC2 and overlapped with subtypes 2 and 3 of FTLD-TDP. The data suggest: FTLD-MND cases have a consistent pathology, variations in the density of NCI in the DG being the major TDP-43-immunoreactive difference between cases, there are considerable similarities in the neuropathology of FTLD-TDP with and without MND, but with greater neuronal loss in FTLD-MND, and FTLD-MND cases are part of the FTLD-TDP 'continuum' overlapping with FTLD-TDP disease subtypes 2 and 3.

Chapter VI- Being a well-establishedand important player in neuronal death, excitotoxicity is a solid basis for understanding selective motor neuron degeneration during amyotrophic lateral sclerosis (ALS). The only available drug for ALS, riluzole, offers patients a moderate increase in survival by targeting this process of excitotoxicity. The overstimulation of glutamate receptors induces calcium influx that leads to detrimental levels of cytosolic calcium, which cause motor neuron loss. Glutamate binds to a number of receptors including the calcium permeable AMPA receptors which facilitate excessive amounts of extracellular calcium to enter the neuron. Glutamate transporters expressed by astrocytes remove this neurotransmitter to limit the effect of glutamate in the synaptic cleft. Interestingly, these processes are impaired or dysregulated in ALS, influencing excitotoxic motor neuron loss. A large number of factors influence excitotoxicity including the inherent characteristics of motor neurons (low intracellular calcium buffering) and their receptors (AMPA receptor subunit combinations), but also their neighbouring cell types, such as astrocytes, play a crucial role. This chapter aims to provide a clear overview of the known players and their interactions and their role in the selective motor neuron loss detected in ALS.

Chapter VII- Amyotrophic lateral sclerosis (ALS) is a neurodegenerative disease where motor neurons within the brain and spinal cord are lost, leading to paralysis and death. Recent studies suggest the involvement of neuronal-glial interactions in ALS pathogenesis where motor neuron degeneration may be due in part to dysfunction of the surrounding astrocyte populations. Stem cells may be able to help in the battle against ALS in many different ways: cell therapy, disease modeling, drug delivery, and drug screening. But how close are we to using these cells to treat ALS? While the obvious use for stem cells would be to make new neurons to replace those that are lost in ALS, a more practical and immediate approach may be to use stem cells to protect the patients' own motor neurons that are undergoing degeneration. Transplantation of different types of stem cells into the spinal cord of either rat or mouse models of ALS have previously resulted in some motor neuron protection and functional improvement. We also demonstrated that transplantation of human stem cells releasing glial cell line-derived neurotrophic factor (GDNF) directly into the spinal cord or skeletal muscle results in robust cellular migration into degenerating regions, efficient delivery of GDNF, and remarkable preservation of host motor neurons. Taken together, ex vivo cell therapy targeting both the skeletal muscles (i.e. nerve terminals of motor neurons) and spinal cord (i.e. cell body) could provide the optimum combination for future human clinical studies.

Chapter VIII- Spinal and bulbar muscular atrophy (SBMA), also known as Kennedy's disease, is an adult-onset, X-linked motor neuron disease characterized by muscle atrophy, weakness, contraction fasciculations and bulbar involvement. SBMA is caused by the expansion of a CAG triplet repeat, encoding a polyglutamine tract within the first exon of the androgen receptor (AR) gene. The histopathological finding in SBMA is the loss of lower motor neurons in the anterior horn of the spinal cord as well as in the brainstem motor nuclei. There is no well-established disease-modifying therapy for SBMA. Animal studies have revealed that the pathogenesis of SBMA depends on the level of serum testosterone, and that androgen deprivation mitigates neurodegeneration through inhibition of nuclear accumulation and/or stabilization of the pathogenic AR. Heat shock proteins, ubiquitin-proteasome system and transcriptional regulation are also potential targets of therapy development for SBMA. Among these therapeutic approaches, androgen deprivation has been translated into clinic. Surgical castration is shown to reverse motor dysfunction in mouse models of SBMA. The luteinizing hormone-releasing hormone analogue, leuprorelin, prevents nuclear translocation of aberrant AR proteins, resulting in a significant improvement of disease phenotype in a mouse model of SBMA. These results of animal studies were verified in a phase 2 clinical trial of leuprorelin, in which the patients treated with this drug exhibited decreased mutant AR accumulation in scrotal skin biopsy and significantly better swallowing parameters than those receiving placebo. An autopsy of one patient who received leuprorelin suggested that androgen deprivation inhibits the nuclear accumulation of mutant AR in the motor neurons of the spinal cord and brainstem. Phase 3 clinical trial showed the possibility that leuprorelin treatment is associated with improved swallowing function particularly in patients with a disease duration less than 10 years. These observations suggest that pharmacological inhibition of the toxic accumulation of mutant AR is a potential therapy for SBMA.

Chapter IX- Motor Neuron Disease (MND) is an adult-onset neurodegenerative disease, which leads to progressive weakness of limb, bulbar and respiratory muscles resulting in death often within three to five years, generally from respiratory failure. The burden of disease of MND upon patients and their caregivers (often family members) is substantial, often beginning long before the actual diagnosis is made, and increasing with worsening disability and the need for medical equipment and assisted care. The course of MND is relentless and in the absence of a cure, management relies mostly on symptomatic, rehabilitative and palliative care. Assistive technology can have a dramatic effect on restoring and maintaining independence, a sense of control and quality of life and is an integral component of the rehabilitative process in the care of persons with MND (pwMND).

The use of assistive technology in MND can be broadly divided into 1) technology that assists with mobility; 2) communication, including computer access, and 3) environmental control units (ECU), with significant overlap and integration amongst the three categories. In a recent stud of 44 pwMND currently receiving multidisciplinary care, limited understanding and availability of assistive technology to facilitate function and decrease reliance on caregivers was identified as an area for improvement. There is a general lack of awareness especially around available environmental control technology even amongst health professionals. It must however also be stressed that, in general, it is essential for patients, families and therapists to work closely together when prescribing and using assistive technology to ensure the correct, safe and optimal use of such aids and equipment; and to anticipate future needs especially with the expense of such technology. Close collaboration with specialised providers of assistive technology that can also supply back-up technical support is also crucial.

Chapter X- Authors reviewed the published documents on application of mechanical ventilation to amyotrophic lateral sclerosis (ALS) patients and analyzed the influential factors of decision making for applying mechanical ventilation by looking into how it is practiced in Japan, the USA, and Europe. In Japan, 29.3% of ALS patients were on invasive ventilation via tracheostomy (TV), 7.2% on non-invasive ventilation (NIV) in 2005. The significant difference in the prevalence of mechanical ventilation was observed among prefectures or hospitals. In the USA, the prevalence rates of TV and NIV were reported to be 3% and 36.2%, respectively, in 2006. NIV is less applied in European nations compared with its usage in Japan and the USA. It is confirmed that the number of patients who choose TV is gradually growing, yet relatively small, in European nations, where an inconsistency in the introduction rate of mechanical ventilation to ALS patients was also observed in accordance with the national, regional and hospital levels. According to the analysis of influential factors in the introduction of mechanical ventilation, it seems that the heavy economic burden is the main factor to decrease the usage rate of mechanical ventilation for ALS patients.

Chapter XI- Unfortunately, the patients with motor neuron disease (MND) might suffer from not only paralytic movements of the body and the limbs, but also motor speech disorder sooner or later during their clinical history. Once speech sound of the patient with MND is affected, progressive course of dysarthria could not only be avoidable, besides but also might be taken away by severely distorted respiratory function. Thus, clinical estimations of the degree and pathophysiological aspects of affected speech sound should be convenient and timely along with the progression of MND. Also the management for the speech disorder of the patient with MND should be considered and coped along with the progression of MND.

In: Motor Neuron Diseases
Editors: Bradley J. Turner and Julie B. Atkin
ISBN: 978-1-61470-101-9
© 2012 Nova Science Publishers, Inc.

Chapter I

MOTOR NEURON DISEASE: CAUSES, CLASSIFICATION AND TREATMENTS

Louisa Ng[*,1,2] *and Fary Khan*[1,2]

[1]Neurological Rehabilitation Physician, Royal Melbourne Hospital,
Parkville, Melbourne VIC 3052, Australia
[2]Department of Rehabilitation Medicine, University of Melbourne, Australia

ABSTRACT

Motor Neuron Disease (MND) is the most common chronic neurodegenerative disorder of the motor system in adults. It is a relatively rare disease with a reported population incidence of between 1.5 and 2.5 per 100,000 per year worldwide. The only established risk factors are age and family history, with age being the most important factor. The disease occurs throughout adult life, with the peak incidence between 50 to 75 years of age. MND occurs more commonly in men than in women in a ratio of 3:2. MND is characterized by the loss of motor neurons in the cortex, brain stem, and spinal cord, manifested by upper and lower motor neuron signs and symptoms affecting bulbar, limb, and respiratory muscles. Death usually results from respiratory failure and follows on average two to four years after onset, but some may survive for a decade or more.

Whilst the aetiology of MND is unknown, current evidence suggests that multiple interacting factors contribute to motor neuron injury in MND. The working hypothesis is that MND, like many other chronic diseases, is a complex genetic condition and the relative contribution of individual environmental and genetic factors is likely to be small. The three key pathogenetic hypotheses are genetic factors, oxidative stress and glutamatergic toxicity, which result in damage to critical target proteins such as neurofilaments and organelles such as mitochondria.

The symptoms in MND are diverse and challenging and include weakness, spasticity, limitations in mobility and activities of daily living, communication deficits and dysphagia, and in those with bulbar involvement, respiratory compromise, fatigue and sleep disorders, pain and psychosocial distress. Hence, the burden of disease and

---

[*] Ph: +61 3 83872000, fax: +61 3 83872222, email: louisa.ng@mh.org.au

economic impact of MND upon patients, their caregivers (often family members) and on society is substantial, often beginning long before the actual diagnosis is made, and increasing with increasing disability and the need for medical equipment and assisted care.

At present, the only approved drug treatment for MND in the USA, Australia and in many European countries is riluzole, which is thought to prolong median survival by about two to three months. In the absence of a cure or indeed any medical intervention, which might stop the progression of MND, the management relies mostly on symptomatic, rehabilitative and palliative therapy, which is the focus of this chapter. An update in the symptomatic and disability management of MND is provided, covering the interface between neurology, rehabilitation and palliative care and incorporates issues encountered over the spectrum of disease, including activity and pain related issues, respiratory and dysphagia issues and psychosocial changes. Recent trends, developments and future research in rehabilitation approaches that maintain and restore functional independence and quality of life will be presented.

1.1. INTRODUCTION

Motor neuron disease (MND), also commonly known as amyotrophic lateral sclerosis (ALS), is a chronic neurodegenerative disorder of the motor system in adults, characterized by the loss of motor neurons in the cortex, brain stem, and spinal cord, manifested by progressive upper and lower motor neuron signs and symptoms affecting bulbar, limb, and respiratory muscles [1]. It was first described by Charcot in the nineteenth century [2] and is also known by the eponym "Lou Gehrig's Disease", after the famous baseball player who was affected with the disease. Death usually results from respiratory failure and follows on average two to four years after onset, but some may survive for a decade or more [3].

MND is a relatively rare disease with a reported population incidence of between 1.5 and 2.5 per 100,000 per year [4] and a prevalence of 2.7-7.4 per 100,000 population [5]. Age is the most important risk factor and the disease occurs throughout adult life, with the peak incidence between 50 to 75 years of age [6]. MND occurs more commonly in men than in women in a ratio of 3:2 [7].

MND is lifelong and persons with MND (pwMND) live with a range of problems that affect every day functional activities. The International Classification of Functioning, Health and Disability (ICF) [8], defines a common language for describing the impact of disease at different levels: impairment (body structure and function), limitation in activity and participation.

Within this framework MND related impairments (weakness, spasticity), can limit 'activity' or function (decreased mobility, self-care, pain) and 'participation' (driving, employment, family, social reintegration). 'Contextual factors', such as environmental (extrinsic) and personal factors (intrinsic) have an impact on the pwMND, their families and the society. MND therefore has personal costs such as reduced quality of life (QoL) and also significant economic costs which may result from increased demand for health care, social services, and caregiver burden.

1.2. IMPACT OF MND

The burden of disease and economic impact of MND upon patients, their caregivers (often family members) and on society is substantial, often beginning long before the actual diagnosis is made, and increasing with increasing disability and the need for medical equipment and assisted care [9]. It has been estimated that basic patient equipment costs (including hospital bed, electric wheelchair, augmentative communication equipment) can cost over USD$40,000 whilst mechanical ventilation costs roughly USD$200,000 a year [9]. These costs do not include earnings loss, therapy costs, and formal and informal care, which often make up the bulk of costs but are often not calculated. Within the Australian healthcare system, provision of care in people with terminal illness largely falls onto informal, unpaid caregivers, usually family and/or friends [10]. In a recent study of Australian pwMND in the community (n=44) [11], 1/3 required help 2-3 times a day for personal care whilst 1/3 required the presence of someone most of the time. A quarter of these 44 pwMND received assistance solely from family. It is therefore not surprising that primary caregivers have been estimated to spend a mean of 9.5 hours a day caring for patients even where there is paid assistance [12]. Whilst the informal care costs for pwMND in the community (by families and others) is not known, these costs account for 43% of total costs in other neurodegenerative conditions [13] (where disability is less marked, such as in multiple sclerosis) and is likely to be as substantial if not more, in MND. Finally, it is well documented that a huge proportion of health care dollars are spent in the last 30 days of a person's life [14]. This is particularly pertinent in a rapidly fatal condition such as MND.

1.3. EPIDEMIOLOGY AND RISK FACTORS

The collection of epidemiological data is challenging due to the low incidence rates of MND. However, the establishment of a number of population-based registers worldwide (mainly in Europe and Australia), has enabled a clearer understanding of MND epidemiology. The incidence and mortality rates of MND have slowly increased over decades [15,16], likely at least partly due to longer life expectancy [17] with improved medical management and supportive care. Incidence rates range between 1.5 and 2.5 per 100,000 per year [4]; whilst prevalence rates range between 2.7-7.4 per 100,000 population [5] which equates to roughly 25,000 in North America [18], 5000 in the UK [19] and 1200 in Australia [20]. The incidence may be higher in Caucasians than in other ethnic groups (African, Asian, Hispanic) but this has been difficult to determine due to methodology variations in studies of non-Caucasian populations [21].

Age and family history are the only well-established risk factors for MND. There is class II evidence that smoking is also a risk factor [22]. Evidence for other risk factors such as physical activity and exposure to heavy metals is conflicting [23-25].

Geographically, the cluster of "Western Pacific ALS" during the 20th century in Guam, the Kii peninsula of Japan and Papua New Guinea has suggested an environmental contribution to MND pathogenesis. However, whilst a number of hypotheses have been proposed, including the dietary consumption of cycad (Cycas circinalis) [26], no definitive cause has been found [27].

The role of genetics is important in MND. Familial MND, more commonly referred to as familial ALS (FALS), accounts for 10% of MND whilst a number of genetic loci have been found to be associated with idiopathic MND (remaining 90%) suggesting genetic susceptibility in pathogenesis [28-30]. At least fifteen chromosomal loci have been linked with familial MND. Familial MND is phenotypically and genetically heterogenous. Majority of familial MND are autosomal dominant in nature and 20% are linked to FALS type 1 or the superoxide dismutase (SOD1) gene [31]. Other autosomal dominant familial MND include FALS types 3 [32], 5 [33], 6 (FUS gene) [34,35], 7 [36], 8 [37], 9 (ANG gene) [38], 10 (TARDBP gene) [39], 11 (FIG4 gene) [40], NF-H gene [41], DAO gene [42], X-linked [43] and MND with FTD [44]. Autosomal recessive familial MND includes FALS 2 [45] and 5 [46].

1.4. Aetiology and Pathogenesis

Although the aetiology of MND remains unknown, current evidence suggests that multiple interacting factors contribute to motor neuron injury in MND. The working hypothesis is that MND, like many other chronic diseases, is a complex genetic condition, and the relative contribution of individual environmental and genetic factors are likely to be relatively small [4]. The three key pathogenetic hypotheses are genetic factors, oxidative stress, and glutamatergic toxicity, which result in damage to critical target proteins such as neurofilaments and organelles such as mitochondria [47-49].

Pathological findings in MND vary depending on the clinical variant. Most patients have the ALS variant where large α-motor neurons in the brainstem and spinal cord degenerate leading to progressive weakness and muscle atrophy whilst loss of upper motor neurones result in spasticity and hyper-reflexia [50]. MND is generally regarded as a multisystem disease -- motor neurons are the earliest and most prominently affected groups of cells but small interneurons in the spinal cord and motor cortex [51], and cortical motor cells are also lost. As a result, retrograde axonal loss and gliosis in the corticospinal tracts occurs, accompanied by involvement of sensory, spinocerebellar pathways and neuropsychological changes [52,53].

Mechanisms of selective motor neuron death are unclear and most current hypotheses are based on animal models [53]. These include: SOD1-mediated toxicity, excitotoxicity, cytoskeletal derangements, mitochondrial dysfunction, apoptosis and others. SOD1 converts superoxide, a toxic by-product of mitochondrial oxidative phosphorylation, to water or hydrogen peroxide. More than 100 mutations are known [31,54,55] and all but one mutation cause dominantly inherited disease. However, how mutant SOD1 leads to motor neuron degeneration is unclear. It is well established though that SOD1-mediated toxicity in MND is not due to loss of function but instead to a gain of toxic properties [56,57] as SOD1 null mice do not develop MND [58]. The role of excitotoxicity in MND is also unclear. The hypothesis is that excessive levels of excitatory neurotransmitter glutamate may initiate a cascade that results in motor neuron death. Lending support to this is the finding that glutamate levels are elevated in a subset of MND patients [59] and that riluzole, an antiglutaminergic drug improves survival in pwMND [60]. Another hypothesis is that SOD1 may induce protein aggregates that are toxic to motor neurons [61]. However, a recent study suggested that accumulation of aggregates were more likely a result of end-stage disease rather than a contributor to MND pathogenesis [62]. Leading on from the abnormal protein aggregation hypothesis however is the cytoskeletal derangement hypothesis. Neurofilament proteins (neuron-specific intermediate filaments) are the most abundant structural protein in mature motor neurons and aggregates of neurofilament proteins are commonly seen in MND. Mitochondrial dysfunction is postulated as another mechanism as mitochrondria in MND patients show abnormal morphology and biochemistry [63].

1.5. CLASSIFICATION

The spectrum of MND can be classified into the following clinical phenotypes:

ALS is the most common form (85%) and includes upper motor neuron (UMN) and lower motor neuron (LMN) pathology.

Progressive muscular atrophy is a progressive LMN disorder and if remains confined to LMN involvement, is consistent with prolonged survival compared with ALS. In the largest study to date (n=962) [64], 91 patients initially diagnosed with progressive muscular atrophy had a longer median survival than 871 patients with ALS (48 versus 36 months). After approximately 80 months, however, the estimated survival in progressive muscular atrophy was about the same as that of ALS. Some individuals with progressive muscular atrophy never develop UMN signs clinically. However, despite the lack of signs, these patients frequently have UMN pathology [65]. In the above study, UMN signs developed in 20 of the 91 patients (22%) initially diagnosed with progressive muscular atrophy [64]. This generally occurs within two years of symptom onset.

Primary lateral sclerosis is a progressive UMN disorder. It progresses the slowest and has the longest survival compared to the other phenotypes [66]. It is also characterized by lack of weight loss, and absence of LMN findings on examination or electromyography in the first four years after symptom onset [67]. Although some individuals never develop clinical LMN signs, most do later in their clinical course [68]. There have been case reports however, of pathological findings of isolated UMN involvement [69].

Progressive bulbar palsy is a progressive UMN and LMN disorder affecting the cranial muscles. Occasionally, only bulbar involvement is seen but more commonly, UMN and LMN signs and symptoms spread to involve other areas (bulbar-onset MND).

The flail arm syndrome is characterized by progressive severe LMN weakness and wasting mainly affecting the arms (particularly proximally). There is a 9:1 male predominance [7] and these patients have a slower rate of progression both to the spread of signs and symptoms in other body segments and to development of respiratory muscle weakness [70].

The flail leg syndrome is characterized by progressive LMN weakness and wasting in the distal leg. These patients also have a slower rate of progression to involvement of other body segments and to the development of respiratory muscle weakness [70].

It is now clear that a proportion of MND patients have additional features such as frontotemporal dementia, autonomic insufficiency, parkinsonism, supranuclear gaze paresis, and/or sensory loss. These patients may be considered to have "ALS plus syndrome" [7].

1.6. DIAGNOSIS

The diagnosis of MND is clinical and includes the presence of UMN and LMN signs, progression of disease and the absence of an alternative explanation. There is no single diagnostic test at present that can confirm or entirely exclude the diagnosis of MND. Clinicians rely mainly on clinical history and examination, supported by electrodiagnostic studies and negative findings in neuroimaging and laboratory studies. Clinically, asymmetric limb weakness is the most common presentation (80%). In upper limb onset, patients may report difficulty with fine-motor tasks such as buttoning or writing. In lower limb onset, patients may report issues resulting from foot drop, such as tripping whilst walking or running. Bulbar onset is next most common (25%) with reports of slurred speech or swallowing difficulties. Occasionally, pain and muscle cramping, fatigue, weight loss, dyspnoea or other respiratory symptoms may be the initial symptoms [71]. Physical findings may confirm UMN involvement (weakness, spasticity, hyperreflexia, slowness of movement, extensor plantar responses) and LMN involvement (fasciculations, muscle wasting, weakness). Electrodiagnostic studies involve electromyography (EMG) and nerve conduction studies. EMG aids identification of LMN loss – the most frequently recognised abnormalities on EMG are fasciculation and spontaneous "denervation" discharges (fibrillation potentials and positive sharp waves) [72]. Nerve conduction studies are important to exclude differential diagnoses. Motor conduction block should be absent in MND and motor and sensory conduction velocity and compound motor action potentials should be (almost) normal in both arm and leg [73]. Differential diagnoses are shown in Box 1.1.

Box 1.1. Differential diagnoses of MND [71]

Disorders that focally involve the spinal cord
• cervical and lumbar spondylosis
• multiple sclerosis, syringomyelia
• tumours
• aterio-venous malformations
• infarction
• congenital dysplasias of the brainstem of spinal cord
Neurogenic and myogenic diseases with LMN symptoms similar to MND
• multifocal motor neuropathy with conduction block
• postpoliomyelities
• muscular atrophy
• Kennedy's disease
• paraneoplastic neuropathy
• inclusion body myositis
Others
• myasthenia gravis
• heavy metal intoxication
• hyperthyroidism
• hyperparathyroidism
• Joseph disease
• hexosaminidase A deficiency

The list of differential diagnoses is rather extensive, yet most other diagnoses can be ruled out through careful history, physical examination, and selective diagnostic testing, which may include MRI of the brain and spine, electrodiagnostic studies, complete blood count, serum chemistries, and thyroid function tests. Heavy metal screen is indicated only if there has been exposure. Antiganglioside antibodies (GM1 antibodies) may be helpful in the setting of multifocal conduction block [71]. The (Revised) El Escorial World Federation of Neurology criteria [74,75] were designed for research purposes but allow an assignment of diagnostic certainty (see box 1.2 and 1.3).

Box 1.2. El Escorial criteria for the diagnosis of MND/ALS [74]

The diagnosis of MND/ALS requires:

A. the presence of:

(A:1) evidence of LMN degeneration by clinical, electrophysiological or neuropathologic examination,

(A:2) evidence of UMN degeneration by clinical examination, and

(A:3) progressive spread of symptoms or signs within a region or to other regions, as determined by history or examination, together with

B. the absence of:

(B:1) electrophysiological and pathological evidence of other disease processes that might explain the signs of LMN and/or UMN degeneration, and

(B:2) neuroimaging evidence of other disease processes that might explain the observed clinical and electrophysiological signs.

Box 1.3. Diagnostic categories based on El Escorial criteria for the diagnosis of MND/ALS [74,75]

Clinically Definite ALS: is defined on clinical evidence alone by the presence of UMN, as well as LMN signs, in three regions.

Clinically Probable ALS: is defined on clinical evidence alone by UMN and LMN signs in at least two regions with some UMN signs necessarily rostral to (above) the LMN signs.

The terms Clinically Probable ALS - Laboratory-supported and Clinically Possible ALS are used to describe these categories of clinical certainty on clinical and laboratory criteria or only clinical criteria:

Clinically Probable - Laboratory-supported ALS: is defined when clinical signs of UMN and LMN dysfunction are in only one region, or when UMN signs alone are present in one region, and LMN signs defined by EMG criteria are present in at least two limbs, with proper application of neuroimaging and clinical laboratory protocols to exclude other causes.

Clinically Possible ALS: is defined when clinical signs of UMN and LMN dysfunction are found together in only one region or UMN signs are found alone in two or more regions; or LMN signs are found rostral to UMN signs and the diagnosis of Clinically Probable - Laboratory-supported ALS cannot be proven by evidence on clinical grounds in conjunction with electrodiagnostic, neurophysiologic, neuroimaging or clinical laboratory studies. Other diagnoses must have been excluded to accept a diagnosis of Clinically possible ALS.

Clinically Suspected ALS: it is a pure LMN syndrome, wherein the diagnosis of ALS could not be regarded as sufficiently certain to include the patient in a research study. Hence, this category is deleted from the revised El Escorial Criteria for the Diagnosis of ALS.

In clinical practice however, the El Escorial criteria are too stringent; as a result early MND is missed and 25% of patients may die from MND without ever meeting the criteria [76,77]. In 2006, a consensus meeting held at Awaji-shima aimed to resolve these issues by recognising the equivalence of clinical and EMG data in detecting chronic neurological change, thus integrating EMG and clinical neurophysiological data into an algorithm [78]. The application of the 'Awaji algorithm' to the revised El Escorial diagnostic criteria for diagnosis of MND appears to increase the sensitivity of the El Escorial criteria for MND diagnosis (95% sensitivity vs 18% using clinical El Escorial criteria and 53% combining clinical and EMG El Escorial criteria)[79] without losing specificity [80]. This increased sensitivity applies in particular to bulbar onset patients (sensitivity improved from 38% to 87%) and for patients with El Escorial "clinically possible ALS" (from 50% to 86%) [78].

1.7. MEASUREMENT TOOLS

There are a number of outcome measurement tools used in MND. They can be broadly divided using the ICF framework [8] into those that measure impairment and activity limitation ("disability") and those that measure participation limitation ("handicap") and quality of life. There is often overlap, however, in the domains as most outcome measures precede the introduction of the ICF framework. Some measures are MND-specific whilst others are generic.

A range of impairment and activity limitation measurement tools are listed in box 1.4. The Amyotrophic Lateral Sclerosis Functional Rating Scale (ALSFRS) is currently the most commonly used. It was developed to enable measurement of a broader range of "disabilities" and minimise inclusion of impairment measurements to allow analysis of disability components [81], and was revised in 1999 to incorporate assessments of respiratory function [82]. The revised version is a 48-point measure with excellent validity and reliability, and can be administered over the phone [83]. It is determined by scoring 0-4 for each of the twelve domains (speech, salivation, swallowing, handwriting, cutting food and handling utensils, dressing and hygiene, turning in bed and adjusting bed clothes, walking, climbing stairs, dyspnoea, orthopnea and respiratory insufficiency). A lower score indicates more disability.

Box 1.4. Impairment and activity limitation measurement tools used in MND

Generic measures [84]
Functional Independence Measure [85]
Barthel Index [86]
Rehabilitation Activities Profile [87]
Frenchay Activities Index [88]
MND-specific measures
Norris Amyotrophic Lateral Sclerosis Scale [89]
Appel Amyotrophic Lateral Sclerosis Scale [90]
ALS Severity Scale [91]
Amyotrophic Lateral Sclerosis Functional Rating Scale [92]

Participation limitation is a significant issue from the perspective of pwMND and their caregivers [11], yet it is poorly covered by existing outcome measurement tools. Given the relentlessly progressive and fatal nature of MND, quality of life is one of the most important areas to address in MND. However, quality of life is a broad concept, and not easily incorporated in a single outcome measurement. Most outcome measures are generic and may not be sensitive to changes specific to a rapidly progressive condition such as MND. Within the generic measurement tools, some measure health-related status (for example, SF-36 or Sickness Impact Profile) whilst others are more specific for measurement of quality of life [eg. McGill Quality of Life Questionnaire, direct-weight version of the Schedule of the Evaluation of Individual Quality of Life (SEIQoLDW)] [93]. The SEIQoLDW [94] is useful as it can be used for both patients and their caregivers. However, this scale is time intensive [95] and whilst it may be of great value in identifying those factors which contribute to the psychosocial well-being of an individual with MND, it does not necessarily reflect aggregate quality of life in pwMND [96]. Although measures specific for MND, such as the ALSAQ-40 [97] have been developed for use, they have yet to be widely taken up. Some are heavily weighted towards physical function (e.g. ALSAQ-40) and do not include an existential element (perception of purpose, meaning of life, capacity for personal growth) relevant for pwMND [93]. Recently, a modified version of the McGill questionnaire was validated as an MND-specific quality of life questionnaire (the ALSSQOL) [98], and a shortened version is currently undergoing validation in a multi-centre study.

Choice of outcome measures is a significant issue in MND clinical trials. The outcome measures used may not capture the entire spectrum of issues in MND, nor reflect change adequately. Whilst survival is clinically important and easy to measure, there are several reasons to consider use of other outcomes [99]. Survival can be influenced by many interventions that do not clearly alter disease progression, such as enteral feeding [100]. The use of survival as an endpoint also mandates large trials that treat patients for long periods of time, thus very few patients will experience the event being measured [99]. Most importantly, the objective of many trials is not to alter the underlying pathology of disease but to reduce symptoms and limitations at the level of activity and participation, and to improve quality of life, hence outcome measures should address these domains.

1.8. PHARMACOLOGICAL MANAGEMENT

Riluzole is the only drug that has been shown to prolong survival (by about two to three months) [60]. Although the precise mechanism of action in MND is unclear [101], riluzole is thought to reduce glutamate-induced excitotoxicity by inhibiting glutamic acid release, blocking NMDA-receptor mediated responses and by direct action on the voltage-dependent sodium channel [102].

A dose of 100mg daily is reasonably safe. The elimination half-life is 12 hours and the recommended dosing is 50mg twice daily. Riluzole is generally well tolerated and the most significant adverse effects are gastrointestinal and hepatic. These are mostly reversible after stopping the drug.

Costs of riluzole are relatively high (approximately $10,000/year in the US)[60] and it is approved only in select countries (eg. USA, Australia, Canada and many European countries).

Current guidelines [103,104] recommend treatment as soon as possible after diagnosis with the following criteria predicting those most likely to benefit: "definite or probable ALS" by El Escorial criteria, symptoms present for less than five years, vital capacity of greater than 60% of predicted and no tracheostomy.

Unproven treatments are an area of increasing interest to physicians and patients alike. It has been estimated that almost 80% of patients take high-dose vitamins, minerals, or other nutriceuticals despite no proof of benefits for any of these in MND (only creatine and vitamin E have been examined for efficacy) [105]. Whilst many drugs have shown promise in preclinical trials, to date none have proven to be of benefit in MND (apart from riluzole) in human clinical trials (see Table 1.1) [106]. A frequently updated list can be found on the ALS Association website (www.alsa.org).

Table 1.1. Drug treatments with unproven outcomes in MND (adapted from [104])

No benefit observed:
– N-Acetylcysteine
– Ciliary neurotrophic factor (CNTF)
– Verapamil
– Gabapentin
– Topiramate
– Lamotrigine
– Celecoxib
– Minocycline [107]
– Coenzyme Q10 [108]
– Insulin-like growth factor (IGF-1)
– Selegiline
– Vitamin E
– Creatine monohydrate
In trial phase:
– Arimoclomol
– Ceftriaxone
– Gene therapy
– Lithium*
– Pramipexole
– Talampanel
– Memantine

*A recent double-blind randomized controlled trial in the United States and Canada was stopped early for futility and it is likely that lithium will not demonstrate therapeutic benefit [109].

Although some of these drugs are currently available for other indications, off-label use in MND is not recommended for a number of reasons [110] including:

- Lack of intensive safety measures outside of a clinical trial. For example, information showing poor outcomes for treated patients in the minocycline and topiramate trials became apparent only after grouped data were studied.

- Using an off-label medication during the conduct of a clinical trial can impede or slow enrolment in a trial, which has the effect of increasing risk to subjects in the trial.

There is also a range of treatments other than drugs with variable safety profiles from "benign" nutritional supplements to potentially dangerous therapies such as chelation, dental amalgam removal, or administration of unknown substances said to be stem cells [110].

MND is a life-threatening disease, but clearly some treatments can reduce quality or length of life; hence it is critical for patients to be given the information they need to avoid these [110].

1.9. MULTIDISCIPLINARY CARE

1.9.1. Definition of Multidisciplinary Care in MND

With no cure currently available, the challenge in MND is to prolong independence, prevent complications and optimise quality of life. This is best met by a multidisciplinary team with a focus on symptomatic, rehabilitative and palliative care [103,104]. The multidisciplinary team (see figure 1.1) comprises of a group of clinical professionals with expertise in MND, directed by a physician, who work as an integrated unit to provide seamless care which is patient-centered, flexible and responsive to the evolving nature of the condition [111], and aims to maximise activity and participation. The literature presented in this review includes all levels of evidence for multidisciplinary care of MND (including randomised and clinical controlled trials, case studies and expert opinion).

1.9.2. Evidence for Multidisciplinary Care in MND

A recent Cochrane review [112] found that in the absence of randomised controlled trials, the 'best' evidence to date (based on five observational studies) suggests some advantage for quality of life without increasing healthcare costs, reduced hospitalisation and improved disability. The evidence for survival is conflicting. However, the absence of proof that multidisciplinary care is effective must not be interpreted as proof that this approach is ineffective. There are multiple, well-defined interventions, such as nutritional support and respiratory support, and interventions by physical, occupational and speech therapists which have individually had significant impact on disease course. Hence, the gap in available trial data showing efficacy when offered simultaneously in a multidisciplinary setting should not at all implicate therapeutic nihilism in the treatment of MND.

1.9.3. Applying the ICF Framework to Multidisciplinary Care in MND

Rehabilitation is defined as 'a problem solving educational process aimed at reducing disability and increasing participation experienced by someone as a result of disease or injury' [113]. Although it is sometimes effective in reducing impairment, its principal focus is to reduce symptoms and limitations at the level of activity and participation, through holistic interventions, which incorporate personal and environmental factors. The rehabilitation perspective is much broader than the 'medical' perspective, and emphasizes the understanding that a person's health and functioning is associated with a condition or disease, and not merely a consequence of it. The rehabilitation model works well with the World Health Organization's ICF framework [114], which is multifaceted. It includes the perspectives of the physicians with regards to the management of complex and interacting symptoms in MND, the therapists' views in terms of managing change in functional status in activities of everyday living and importantly, also the perspective of the pwMND and their caregivers, which may differ from the others.

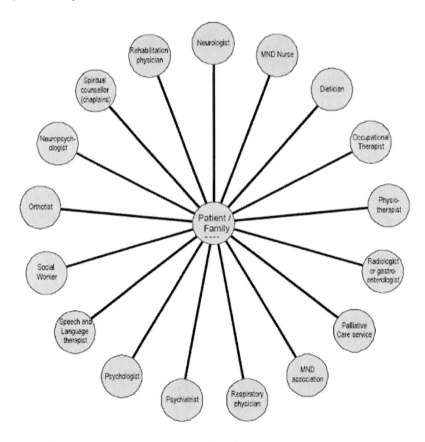

Figure 1.1. The multidisciplinary team in MND (adapted from [111]).

The aim of the ICF classification system is to provide a common language and framework for the description of health and health-related states. The domains in the ICF are divided into a) Body Functions and Structures; and b) Activities and Participation. These terms replace the previously used terms 'impairments' and 'handicap'. The ICF domains for people with a health condition such as MND describe what a pwMND can do or does do. 'Functioning' is an umbrella term encompassing all body functions, activities and participation; similarly 'Disability' includes impairments, activity limitations or restriction in participation. The ICF acknowledges that environmental factors (physical, social and attitudinal environment in which people live and conduct their lives) and personal factors (intrinsic influences such as self-efficacy, positive adaptation) interact with all the other constructs within the ICF (see figure 1.2).

A pwMND can therefore present to rehabilitation with various combinations of deficits, which can be classified according to the ICF:

- "Impairments" are problems with body (anatomical) structures or (physiological) function (such as weakness, spasticity, dysphagia).
- "Activity limitation" (disability) describes the difficulties that a person may have in executing everyday tasks (reduced mobility and self care, pain).
- "Restriction in participation" relates to problems experienced by a person with involvement in societal participation and life situations (driving, work, family,
- psychosocial activities).
- "Contextual factors" include:
  o 'environmental' factors (such as access to medical care); and
  o 'personal factors' including gender, race, self-efficacy, coping style and social and educational background.

All these constructs combine to affect the person's experience of living with their condition.

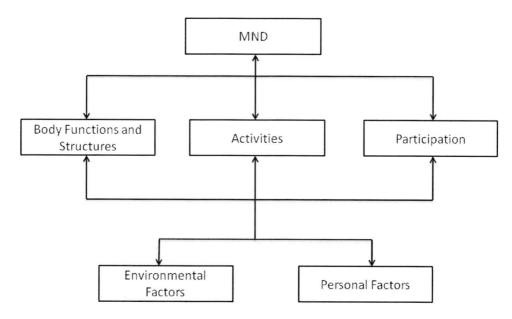

Figure 1.2. The interactions between the various components of the ICF (adapted from [114]).

The ICF can be used to further facilitate and optimise clinical care through the development of "core sets". These are ICF categories selected by experts (patients, caregivers, clinicians) that list issues in impairment, disability, participation environmental factors that need to be addressed in multidisciplinary care settings. This has been done in other neurological conditions such as stroke [115], multiple sclerosis [116] and Guillain-Barré syndrome [117]. A set of relevant ICF categories has not been identified in MND and would be very useful in both clinical and research settings given the rare incidence of MND and diverse and challenging nature of the symptoms. It has also been highlighted that current outcome measures do not capture the entire spectrum of issues in MND (see section 1.7 Measurement Tools); use of the ICF could contribute towards development of appropriate outcome measures for MND.

1.9.4. Service Models and Standards: Interface between Neurology, Rehabilitation and Palliative Care

MND is a 'progressive' long-term neurological condition. The symptoms in MND are diverse and challenging and include: weakness, spasticity, imitations in mobility and activities of daily living, communication deficits and dysphagia, respiratory compromise, fatigue and sleep disorders, pain and psychosocial distress [1]. The National Service Framework [118] was developed by the department of Health in the UK to provide quality requirements for the inspection authorities (the Healthcare Commission and the Commission for Social Care Inspection) to use in measuring local progress for long-term neurological conditions. It advocates the need for integrated care and joined-in services in the delivery of multidisciplinary care. Included within its guidelines are 11 Quality Requirements, which make recommendations for specialist neurology, rehabilitation, and palliative care services to support pwMND to the end of their lives. The interface between neurology, rehabilitation and palliative care ensures co-ordinated care for pwMND rather than duplicating services.

Current guidelines [103] state that specialized multidisciplinary clinical referral should be considered for pwMND to enable optimal health care delivery. However, even within multidisciplinary clinics, there is a shortfall in service provision from the perspective of pwMND and their caregivers. A recent study (n=44 pwMND, n=37 caregivers of pwMND) [11] showed that despite a universal health system (Medicare) and accessibility to a specialised MND multidisciplinary clinic, gaps included a) the limited understanding and availability of assistive technology to facilitate function and decrease reliance on caregivers, b) advice regarding employment and driving and c) limited psychosocial support from the caregivers' perspective. In a different study also based in Australia (patient n=503, caregiver n=373) comparing the extent to which existing supportive service models met the needs of four neurodegenerative disorders (MND, multiple sclerosis, Parkinsons' disease, Huntington's disease), the caregivers of pwMND reported the lowest quality of life and were most distressed by fatigue and tiredness [119].

The gaps in service most likely relate to a) variations in service by local community providers compounded by the absence of care by rehabilitation or palliative care physicians, b) lack of consensus about what issues should be addressed in multidisciplinary care programs for pwMND that incorporates the patients', caregivers', and treating clinicians' perspective and c) poor understanding of allied health roles. The healthcare needs of pwMND can be difficult to determine due to variable MND disease severity and progression. The limitations in activity and participation can be subjective and are not always easy to quantify with the differing perspectives of the pwMND, their caregiver, treating health professionals and by the community as a whole. The 'insider' lived experience of disablement is important in the context of providing effective clinical care. Information from such insights can guide service policy, planning, development and resource utilization. Use of the ICF for this purpose has been discussed in Section 1.9.3.

The recent guidelines for persons with long-term neurological conditions (including MND) recommend the interface between neurology, rehabilitation and palliative care to address the diagnostic, restorative and palliative phases of illness [120]. Neurologists assess, diagnose and manage disease. Involvement of palliative care physicians at an earlier stage of disease is important for management of distressing symptoms (such as nausea, vomiting and breathlessness). While rehabilitation physicians can contribute to care by assisting with disability management and adaptive equipment provision (such as strategies and aids for communication, mobility and ability to perform activities of daily living; procedures for spasticity, pain control; and behaviour management), they can struggle as disease advances, while palliative care teams may struggle at stages where disease is not advancing. These issues may be addressed by cross-referral and closer collaboration between different services.

A proposed model for service interaction in caring for persons with MND shows involvement of neurologists and palliative care teams in the acute and terminal phases of care, with a relatively smaller role for rehabilitation physicians. However rehabilitation plays a major role in long-term care and support (over years) in the more slowly progressive phase [120].

Early rehabilitation intervention and treatment has much to contribute to improve health and quality of life prior to accumulation of disability through symptomatic and supportive therapies to enhance functional independence and community integration and reduce barriers (such as lack of knowledge about treatment, economic constraints) [121]. Disability management in MND should also be planned, with deficits should be anticipated (over time) to avoid 'crisis management'. Early palliative care intervention too has much to offer particularly in symptom management, respite care, and in addressing the psychological and spiritual issues that have been shown to have a greater bearing on quality of life in MND than physical functioning. An earlier palliative care referral allows the development of a relationship of trust while communication is generally easier, and mutual education and support of treating physicians and other disciplines in issues around communication and dying [122].

As patients deteriorate the rehabilitation and palliative care approaches can overlap, i.e. 'neuropalliative rehabilitation'. Key skills in neuropalliative rehabilitation include: understanding disease progression, symptom control, managing expectations, issues relating to communication, addressing end of life issues, legal issues (mental capacity, wills), specialist interventions (ventilation), equipment needs, counselling and support, and welfare advice [120].

The gaps and deficiencies in MND care and services need to be addressed by collaborative work practice - clinicians need to respect others with expertise in related areas; co-ordination should occur between services; communication between specialties and between specialist and local services needs to improve [123,124].

1.10. Multidisciplinary Care Issues in MND

MND is a fatal disease with a challenging progressive course that results in a broad and ever-changing spectrum of care needs. Symptoms are varied (see box 1.5) and need to be carefully assessed and managed. The timing of provision of appropriate care is important as whilst information needs to be provided when patients are psychologically in the right frame of mind, the options of certain interventions may be time-limited as the disease continues to progress.

Box 1.5. Symptoms experienced by MND patients (adapted from [125])

Weakness 94%
Dysphagia 90%
Dyspnoea 85%
Pain 73%
Weight loss 71%
Speech issues 71%
Constipation 54%
Cough 48%
Sleep issues 29%
Emotional lability 27%
Drooling 25%

1.10.1. Respiratory Management

Most deaths in MND are due to respiratory failure as a consequence of respiratory muscle weakness, hence the diagnosis and management of respiratory symptoms is important (figure 1.3) [105]. Counselling may be initiated at the time of diagnosis especially if respiratory symptoms are present and/or forced vital capacity (FVC) is <60% of predicted. Early symptoms may be suggestive of nocturnal hypoventilation (eg. frequent arousals, morning headaches, excessive daytime sleepiness, vivid dreams) rather than overt dyspnoea [105]. It is important to discuss the options of respiratory choices, including tracheostomy and ventilatory support well before these are clinically indicated to enable advance planning or directives. It is also important to offer patients information about the terminal stages of MND and reassure regarding terminal hypercapnoeic coma and resulting peaceful death, as many may fear "choking to death" [126].

Respiratory function should be evaluated every three months from the time of diagnosis. Whilst FVC is the most commonly used [127] and significantly predicts survival [128], it can be insensitive to slight changes in muscle strength [129]. The maximal inspiratory pressure (MIP) also requires a mouthpiece. The maximal sniff nasal inspiratory force or sniff nasal pressure (SNP) may be more appropriate especially in those with bulbar weakness (no mouthpiece) and has been found to be more sensitive to changes in diaphragmatic and respiratory muscle strength [130,131]. It is also more reliably recorded in the later stages of MND and is more sensitive, although less specific than FVC for predicting six-month mortality [132].

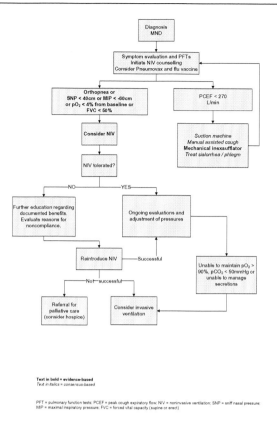

Figure 1.3. Respiratory management algorithm in MND (adapted from [105]).

Initial management can include chest physiotherapy and postural drainage, especially if the patient has difficulty clearing secretions from the chest [133]. A suction machine may also be helpful for this purpose. Preventing respiratory infections is a primary goal and pneumococcal and influenza vaccines should be administered. Respiratory muscle exercise can be instituted and may delay the onset of ventilatory failure [134].

Non-invasive ventilation (NIV) should be considered for patients with respiratory insufficiency (see figure 1.3 for criteria) and is especially helpful overnight for symptomatic nocturnal respiratory compromise although it is also often used in addition, during the day as the disease progresses. A recent Cochrane review concluded that NIV significantly improves quality of life when tolerated and may prolong survival in those with normal to moderately impaired bulbar function especially if used for $\geq$ 4 hours a day [135]. Successful use of NIV is dependent on respiratory therapists and patients working closely and patiently through the adjustment phase of NIV, especially with selection and tolerance of face masks. A small dose of anxiolytic may assist with the process in select patients. Bulbar involvement and executive dysfunction may also impact negatively on compliance [105].

Invasive ventilation should be offered when longer-term survival is the goal. Careful counselling is necessary with regards to benefits and burden (expense, intensive physical support with suctioning and nursing care, high caregiver burden) as many may not be able to manage invasive ventilation at home, thus requiring residential care (nursing home) placement [105,136]. Not all residential facilities manage invasive ventilation, which might further restrict options of placement. Approximately 10-20% of pwMND elect invasive ventilation. However, of those who do undergo invasive ventilation (including those administered at the time of acute respiratory failure without advance discussion), there appears to be good acceptance and satisfactory quality of life [137].

1.10.2. Communication

Dysarthria is common as a result of bulbar involvement and can be a source of significant frustration to the pwMND and their families. Early changes include nasality or reduced vocal volume and changes in oral movement rates and speech rates [138]. As weakness and spasticity of the oral and laryngeal muscles increase, imprecise consonant production, hypernasality, harsh vocal quality, slowed rate of speech and breath volumes affect intelligibility [139]. Speech pathologists can teach the patient to slow speech rate, exaggerate articulation and improve respiratory efficiency through phrasing [1]. Palatal lift and palatal augmentation prostheses may also be of some use to reduce the hypernasal aspect of dysarthria [140]. As intelligibility worsens, augmentation of communication may be achieved with devices ranging from simple pen and paper or alphabet/word communication boards to more high-tech keyboard-based and computerised instruments. Environmental control units that use movement input from any part of the body (eg. eye gaze) can be used in very advanced disease [141]. Whilst some of these devices can be expensive, they help the patient and caregivers stay connected, respond to their need and discuss complex important issues, including medical information [142]. For those who have no voluntary motor control for communication, brain-computer interface that use electroencephalogram signals are being researched [143].

1.10.2. Swallowing and Nutrition

Dysphagia affects a third of pwMND at onset and the majority by late disease [144]. It increases the risk of suboptimal caloric and fluid intake and can worsen weakness and fatigue [145]. Aspiration pneumonia (13%) is a contributor to respiratory complications and is associated with increased mortality with mean survival time post-infection of 2 months [146].

More than 50% of pwMND report difficulties in the oral preparatory stage of swallowing (preparation of food for propulsion to the pharynx) [147]. Symptoms include jaw weakness, fatigue, drooling, choking on food and slow eating. In addition, loss of upper limb function and fear of choking or depression can further impact on self-feeding abilities and oral intake [148]. A speech pathologist can perform a bed-side assessment and/or further imaging (eg videofluroscopy) to evaluate the degree of dysphagia. Mild dysphagia can be managed with specific interventions such a alteration of food consistency, upright positioning, small bolus size, soft collar for neck extensor weakness and the chin-tuck technique, in which the person flexes their neck to the anterior chest wall as they swallow, narrowing the inlet to the larynx and reducing the chance of food aspiration. Dieticians monitor nutritional status through body weight, percentage weight loss and body mass index. Common advice includes high calorie diets, texture modification and prescription of nutritional supplements [149]. Patients may show nutritional compromise even before bulbar symptoms become significant [148] as in addition to muscle wasting, pwMND at all stages of disease often do not meet their energy requirements [150]. Dehydration is also a common and important problem contributing to fatigue and thickened secretions [1].

As dysphagia progresses, evidence (Level B) suggests a percutaneous endoscopic gastrostomy (PEG) or equivalent (eg. radiologically inserted gastrostomy) is indicated to supplement oral intake (as long as this remains safe) for weight maintenance [151]. PEGs prolong survival but there is currently little evidence regarding the impact of PEG on quality of life [100]. Timing of a PEG can be challenging. Weight loss (a loss of 5-10% of body weight implies nutritional risk [1]) and FVC should be considered (PEGs should be placed before FVC falls below 50% of predicted [152] as risks of largyngeal spasm, localized infection, gastric haemorrhage, technical difficulties of PEG placement and respiratory arrest increase [153,154]).

Sialorrhoea can be a significant issue in MND and is generally not related to increased saliva production but rather to impaired ability to swallow saliva, combined with facial weakness causing labial incompetence and neck weakness causing the head to tip forward [1]. Improved positioning, use of a cervical collar and orolingual exercises may be helpful. Medications such as anticholinergics and tricyclics can also be trialled [155], as can suction machines. In the US, most commonly used medications are amitriptyline, glycopyrrolate, atropine and propantheline [156]. However, medications may further thicken secretions, hence should be used with caution in those with respiratory insufficiency or poor cough. More recently, botulinum toxin injected into the salivary glands (parotid, submandibular) appears to be safe and has been used to treat sialorrhea with beneficial effects lasting approximately 3 months [157,158]. Thick oropharyngeal secretions may be treated with increased fluid intake, humidification of air, cough augmentation, suction machines and guaifenesin [156].

1.10.3. Exercise

The effects of exercise and safe therapeutic range in MND are poorly understood. It is generally accepted that weakness and muscle fibre degeneration may be accelerated by overwork or heavy exercise as it is already functioning close to its maximal limits [159]. However, inactivity leads to deconditioning and disuse weakness. In addition, muscle and joint spasticity can cause pain, contractures and further loss of function. A recent Cochrane review [160] identified two trials (n = 52), which addressed therapeutic exercise in MND. The trials examined the effects of moderate intensity, endurance type exercise on spasticity, and effects of moderate intensity resistance type exercises in MND. Although one of the trials reported improvement in function and quality of life, both trials were too small to determine to what extent strengthening exercises were beneficial or harmful in this population [160]. In view of the paucity of evidence to guide exercise prescription, the current recommendations are [161]:

- Stretching exercise to improve flexibility to maintain muscle length and joint mobility and prevent contractures.
- Strengthening exercise of sub-maximal (low, non-fatiguing) intensity, with degree of resistance tailored to muscle strength.

- Aerobic/endurance exercise may improve cardio-respiratory fitness and is probably safe but adequate oxygenation, aeration and carbohydrate load is important to reduce oxidative stress load.

1.10.4. Mobility and Activities of Daily Living

In early stages of disease, rehabilitation aims to prolong independence in mobility and activities of daily living, prevent complications such as falls, contractures, and musculoskeletal pain, maintain strength, range of movement and conditioning through an appropriate exercise program, educate the patient and family about the disease, provide psychological support, evaluate the home for safety and teach energy conservation techniques [162].

As weakness worsens, the physiotherapist can instruct the patient and family in safe transfer techniques (eg. between bed and chair, in and out of cars), optimise gait pattern and provide gait re-training with appropriate gait aids (eg. walking frame, sticks) and orthoses (ankle-foot orthosis to facilitate foot clearance during gait and stabilise knee to prevent falls). Occupational therapists can fabricate with upper limb orthoses to assist with fine motor function. For example, patients with distal weakness can improve hand function with wrists braced in 30° extension which improves efficiency of grip and addition of a universal cuff can assist those with weak grasp in feeding and typing [1]. Other adaptive equipment is also provided, such as built-up cutlery for eating, Velcro fasteners for dressing, long-handled aids, and bathroom equipment (rails, over-the-toilet frames, bath boards, shower chairs, commodes).

Wheelchairs are generally eventually required although introduction of a wheelchair whilst a patient is still ambulant, for intermittent community use, is important to enhance energy conservation. Future needs should be anticipated and considered when prescribing a powered wheelchair (eg. reclining, tilt-in-space, custom seating, and modifiable control system) to optimise independence and social interaction whilst preventing contractures, compression nerve palsies, skin breakdown and aspiration. A motorised scooter may be more appropriate for some patients [1]. Other equipment such as hospital beds with pressure-relieving mattress and hoists for lifting might also be required. Caregiver training in the use of hoists is important to prevent injury.

1.10.5. Bladder, Bowel and Sexuality

Although bowel and bladder sphincters are generally spared, bowel, bladder and sexual dysfunction may be much more common (30%) than reported to health professionals by pwMND [11,163]. These areas are in general poorly studied in MND. Constipation is likely to be common with inactivity and poor nutritional intake and can be treated with a regular bowel program with intake of fibre/bulking agents and adequate fluids. Suppositories, stool softeners and enemas may be required. In a group of 38 pwMND who underwent urological evaluations, 47% had micturition symptoms and urodynamics studies found a range of UMN abnormalities [164]. Where urinary urgency is an issue, oxybutinin may be helpful.

Contributory factors to incontinence, such as urinary tract infections, drinking large amount of fluids late in the day and dependent oedema causing nocturia when the legs are elevated overnight should be considered and treated. Wasner et al [165] suggested a prevalence of 62% (n=62) in sexual dysfunction with issues including decreased libido and passivity of the patient and partner due to physical weakness and the body image changes. The wide variation in reported prevalence in bowel, bladder and sexual dysfunction suggests that patients may not volunteer this information; hence its inclusion in routine enquiries might help to encourage reporting and thus the facilitation of appropriate treatment, such as sexual counselling and suggestion of specific techniques.

1.10.6. Pain

Pain is common in MND, especially in the later stages. Musculoskeletal pain from weakness and resulting postural changes can be ameliorated with range of motion exercises, adequate support in sitting and supine positions and proper lifting and transfer techniques to prevent undue traction on weakened joints. Fatigue and depressive symptoms may also worsen a patient's experience of pain.

Spasticity and muscle spasms are not an uncommon source of pain and with the current paucity of supporting evidence, this is often treated with stretching exercises in combination with a muscle relaxant (baclofen is the drug of choice) [166]. Baclofen should be started at low doses (5mg twice to three times daily) and slowly increased (up to 100mg a day in divided doses). Baclofen however can be associated with muscle weakness. Tizanidine (2mg twice daily up to 24 mg a day) is likely as efficacious but it is associated with dry mouth. Other options include clonidine (25 µg twice a day) which can cause hypotension, drowsiness and bradycardia and benzodiazepines which can cause sedation and habituation and respiratory depression. Dantrolene is not recommended as it can cause excessive muscle weakness in MND [167]. Intrathecal baclofen is rarely required but may be indicated in those with intractable spasticity, needing more than the maximum oral dose [168]. There are few reports of use of botulinum toxin for spasticity in MND in literature. Caution is advised as pwMND may be more prone to developing generalised weakness after being injected with botulinum toxin A to treat spasticity [169].

Muscle cramps can cause severe pain and discomfort and are a result of spontaneous activity of motor units induced by contraction of shortened muscles [170]. The list of potentially useful drugs for cramps is extensive, implying efficacy of individual agents is low and variable and the evidence base weak. In the US, quinine (35%), baclofen (19%), phenytoin (10%), and gabapentin (7%) were the preferred agents [156]; in Europe, choices were quinine (58%), benzodiazepines (40%), magnesium (25%) and carbamazepine (23%) [171]. In 2006 however, the US Food and Drug admininstration restricted the use of quinine sulfate in the US to treatment of malaria faciparum because of concerns regarding severe adverse events, including cardiaarthymias, thrombocytopaenia, severe hypersentivity reactions and serious drug interaction [172].

In advanced disease, pain often results due to immobility. Adequate mattress support, range of motion exercise and frequent turning of the patient are essential. Equipment such as motorized beds that slowly rotate from the side to side can be useful for reducing caregiver burden [1]. Analgesia such as nonsteroidal anti-inflammatory drugs or narcotics (oral or sublingual) may also be required (with careful respiratory status monitoring in the latter). Intramuscular delivery of medications should be avoided due to muscle wasting [141].

1.10.7. Fatigue and Sleep Disorders

Fatigue is a common disability in MND – 77-83% in recent studies [11,173] but understudied and often overlooked by clinicians [174]. It is unrelated to clinical strength as a large component of fatigue in MND has a central origin [175]. Fatigue in MND does not correlate directly with gender, educational level, disease duration, physical function, quality of life, dyspnoea, depression or sleepiness [173]. However, contributory factors may include sepsis (including aspiration), depression and/or anxiety, pain, hypoventilation, positioning, sleep disruption and effortful activity and these should be treated where possible. It may manifest as reduced energy, difficulty in maintaining sustained attention and increased motor weakness, incoordination and gait difficulties. No double-blind, placebo-controlled trials have been performed for treatment of fatigue. Physostigmine is sometimes prescribed but not necessarily effective [176]. Modafinil appears to be well-tolerated in a recent small open-label study (n=15) and may reduce symptoms of fatigue [177]. Rehabilitation strategies involve pacing activities (regular rest breaks), energy conservation and fatigue management strategies, addressing sleep disorders, consideration of exercise to improve fitness if appropriate and treating other exacerbating factors.

High incidence of sleep disturbance in MND has been reported with pain, micturition, and choking listed by patients as the most common causes for awakening [178]. Other contributors to poor sleep include abnormal nocturnal movements such as periodic leg movements or fragmentary myoclonus, which was demonstrated on polysomnography in almost all patients with fatigue [178]. Such movements may be treated with controlled release carbidopa-levodopa (Sinemet CR) [179]. Antihistamines (eg. diphenhydramine) and other sedatives (eg. Chloral hydrate 250-500mg, benzodiazepines) can also be considered once respiratory causes for sleep disturbance have been ruled out (see section 1.10.1 for the treatment of respiratory-related sleep disturbance).

1.10.8. Cognition and Behavioural Impairment

Cognitive impairment is increasingly recognised in MND -- 50% are thought to have frontal executive deficits (see box 1.6) [180]. Visuospatial function, praxis and memory storage are usually spared [181-183]. Use of memory aids such as diaries, planners and structured daily routine is encouraged. Other conditions (depression, anxiety, fatigue) and medications (anticholinergics, benzodiazepines) should be monitored as they can worsen cognitive function.

Behavioural changes unrelated to mood or cognition has also been noted although estimates of prevalence vary widely [184]. Marked apathy occurs in an estimated 55% of pwMND [185].This correlates with deficits in verbal fluency but not depression, disease duration, FVC or ALSFRS scores and may be related to fatigue, respiratory weakness, impaired sleep, anxiety or medication [184]. It may also be a psychological coping mechanism [184].

In a subset of pwMND (approximately 5%), clear fronto-temporal dementia (also known as fronto-temporal lobar degeneration) is the presenting picture with severe behavioural dysfunction (insidious onset with gradual progression, altered social conduct, impaired regulation of personal conduct, emotional blunting, loss of insight) that begins before motor weakness becomes obvious [184]. In addition, those with fronto-temporal dementia may exhibit disinhibition, restlessness, reduced empathy, lack of foresight, impulsiveness, social withdrawal, verbal stereotypes, verbal or motor perseveration and/or sexual hyperactivity [186].

Management of behavioural and cognitive deficits can be challenging and begins with the identification of these issues. An assessment by a neuropsychologist is often helpful in terms of defining the deficits and provision of cognitive and behavioural remediation strategies. Education and counselling of the patient and family is important. No trials have been conducted in efficacy of pharmacological interventions in this area; however the use of antidepressants and antipsychotics may be considered.

Box 1.6. Cognitive deficits in MND (adapted from [184])

Attention and concentration
Working memory
Cognitive flexibility (rigidity)
Response inhibition
Planning/problem/solving/abstract reasoning
Visual-perceptual skills
Memory
Word generation (fluency)

1.10.9. Pseudobulbar Affect

Pseudobulbar affect describes sudden uncontrollable outbursts of laughter or tearfulness and is a result of bilateral corticobulbar tract degeneration [187]. It is common, affecting between 50-70% of pwMND [188] especially those with the bulbar form of MND. Pseudobulbar affect can have a significant impact on anxiety and emotional frailty [188], social functioning and relationships in pwMND as these sudden, frequent, extreme, uncontrollable emotional outbursts may lead to severe embarrassment and social withdrawal [189].

Despite the prevalence of this issue, less than 15% ask for treatment [190]. Education of the pwMND and their family and friends assists with understanding and acceptance of these pathological and involuntary outbursts and is an important component of the appropriate treatment of pseudobulbar affect. Crying associated with pseudobulbar affect is easily incorrectly interpreted as depression; laughter may be embarrassing. Pharmacological treatment can include amitryiptiline (10-150mg nocte, starting with 10mg and slowly increasing the dose) which also has the positive benefit on weight loss and loss of appetite [190] or fluvoxamine (100-200mg daily). A more recent study (n=140) showed that dextromethorphan and quinidine in combination appears to be more effective in reducing the frequency and severity of psudobulbar affect and to improve quality of life) [191]. However, side effects are also more common (nausea, dizziness, gastrointestinal complaints) [191].

1.10.10. Psychosocial Issues

MND is a devastating condition, which takes its toll on the patient and family especially as the disease progresses, and loss of independence occurs. Rates of depression and anxiety are reported to be 0-44% and 0-30% respectively in pwMND [192] and depression does not appear to increase in more advanced disease [193]. Quality of life also appears to be more dependent on psychological and existential factors than physical factors [194,195]. Amongst caregivers, 23% are depressed [196] and caregiver strain is often significant as a result of increased caregiving time, cognitive impairments in pwMND, emotional labour and socio-economic considerations [12,197,198]. Hence, referrals to support groups and counselling and education of patients and their families (often their caregivers) are essential. Frank discussions facilitate understanding of the disease and improve coping skills. Carer support (both physical and emotional) and respite care should be discussed. Referrals to the local MND associations are also recommended as these provide patients and families with ongoing support, resources and equipment needs. Psychotherapy should also be considered to assist with coping strategies [199]. Antidepressants such as amitriptyline and selective serotonin reuptake inhibitors may be used, the former being also useful for other symptoms such as drooling, pseudobulbar affect and insomnia. Anxiety is difficult to measure due to physical confounding symptoms such as shortness of breath, muscle cramps and restlessness. Anxiety can be treated with psychotherapy and training in relaxation and breathing techniques, as well as participation in support groups. It is generally thought that the rates of anxiety increase in the pre-terminal stage [192], hence anxiolytics at this time such as benzodiazepines should be offered. With good support, mental health and quality of life can remain stable despite deteriorating physical health [200].

1.10.11. End of Life Issues

It is important to establish an open environment of communication with pwMND and their families from the time of diagnosis. Specialist palliative care providers should be involved as early as possible. Discussions should take place early, well before specific decisions need to be made. The actual timing of when to introduce these discussions however can be challenging and will depend on a number of factors including coping skills, depression and anxiety, cultural issues and functional status [201]. Some triggers may include the patient or family initiation of discussion, severe psychosocial distress, pain requiring high dosages of analgesia, dysphagia, dyspnoea and functional loss in two body regions [201]. Given the progressive nature of the disease, the patient eventually has to choose between life-sustaining therapies (respiratory assistance, feeding tubes) and terminal palliative care whilst considering issues relating to quality of life, burden of therapies, their own wishes and those of their family. It is important that clinicians caring for MND patients and their families appreciate and communicate the significance of life-threatening symptoms, monitor decision-making capacity, ensure that multiple possible end of life scenarios are anticipated and managed with all options provided (including hospice care), review advance care directives and comprehensively consider and aggressively manage symptoms [202].

Medications should be available for all patients who are deteriorating and may be approaching the terminal phase, although the terminal phase may be difficult to recognise as there is usually slow deterioration until a quicker change leads to death within a few days or less [203]. Medications should include morphine to relieve dyspnoea and pain, midazolam to relieve distress and agitation and glycopyrronium bromide or hyoscine hydrobromide to reduce chest secretions, delivered parenterally [203]. Cultural and spiritual issues should also be addressed [201,204]. Although many pwMND fear the terminal stages of MND, with good palliative care, the later stages can be a time of fulfilment and peace for both pwMND and their families [203].

Bereavement in MND occurs in both the patient and their family and continues, in families, after the death of the patient. Some families feel relieved of their caregiver burden and the burden of losses for the patient but also have feelings of guilt that they feel these emotions; hence support is vital in this area [205].

CONCLUSION

MND is a complex and challenging condition with no cure. As such, integrated and coordinated health care delivery and services are needed for comprehensive care for pwMND using the neuropalliative rehabilitation model with the aim of maximising activity and participation and optimising quality of life. Many areas in MND are poorly understood, with research often further hindered by the logistical and ethical difficulties. Further research is needed into appropriate study designs; outcome measurement; the evaluation of optimal settings, type, intensity or frequency and cost-effectiveness of multidisciplinary care; and the different phases of MND, covering the spectrum of care required for this patient population. The interface between neurological, rehabilitative and palliative components of care, and caregiver needs should be explored and developed to provide long-term support for this population.

REFERENCES

[1] Francis K, Bach JR, DeLisa JA. Evaluation and rehabilitation of patients with adult motor neuron disease. *Arch. Phys. Med. Rehabil.* 1999 Aug;80(8):951-63.

[2] Rowland LP. How amyotrophic lateral sclerosis got its name: the clinical-pathologic genius of Jean-Martin Charcot. *Arch. Neurol.* 2001 Mar;58(3):512-5.

[3] Forsgren L, Almay BG, Holmgren G, Wall S. Epidemiology of motor neuron disease in northern Sweden. *Acta Neurol. Scand.* 1983 Jul;68(1):20-9.

[4] Logroscino G, Traynor BJ, Hardiman O, Chio A, Couratier P, Mitchell JD, et al. Descriptive epidemiology of amyotrophic lateral sclerosis: new evidence and unsolved issues. *J. Neurol. Neurosurg Psychiatry.* 2008 Jan;79(1):6-11.

[5] Worms PM. The epidemiology of motor neuron diseases: a review of recent studies. *J. Neurol. Sci.* 2001 Oct 15;191(1-2):3-9.

[6]   Rocha JA, Reis C, Simoes F, Fonseca J, Mendes Ribeiro J. Diagnostic investigation and multidisciplinary management in motor neuron disease. *J. Neurol.* 2005 Dec;252(12):1435-47.

[7]   Turner MR, Al-Chalabi A. Clinical phenotypes. In: Kiernan M, editor. *The Motor Neurone Disease Handbook.* Prymont: Australasian Medical Publishing Company Limited; 2007. p. 56-73.

[8]   World Health Organization. International Classification of Functioning, Disability, and Health (ICF). Geneva2001.

[9]   Klein LM, Forshew DA. The economic impact of ALS. *Neurology.* 1996 Oct;47(4 Suppl 2):S126-9.

[10]   Rhodes P, Shaw S. Informal care and terminal illness. *Health Soc Care Community.* 1999 Jan;7(1):39-50.

[11]   Ng L, Talman P, Khan F. Motor Neurone Disease: Disability profile and service needs in an Australian cohort. *Int. J. Rehabil. Res.* 2011;in press.

[12]   Chio A, Gauthier A, Vignola A, Calvo A, Ghiglione P, Cavallo E, et al. Caregiver time use in ALS. *Neurology.* 2006 Sep 12;67(5):902-4.

[13]   Acting positively: strategic implications of the economic costs of multiple sclerosis in Australia. Sydney, Australia: Access Economics2005

[14]   Emanuel EJ, Emanuel LL. The economics of dying. The illusion of cost savings at the end of life. *N. Engl. J. Med.* 1994 Feb 24;330(8):540-4.

[15]   Chancellor AM, Warlow CP. Adult onset motor neuron disease: worldwide mortality, incidence and distribution since 1950. *J. Neurol. Neurosurg. Psychiatry.* 1992 Dec;55(12):1106-15.

[16]   Murphy M, Quinn S, Young J, Parkin P, Taylor B. Increasing incidence of ALS in Canterbury, New Zealand: a 22-year study. *Neurology.* 2008 Dec 2;71(23):1889-95.

[17]   Chio A, Magnani C, Schiffer D. Gompertzian analysis of amyotrophic lateral sclerosis mortality in Italy, 1957-1987; application to birth cohorts. *Neuroepidemiology.* 1995;14(6):269-77.

[18]   McGuire D, Garrison L, Armon C, Barohn R, Bryan W, Miller R, et al. Relationship of the Tufts Quantitative Neuromuscular Exam (TQNE) and the Sickness Impact Profile (SIP) in measuring progression of ALS. SSNJV/CNTF ALS Study Group. *Neurology.* 1996 May;46(5):1442-4.

[19]   Motor Neurone Disease Association. *Research Strategy 2006-2012.* Northampton, UK: Motor Neurone Disease Association2007.

[20]   AMNDR Steering Committee. Australian Motor Neurone Disease Registry (poster): World Federation of Neurology Meeting2005.

[21]   Cronin S, Hardiman O, Traynor BJ. Ethnic variation in the incidence of ALS: a systematic review. *Neurology.* 2007 Mar 27;68(13):1002-7.

[22]   Armon C. Smoking may be considered an established risk factor for sporadic ALS. *Neurology.* 2009 Nov 17;73(20):1693-8.

[23]   Chio A, Benzi G, Dossena M, Mutani R, Mora G. Severely increased risk of amyotrophic lateral sclerosis among Italian professional football players. *Brain.* 2005 Mar;128(Pt 3):472-6.

[24]   Veldink JH, Kalmijn S, Groeneveld GJ, Titulaer MJ, Wokke JH, van den Berg LH. Physical activity and the association with sporadic ALS. *Neurology.* 2005 Jan 25;64(2):241-5.

[25] Rowland LP, Shneider NA. Amyotrophic lateral sclerosis. *N. Engl. J. Med.* 2001 May 31;344(22):1688-700.

[26] Spencer PS, Nunn PB, Hugon J, Ludolph AC, Ross SM, Roy DN, et al. Guam amyotrophic lateral sclerosis-parkinsonism-dementia linked to a plant excitant neurotoxin. *Science*. 1987 Jul 31;237(4814):517-22.

[27] Steele JC, McGeer PL. The ALS/PDC syndrome of Guam and the cycad hypothesis. *Neurology*. 2008 May 20;70(21):1984-90.

[28] Dunckley T, Huentelman MJ, Craig DW, Pearson JV, Szelinger S, Joshipura K, et al. Whole-genome analysis of sporadic amyotrophic lateral sclerosis. *N. Engl. J. Med.* 2007 Aug 23;357(8):775-88.

[29] van Es MA, Van Vught PW, Blauw HM, Franke L, Saris CG, Andersen PM, et al. ITPR2 as a susceptibility gene in sporadic amyotrophic lateral sclerosis: a genome-wide association study. *Lancet Neurol*. 2007 Oct;6(10):869-77.

[30] van Es MA, van Vught PW, Blauw HM, Franke L, Saris CG, Van den Bosch L, et al. Genetic variation in DPP6 is associated with susceptibility to amyotrophic lateral sclerosis. *Nat. Genet*. 2008 Jan;40(1):29-31.

[31] Rosen DR. Mutations in Cu/Zn superoxide dismutase gene are associated with familial amyotrophic lateral sclerosis. *Nature*. 1993 Jul 22;364(6435):362.

[32] Hand CK, Khoris J, Salachas F, Gros-Louis F, Lopes AA, Mayeux-Portas V, et al. A novel locus for familial amyotrophic lateral sclerosis, on chromosome 18q. *Am. J. Hum. Genet*. 2002 Jan;70(1):251-6.

[33] Chance PF, Rabin BA, Ryan SG, Ding Y, Scavina M, Crain B, et al. Linkage of the gene for an autosomal dominant form of juvenile amyotrophic lateral sclerosis to chromosome 9q34. *Am. J. Hum. Genet*. 1998 Mar;62(3):633-40.

[34] Kwiatkowski TJ, Jr., Bosco DA, Leclerc AL, Tamrazian E, Vanderburg CR, Russ C, et al. Mutations in the FUS/TLS gene on chromosome 16 cause familial amyotrophic lateral sclerosis. *Science*. 2009 Feb 27;323(5918):1205-8.

[35] Yan J, Deng HX, Siddique N, Fecto F, Chen W, Yang Y, et al. Frameshift and novel mutations in FUS in familial amyotrophic lateral sclerosis and ALS/dementia. *Neurology*. 2010 Aug 31;75(9):807-14.

[36] Sapp PC, Hosler BA, McKenna-Yasek D, Chin W, Gann A, Genise H, et al. Identification of two novel loci for dominantly inherited familial amyotrophic lateral sclerosis. *Am. J. Hum. Genet*. 2003 Aug;73(2):397-403.

[37] Nishimura AL, Mitne-Neto M, Silva HC, Oliveira JR, Vainzof M, Zatz M. A novel locus for late onset amyotrophic lateral sclerosis/motor neurone disease variant at 20q13. *J. Med. Genet*. 2004 Apr;41(4):315-20.

[38] Greenway MJ, Andersen PM, Russ C, Ennis S, Cashman S, Donaghy C, et al. ANG mutations segregate with familial and 'sporadic' amyotrophic lateral sclerosis. *Nat. Genet*. 2006 Apr;38(4):411-3.

[39] Sreedharan J, Blair IP, Tripathi VB, Hu X, Vance C, Rogelj B, et al. TDP-43 mutations in familial and sporadic amyotrophic lateral sclerosis. *Science*. 2008 Mar 21;319(5870):1668-72.

[40] Chow CY, Landers JE, Bergren SK, Sapp PC, Grant AE, Jones JM, et al. Deleterious variants of FIG4, a phosphoinositide phosphatase, in patients with ALS. *Am. J. Hum. Genet*. 2009 Jan;84(1):85-8.

[41] Al-Chalabi A, Andersen PM, Nilsson P, Chioza B, Andersson JL, Russ C, et al. Deletions of the heavy neurofilament subunit tail in amyotrophic lateral sclerosis. *Hum. Mol. Genet.* 1999 Feb;8(2):157-64.

[42] Mitchell J, Paul P, Chen HJ, Morris A, Payling M, Falchi M, et al. Familial amyotrophic lateral sclerosis is associated with a mutation in D-amino acid oxidase. *Proc. Natl. Acad. Sci. USA.* 2010 Apr 20;107(16):7556-61.

[43] Figlewicz DA, Orrell RW. The genetics of motor neuron diseases. *Amyotroph Lateral Scler Other Motor Neuron Disord.* 2003 Dec;4(4):225-31.

[44] Hosler BA, Siddique T, Sapp PC, Sailor W, Huang MC, Hossain A, et al. Linkage of familial amyotrophic lateral sclerosis with frontotemporal dementia to chromosome 9q21-q22. *JAMA.* 2000 Oct 4;284(13):1664-9.

[45] Eymard-Pierre E, Lesca G, Dollet S, Santorelli FM, di Capua M, Bertini E, et al. Infantile-onset ascending hereditary spastic paralysis is associated with mutations in the alsin gene. *Am. J. Hum. Genet.* 2002 Sep;71(3):518-27.

[46] Hentati A, Ouahchi K, Pericak-Vance MA, Nijhawan D, Ahmad A, Yang Y, et al. Linkage of a commoner form of recessive amyotrophic lateral sclerosis to chromosome 15q15-q22 markers. *Neurogenetics.* 1998 Dec;2(1):55-60.

[47] Brown RH, Jr. Amyotrophic lateral sclerosis: recent insights from genetics and transgenic mice. *Cell.* 1995 Mar 10;80(5):687-92.

[48] Cookson MR, Shaw PJ. Oxidative stress and motor neurone disease. *Brain Pathol.* 1999 Jan;9(1):165-86.

[49] Shaw PJ, Ince PG. Glutamate, excitotoxicity and amyotrophic lateral sclerosis. *J. Neurol.* 1997 May;244 Suppl 2:S3-14.

[50] Majoor-Krakauer D, Willems PJ, Hofman A. Genetic epidemiology of amyotrophic lateral sclerosis. *Clin. Genet.* 2003 Feb;63(2):83-101.

[51] Cleveland DW, Rothstein JD. From Charcot to Lou Gehrig: deciphering selective motor neuron death in ALS. *Nat. Rev. Neurosci.* 2001 Nov;2(11):806-19.

[52] Shaw PJ. Molecular and cellular pathways of neurodegeneration in motor neurone disease. *J. Neurol. Neurosurg Psychiatry.* 2005 Aug;76(8):1046-57.

[53] Bruijn LI, Miller TM, Cleveland DW. Unraveling the mechanisms involved in motor neuron degeneration in ALS. *Annu. Rev. Neurosci.* 2004;27:723-49.

[54] Andersen PM. Genetic factors in the early diagnosis of ALS. *Amyotroph Lateral Scler Other Motor Neuron Disord.* 2000 Mar;1 Suppl 1:S31-42.

[55] Andersen PM, Spitsyn VA, Makarov SV, Nilsson L, Kravchuk OI, Bychkovskaya LS, et al. The geographical and ethnic distribution of the D90A CuZn-SOD mutation in the Russian Federation. *Amyotroph. Lateral Scler. Other Motor Neuron Disord.* 2001 Jun;2(2):63-9.

[56] Gurney ME. Transgenic-mouse model of amyotrophic lateral sclerosis. *N. Engl. J. Med.* 1994 Dec 22;331(25):1721-2.

[57] Gurney ME. Transgenic animal models of familial amyotrophic lateral sclerosis. *J. Neurol.* 1997 May;244 Suppl 2:S15-20.

[58] Reaume AG, Elliott JL, Hoffman EK, Kowall NW, Ferrante RJ, Siwek DF, et al. Motor neurons in Cu/Zn superoxide dismutase-deficient mice develop normally but exhibit enhanced cell death after axonal injury. *Nat. Genet.* 1996 May;13(1):43-7.

[59] Shaw PJ, Forrest V, Ince PG, Richardson JP, Wastell HJ. CSF and plasma amino acid levels in motor neuron disease: elevation of CSF glutamate in a subset of patients. *Neurodegeneration*. 1995 Jun;4(2):209-16.

[60] Miller RG, Mitchell JD, Lyon M, Moore DH. Riluzole for amyotrophic lateral sclerosis (ALS)/motor neuron disease (MND). *Cochrane Database Syst. Rev.* 2007(1):CD001447.

[61] Cleveland DW, Liu J. Oxidation versus aggregation - how do SOD1 mutants cause ALS? *Nat. Med.* 2000 Dec;6(12):1320-1.

[62] Karch CM, Prudencio M, Winkler DD, Hart PJ, Borchelt DR. Role of mutant SOD1 disulfide oxidation and aggregation in the pathogenesis of familial ALS. *Proc. Natl. Acad. Sci. USA*. 2009 May 12;106(19):7774-9.

[63] Manfredi G, Xu Z. Mitochondrial dysfunction and its role in motor neuron degeneration in ALS. *Mitochondrion*. 2005 Apr;5(2):77-87.

[64] Kim WK, Liu X, Sandner J, Pasmantier M, Andrews J, Rowland LP, et al. Study of 962 patients indicates progressive muscular atrophy is a form of ALS. *Neurology*. 2009 Nov 17;73(20):1686-92.

[65] Ince PG, Evans J, Knopp M, Forster G, Hamdalla HH, Wharton SB, et al. Corticospinal tract degeneration in the progressive muscular atrophy variant of ALS. *Neurology*. 2003 Apr 22;60(8):1252-8.

[66] Talman P, Forbes A, Mathers S. Clinical phenotypes and natural progression for motor neuron disease: analysis from an Australian database. *Amyotroph Lateral Scler*. 2009 Apr;10(2):79-84.

[67] Gordon PH, Cheng B, Katz IB, Mitsumoto H, Rowland LP. Clinical features that distinguish PLS, upper motor neuron-dominant ALS, and typical ALS. *Neurology*. 2009 Jun 2;72(22):1948-52.

[68] Gordon PH, Cheng B, Katz IB, Pinto M, Hays AP, Mitsumoto H, et al. The natural history of primary lateral sclerosis. *Neurology*. 2006 Mar 14;66(5):647-53.

[69] Tan CF, Kakita A, Piao YS, Kikugawa K, Endo K, Tanaka M, et al. Primary lateral sclerosis: a rare upper-motor-predominant form of amyotrophic lateral sclerosis often accompanied by frontotemporal lobar degeneration with ubiquitinated neuronal inclusions? Report of an autopsy case and a review of the literature. *Acta Neuropathol*. 2003 Jun;105(6):615-20.

[70] Wijesekera LC, Mathers S, Talman P, Galtrey C, Parkinson MH, Ganesalingam J, et al. Natural history and clinical features of the flail arm and flail leg ALS variants. *Neurology*. 2009 Mar 24;72(12):1087-94.

[71] Bryant PR, Geis CC, Moroz A, O'Neill B J, Bogey RA. Stroke and neurodegenerative disorders. 4. Neurodegenerative disorders. *Arch. Phys. Med. Rehabil.* 2004 Mar;85(3 Suppl 1):S21-33.

[72] Eisen A, Swash M. Clinical neurophysiology of ALS. *Clin. Neurophysiol.* 2001 Dec;112(12):2190-201.

[73] Krivickas LS. Amyotrophic lateral sclerosis and other motor neuron diseases. *Phys. Med. Rehabil. Clin. N Am.* 2003 May;14(2):327-45.

[74] Brooks BR. El Escorial World Federation of Neurology criteria for the diagnosis of amyotrophic lateral sclerosis. Subcommittee on Motor Neuron Diseases/Amyotrophic Lateral Sclerosis of the World Federation of Neurology Research Group on

Neuromuscular Diseases and the El Escorial "Clinical limits of amyotrophic lateral sclerosis" workshop contributors. *J. Neurol. Sci.* 1994 Jul;124 Suppl:96-107.

[75] Brooks BR, Miller RG, Swash M, Munsat TL. El Escorial revisited: revised criteria for the diagnosis of amyotrophic lateral sclerosis. *Amyotroph Lateral Scler Other Motor Neuron Disord.* 2000 Dec;1(5):293-9.

[76] Ross MA, Miller RG, Berchert L, Parry G, Barohn RJ, Armon C, et al. Toward earlier diagnosis of amyotrophic lateral sclerosis: revised criteria. rhCNTF ALS Study Group. *Neurology.* 1998 Mar;50(3):768-72.

[77] Traynor BJ, Codd MB, Corr B, Forde C, Frost E, Hardiman OM. Clinical features of amyotrophic lateral sclerosis according to the El Escorial and Airlie House diagnostic criteria: A population-based study. *Arch. Neurol.* 2000 Aug;57(8):1171-6.

[78] de Carvalho M, Dengler R, Eisen A, England JD, Kaji R, Kimura J, et al. Electrodiagnostic criteria for diagnosis of ALS. *Clin. Neurophysiol.* 2008 Mar;119(3):497-503.

[79] Carvalho MD, Swash M. Awaji diagnostic algorithm increases sensitivity of El Escorial criteria for ALS diagnosis. *Amyotroph. Lateral Scler.* 2009 Feb;10(1):53-7.

[80] Boekestein WA, Kleine BU, Hageman G, Schelhaas HJ, Zwarts MJ. Sensitivity and specificity of the 'Awaji' electrodiagnostic criteria for amyotrophic lateral sclerosis: retrospective comparison of the Awaji and revised El Escorial criteria for ALS. *Amyotroph. Lateral Scler.* 2010 Dec;11(6):497-501.

[81] Brooks B. Amyotrophic Lateral Sclerosis Clinimetric Scales - Guidelines for Administration and Scoring. In: Herndon RM, editor. *Handbook of Neurologic Rating Scales.* 2nd ed. New York: Demos Medical Publishing; 2006. p. 93-144.

[82] Cedarbaum JM, Stambler N, Malta E, Fuller C, Hilt D, Thurmond B, et al. The ALSFRS-R: a revised ALS functional rating scale that incorporates assessments of respiratory function. BDNF ALS Study Group (Phase III). *J. Neurol. Sci.* 1999 Oct 31;169(1-2):13-21.

[83] Kaufmann P, Levy G, Montes J, Buchsbaum R, Barsdorf AI, Battista V, et al. Excellent inter-rater, intra-rater, and telephone-administered reliability of the ALSFRS-R in a multicenter clinical trial. *Amyotroph. Lateral Scler.* 2007 Feb;8(1):42-6.

[84] De Groot IJ, Post MW, Van Heuveln T, Van Den Berg LH, Lindeman E. Measurement of decline of functioning in persons with amyotrophic lateral sclerosis: responsiveness and possible applications of the Functional Independence Measure, Barthel Index, Rehabilitation Activities Profile and Frenchay Activities Index. *Amyotroph. Lateral Scler.* 2006 Sep;7(3):167-72.

[85] Granger CV. The emerging science of functional assessment: our tool for outcomes analysis. *Arch. Phys. Med. Rehabil.* 1998 Mar;79(3):235-40.

[86] Mahoney FI, Barthel DW. Functional Evaluation: The Barthel Index. Md. *State Med. J..* 1965 Feb;14:61-5.

[87] van Bennekom CA, Jelles F, Lankhorst GJ, Bouter LM. The Rehabilitation Activities Profile: a validation study of its use as a disability index with stroke patients. Arch Phys Med Rehabil. 1995 Jun;76(6):501-7.

[88] Wade DT, Legh-Smith J, Langton Hewer R. Social activities after stroke: measurement and natural history using the Frenchay Activities Index. *Int. Rehabil. Med.* 1985;7(4):176-81.

[89]   Norris FH, Jr., Calanchini PR, Fallat RJ, Panchari S, Jewett B. The administration of guanidine in amyotrophic lateral sclerosis. *Neurology.* 1974 Aug;24(8):721-8.

[90]   Appel V, Stewart SS, Smith G, Appel SH. A rating scale for amyotrophic lateral sclerosis: description and preliminary experience. *Ann. Neurol.* 1987 Sep;22(3):328-33.

[91]   Hillel AD, Miller RM, Yorkston K, McDonald E, Norris FH, Konikow N. Amyotrophic lateral sclerosis severity scale. *Neuroepidemiology.* 1989;8(3):142-50.

[92]   The Amyotrophic Lateral Sclerosis Functional Rating Scale. Assessment of activities of daily living in patients with amyotrophic lateral sclerosis. The ALS CNTF treatment study (ACTS) phase I-II Study Group. *Arch. Neurol.* 1996 Feb;53(2):141-7.

[93]   Bromberg MB. Quality of life in amyotrophic lateral sclerosis. *Phys. Med. Rehabil. Clin. N. Am.* 2008 Aug;19(3):591-605, x-xi.

[94]   Hickey AM, Bury G, O'Boyle CA, Bradley F, O'Kelly FD, Shannon W. A new short form individual quality of life measure (SEIQoL-DW): application in a cohort of individuals with HIV/AIDS. *BMJ.* 1996 Jul 6;313(7048):29-33.

[95]   Mountain LA, Campbell SE, Seymour DG, Primrose WR, Whyte MI. Assessment of individual quality of life using the SEIQoL-DW in older medical patients. *QJM.* 2004 Aug;97(8):519-24.

[96]   Felgoise SH, Stewart JL, Bremer BA, Walsh SM, Bromberg MB, Simmons Z. The SEIQoL-DW for assessing quality of life in ALS: Strengths and limitations. *Amyotroph Lateral Scler.* 2008 Oct 7:1-7.

[97]   Jenkinson C, Fitzpatrick R, Brennan C, Bromberg M, Swash M. Development and validation of a short measure of health status for individuals with amyotrophic lateral sclerosis/motor neurone disease: the ALSAQ-40. *J. Neurol.* 1999 Nov;246 Suppl 3:III16-21.

[98]   Simmons Z, Felgoise SH, Bremer BA, Walsh SM, Hufford DJ, Bromberg MB, et al. The ALSSQOL: balancing physical and nonphysical factors in assessing quality of life in ALS. *Neurology.* 2006 Nov 14;67(9):1659-64.

[99]   Shefner JM. Designing clinical trials in amyotrophic lateral sclerosis. *Phys. Med. Rehabil. Clin. N Am.* 2008 Aug;19(3):495-508, ix.

[100] Langmore SE, Kasarskis EJ, Manca ML, Olney RK. Enteral tube feeding for amyotrophic lateral sclerosis/motor neuron disease. *Cochrane Database Syst. Rev.* 2006(4):CD004030.

[101] Kennel P, Revah F, Bohme GA, Bejuit R, Gallix P, Stutzmann JM, et al. Riluzole prolongs survival and delays muscle strength deterioration in mice with progressive motor neuronopathy (pmn). *J. Neurol. Sci.* 2000 Nov 1;180(1-2):55-61.

[102] Riviere M, Meininger V, Zeisser P, Munsat T. An analysis of extended survival in patients with amyotrophic lateral sclerosis treated with riluzole. *Arch. Neurol.* 1998 Apr;55(4):526-8.

[103] Miller RG, Jackson CE, Kasarskis EJ, England JD, Forshew D, Johnston W, et al. Practice parameter update: The care of the patient with amyotrophic lateral sclerosis: multidisciplinary care, symptom management, and cognitive/behavioral impairment (an evidence-based review): report of the Quality Standards Subcommittee of the American Academy of Neurology. *Neurology.* 2009 Oct 13;73(15):1227-33.

[104] Andersen PM, Borasio GD, Dengler R, Hardiman O, Kollewe K, Leigh PN, et al. Good practice in the management of amyotrophic lateral sclerosis: clinical guidelines. An

44 Louisa Ng and Fary Khan

evidence-based review with good practice points. EALSC Working Group. *Amyotroph Lateral Scler.* 2007 Aug;8(4):195-213.

[105] Miller RG, Jackson CE, Kasarskis EJ, England JD, Forshew D, Johnston W, et al. Practice parameter update: The care of the patient with amyotrophic lateral sclerosis: drug, nutritional, and respiratory therapies (an evidence-based review): report of the Quality Standards Subcommittee of the American Academy of Neurology. *Neurology.* 2009 Oct 13;73(15):1218-26.

[106] Mitsumoto H. [A strategy to develop effective ALS therapy]. *Brain Nerve.* 2007 Apr;59(4):383-91.

[107] Gordon PH, Moore DH, Miller RG, Florence JM, Verheijde JL, Doorish C, et al. Efficacy of minocycline in patients with amyotrophic lateral sclerosis: a phase III randomised trial. *Lancet Neurol.* 2007 Dec;6(12):1045-53.

[108] Kaufmann P, Thompson JL, Levy G, Buchsbaum R, Shefner J, Krivickas LS, et al. Phase II trial of CoQ10 for ALS finds insufficient evidence to justify phase III. *Ann. Neurol.* 2009 Aug;66(2):235-44.

[109] Aggarwal SP, Zinman L, Simpson E, McKinley J, Jackson KE, Pinto H, et al. Safety and efficacy of lithium in combination with riluzole for treatment of amyotrophic lateral sclerosis: a randomised, double-blind, placebo-controlled trial. *Lancet Neurol.* 2010 May;9(5):481-8.

[110] Shefner J, Cudkowicz M. ALS and Unproven Treatments: What Should Patients and Physicians Do? *Neurology Today.* 2008;8(18):5-7.

[111] Hardiman O. Multidisciplinary care in motor neurone disease. In: Kiernan M, editor. *The Motor Neurone Disease Handbook.* Prymont: Australasian Medical Publishing Company Limited; 2007. p. 164.

[112] Ng L, Khan F, Mathers S. Multidisciplinary care for adults with amyotrophic lateral sclerosis or motor neuron disease. *Cochrane Database Syst. Rev. 2009*(4):CD007425.

[113] Wade DT. *Measurement in Neurology Rehabilitation.* Oxford: Oxford University Press; 1992.

[114] Organization WH. *International Classification of Functioning, Disability and Health* (ICF). Geneva: World Health Organization2001.

[115] Geyh S, Cieza A, Schouten J, Dickson H, Frommelt P, Omar Z, et al. ICF Core Sets for stroke. *J. Rehabil. Med.* 2004 Jul(44 Suppl):135-41.

[116] Khan F, Pallant JF. Use of the International Classification of Functioning, Disability and Health (ICF) to identify preliminary comprehensive and brief core sets for multiple sclerosis. *Disabil. Rehabil.* 2007c Feb 15;29(3):205-13.

[117] Khan F, Pallant JF. Use of the International Classification of Functioning, Disability and Health (ICF) to identify preliminary comprehensive and brief core sets for Guillain Barre syndrome. *Disabil. Rehabil.* 2010a;in press (accepted September 2010).

[118] Department of Health. *The National Service Framework (NSF)* for Long-term conditions. London, U.K.2005.

[119] Kristjanson LJ, Aoun SM, Yates P. Are supportive services meeting the needs of Australians with neurodegenerative conditions and their families? *J. Palliat Care.* 2006 Autumn;22(3):151-7.

[120] Royal college of Physicians National Council for palliative Care BSoRM. Long Term Neurological Conditions: Management at the interface between neurology, rehabilitation and palliative care. London: RCP2008.

[121] Kemp BJ. What the rehabilitation professional and the consumer need to know. *Phys. Med. Rehabil. Clin. N Am.* 2005 Feb;16(1):1-18, vii.

[122] McKenna C, MacLeod R. Access to palliative care for people with motor neurone disease in New Zealand. *N Z Med. J.* 2005 Sep 16;118(1222):U1667.

[123] Traue DC, Ross JR. Palliative care in non-malignant diseases. *J. R. Soc. Med.* 2005 Nov;98(11):503-6.

[124] Turner-Stokes L, Sykes N, Silber E, Khatri A, Sutton L, Young E. From diagnosis to death: exploring the interface between neurology, rehabilitation and palliative care in managing people with long-term neurological conditions. *Clin. Med.* 2007 Apr;7(2):129-36.

[125] Oliver D. The quality of care and symptom control--the effects on the terminal phase of ALS/MND. *J. Neurol. Sci.* 1996 Aug;139 Suppl:134-6.

[126] Borasio GD, Voltz R, Miller RG. Palliative care in amyotrophic lateral sclerosis. *Neurol. Clin.* 2001 Nov;19(4):829-47.

[127] Melo J, Homma A, Iturriaga E, Frierson L, Amato A, Anzueto A, et al. Pulmonary evaluation and prevalence of non-invasive ventilation in patients with amyotrophic lateral sclerosis: a multicenter survey and proposal of a pulmonary protocol. *J. Neurol. Sci.* 1999 Oct 31;169(1-2):114-7.

[128] Czaplinski A, Yen AA, Appel SH. Forced vital capacity (FVC) as an indicator of survival and disease progression in an ALS clinic population. *J. Neurol. Neurosurg Psychiatry.* 2006 Mar;77(3):390-2.

[129] Fitting JW, Paillex R, Hirt L, Aebischer P, Schluep M. Sniff nasal pressure: a sensitive respiratory test to assess progression of amyotrophic lateral sclerosis. *Ann. Neurol.* 1999 Dec;46(6):887-93.

[130] Stefanutti D, Benoist MR, Scheinmann P, Chaussain M, Fitting JW. Usefulness of sniff nasal pressure in patients with neuromuscular or skeletal disorders. *Am. J. Respir. Crit. Care Med.* 2000 Oct;162(4 Pt 1):1507-11.

[131] Lyall RA, Donaldson N, Polkey MI, Leigh PN, Moxham J. Respiratory muscle strength and ventilatory failure in amyotrophic lateral sclerosis. *Brain.* 2001 Oct;124(Pt 10):2000-13.

[132] Morgan RK, McNally S, Alexander M, Conroy R, Hardiman O, Costello RW. Use of Sniff nasal-inspiratory force to predict survival in amyotrophic lateral sclerosis. *Am. J. Respir. Crit. Care Med.* 2005 Feb 1;171(3):269-74.

[133] Shaw P. Motor neurone disease. In: Greenwood RJ, Barnes MP, McMillan TM, al. E, editors. *Handbook of neurological rehabilitation.* 2nd ed. New York: Psychology Press; 2003. p. 641-61.

[134] Schiffman PL. Pulmonary function and respiratory management of the ALS patient. In: Belsh JM, Schiffman PL, editors. *Amyotrophic Lateral Sclerosis: diagnosis and management for the clinician.* Armonk (NY): Futura Publishing Company; 1996. p. 333-55.

[135] Radunovic A, Annane D, Jewitt K, Mustfa N. Mechanical ventilation for amyotrophic lateral sclerosis/motor neuron disease. *Cochrane Database Syst. Rev.* 2009(4):CD004427.

[136] Kaub-Wittemer D, Steinbuchel N, Wasner M, Laier-Groeneveld G, Borasio GD. Quality of life and psychosocial issues in ventilated patients with amyotrophic lateral sclerosis and their caregivers. *J. Pain Symptom Manage.* 2003 Oct;26(4):890-6.

[137] Vianello A, Arcaro G, Palmieri A, Ermani M, Braccioni F, Gallan F, et al. Survival and quality of life after tracheostomy for acute respiratory failure in patients with amyotrophic lateral sclerosis. *J. Crit. Care.* 2010 Jul 22.

[138] Yorkston KM, Strand E, Miller R, Hillel A, Smith K. Speech deterioration in amyotrophic lateral sclerosis: implications for the timing of intervention. *J. Med. Speech-Language pathol.* 1993;1:35-46.

[139] Hillel AD, Miller R. Bulbar amyotrophic lateral sclerosis: patterns of progression and clinical management. *Head Neck.* 1989 Jan-Feb;11(1):51-9.

[140] Esposito SJ, Mitsumoto H, Shanks M. Use of palatal lift and palatal augmentation prostheses to improve dysarthria in patients with amyotrophic lateral sclerosis: a case series. *J.Prosthet Dent.* 2000 Jan;83(1):90-8.

[141] Mayadev AS, Weiss MD, Distad BJ, Krivickas LS, Carter GT. The amyotrophic lateral sclerosis center: a model of multidisciplinary management. *Phys. Med. Rehabil. Clin. N. Am.* 2008 Aug;19(3):619-31, xi.

[142] Fried-Oken M, Fox L, Rau MT, Tullman J, Baker G, Hindal M, et al. Purposes of AAC device use for persons with ALS as reported by caregivers. *Augment Altern Commun.* 2006 Sep;22(3):209-21.

[143] Kubler A, Nijboer F, Mellinger J, Vaughan TM, Pawelzik H, Schalk G, et al. Patients with ALS can use sensorimotor rhythms to operate a brain-computer interface. *Neurology.* 2005 May 24;64(10):1775-7.

[144] Higo R, Tayama N, Nito T. Longitudinal analysis of progression of dysphagia in amyotrophic lateral sclerosis. *Auris Nasus Larynx.* 2004 Sep;31(3):247-54.

[145] Borasio GD. Palliative care in ALS: searching for the evidence base. *Amyotroph. Lateral Scler Other Motor Neuron Disord.* 2001 Mar;2 Suppl 1:S31-5.

[146] Sorenson EJ, Crum B, Stevens JC. Incidence of aspiration pneumonia in ALS in Olmsted County, MN. *Amyotroph. Lateral Scler.* 2007 Apr;8(2):87-9.

[147] Mayberry JF, Atkinson M. Swallowing problems in patients with motor neuron disease. *J. Clin. Gastroenterol.* 1986 Jun;8(3 Pt 1):233-4.

[148] Slowie LA, Paige MS, Antel JP. Nutritional considerations in the management of patients with amyotrophic lateral sclerosis (ALS). *J. Am. Diet Assoc.* 1983 Jul;83(1):44-7.

[149] Rio A, Cawadias E. Nutritional advice and treatment by dietitians to patients with amyotrophic lateral sclerosis/motor neurone disease: a survey of current practice in England, Wales, Northern Ireland and Canada. *J. Hum. Nutr. Diet.* 2007 Feb;20(1):3-13.

[150] Kasarskis EJ, Neville HE. Management of ALS: nutritional care. *Neurology.* 1996 Oct;47(4 Suppl 2):S118-20.

[151] Loser C, Aschl G, Hebuterne X, Mathus-Vliegen EM, Muscaritoli M, Niv Y, et al. ESPEN guidelines on artificial enteral nutrition--percutaneous endoscopic gastrostomy (PEG). *Clin. Nutr.* 2005 Oct;24(5):848-61.

[152] Kasarskis EJ, Scarlata D, Hill R, Fuller C, Stambler N, Cedarbaum JM. A retrospective study of percutaneous endoscopic gastrostomy in ALS patients during the BDNF and CNTF trials. *J. Neurol. Sci.* 1999 Oct 31;169(1-2):118-25.

[153] Mazzini L, Corra T, Zaccala M, Mora G, Del Piano M, Galante M. Percutaneous endoscopic gastrostomy and enteral nutrition in amyotrophic lateral sclerosis. *J. Neurol.* 1995 Oct;242(10):695-8.

[154] Mathus-Vliegen LM, Louwerse LS, Merkus MP, Tytgat GN, Vianney de Jong JM. Percutaneous endoscopic gastrostomy in patients with amyotrophic lateral sclerosis and impaired pulmonary function. *Gastrointest Endosc.* 1994 Jul-Aug;40(4):463-9.

[155] Schiffman PL, Belsh JM. Overall management of the ALS patient. In: Belsh JM, Schiffman PL, editors. *Amyotrophic lateral sclerosis: diagnosis and management for the clinician.* Armonk (NY): Futura Publishing Company; 1996. p. 271-301.

[156] Forshew DA, Bromberg MB. A survey of clinicians' practice in the symptomatic treatment of ALS. *Amyotroph. Lateral Scler Other Motor Neuron Disord.* 2003 Dec;4(4):258-63.

[157] Verma A, Steele J. Botulinum toxin improves sialorrhea and quality of living in bulbar amyotrophic lateral sclerosis. *Muscle Nerve.* 2006 Aug;34(2):235-7.

[158] Contarino MF, Pompili M, Tittoto P, Vanacore N, Sabatelli M, Cedrone A, et al. Botulinum toxin B ultrasound-guided injections for sialorrhea in amyotrophic lateral sclerosis and Parkinson's disease. *Parkinsonism Relat Disord.* 2007 Jul;13(5):299-303.

[159] Johnson EW, Braddom R. Over-work weakness in facioscapulohuumeral muscular dystrophy. *Arch. Phys. Med. Rehabil.* 1971 Jul;52(7):333-6.

[160] Dalbello-Haas V, Florence JM, Krivickas LS. Therapeutic exercise for people with amyotrophic lateral sclerosis or motor neuron disease. *Cochrane Database Syst. Rev.* 2008(2):CD005229.

[161] Chen A, Montes J, Mitsumoto H. The role of exercise in amyotrophic lateral sclerosis. *Phys. Med. Rehabil. Clin. N Am.* 2008 Aug;19(3):545-57, ix-x.

[162] Khanna P, Nations SP, Trivedi JR. Motor Neuron Diseases. In: Braddom R, editor. *Physical Medicine and Rehabilitation.* 3rd ed. Philadelphia: Saunders Elsevier; 2007.

[163] Ng L, Khan F. Use of the International Classification of Functioning, Disability and Health to describe patient-reported disability: A comparison of Motor Neurone Disease, Guillain-Barré Syndrome and Multiple Sclerosis in an Australian cohort. *Journal of Rehabilitation Medicine.* 2011; under review.

[164] Hattori T, Hirayama K, Yasuda K, Shimazaki J. [Disturbance of micturition in amyotrophic lateral sclerosis]. Rinsho Shinkeigaku. 1983 Mar;23(3):224-7.

[165] Wasner M, Bold U, Vollmer TC, Borasio GD. Sexuality in patients with amyotrophic lateral sclerosis and their partners. *J. Neurol.* 2004 Apr;251(4):445-8.

[166] Ashworth NL, Satkunam LE, Deforge D. Treatment for spasticity in amyotrophic lateral sclerosis/motor neuron disease. *Cochrane Database Syst. Rev.* 2006(1):CD004156.

[167] Krivickas LS, Carter GT. Motor neuron disease. In: J.A. D, Gans BM, Walsh NE, editors. *Physical medicine and rehabilitation: principles and practice.* 4th ed. Philadelphia: Lippincott Williams and Wilkins; 2005.

[168] Marquardt G, Seifert V. Use of intrathecal baclofen for treatment of spasticity in amyotrophic lateral sclerosis. *J. Neurol. Neurosurg. Psychiatry.* 2002;72:275-6.

[169] Mezaki T, Kaji R, Kohara N, Kimura J. Development of general weakness in a patient with amyotrophic lateral sclerosis after focal botulinum toxin injection. *Neurology.* 1996 Mar;46(3):845-6.

[170] Norris FH, Jr., Gasteiger EL, Chatfield PO. An electromyographic study of induced and spontaneous muscle cramps. *Electroencephalogr Clin. Neurophysiol.* 1957 Feb;9(1):139-47.

[171] Borasio GD, Shaw PJ, Hardiman O, Ludolph AC, Sales Luis ML, Silani V. Standards of palliative care for patients with amyotrophic lateral sclerosis: results of a European survey. *Amyotroph. Lateral Scler Other Motor Neuron Disord.* 2001 Sep;2(3):159-64.

[172] U.S. Food and Drug Administration. FDA advances effort against marketed unapproved drugs. FDA orders unapproved quinine drugs from the market and cautions consumers about "off-label" use of quinine to treat leg cramps. 2006 [cited 2011 January]; Available from: http://www.fda.gov/NewsEvents/Newsroom/PressAnnouncements /2006/ucm108799.htm.

[173] Ramirez C, Piemonte ME, Callegaro D, Da Silva HC. Fatigue in amyotrophic lateral sclerosis: frequency and associated factors. *Amyotroph. Lateral Scler.* 2008 Apr;9(2):75-80.

[174] Lou JS. Fatigue in amyotrophic lateral sclerosis. *Phys. Med. Rehabil Clin. N Am.* 2008 Aug;19(3):533-43, ix.

[175] Kent-Braun JA, Miller RG. Central fatigue during isometric exercise in amyotrophic lateral sclerosis. *Muscle Nerve.* 2000 Jun;23(6):909-14.

[176] Norris FH, Tan Y, Fallat RJ, Elias L. Trial of oral physostigmine in amyotrophic lateral sclerosis. *Clin. Pharmacol Ther.* 1993 Dec;54(6):680-2.

[177] Carter GT, Weiss MD, Lou JS, Jensen MP, Abresch RT, Martin TK, et al. Modafinil to treat fatigue in amyotrophic lateral sclerosis: an open label pilot study. *Am. J. Hosp. Palliat Care.* 2005 Jan-Feb;22(1):55-9.

[178] Kinnear W, Scriven N, Orpe V, Jefferson D. *Prevalence of symptoms of sleep disturbance in patients with motor neurone disease* [abstract]. 8th International Symposium on ALS/MND; Glasgow1997 Nov 3-5.

[179] Sufit R. Symptomatic treatment of ALS *Neurology.* 1997;48:15S-22S.

[180] Lomen-Hoerth C, Murphy J, Langmore S, Kramer JH, Olney RK, Miller B. Are amyotrophic lateral sclerosis patients cognitively normal? *Neurology.* 2003 Apr 8;60(7):1094-7.

[181] Massman PJ, Sims J, Cooke N, Haverkamp LJ, Appel V, Appel SH. Prevalence and correlates of neuropsychological deficits in amyotrophic lateral sclerosis. *J. Neurol. Neurosurg. Psychiatry.* 1996 Nov;61(5):450-5.

[182] Abrahams S, Leigh PN, Goldstein LH. Cognitive change in ALS: a prospective study. *Neurology.* 2005 Apr 12;64(7):1222-6.

[183] Ringholz GM, Appel SH, Bradshaw M, Cooke NA, Mosnik DM, Schulz PE. Prevalence and patterns of cognitive impairment in sporadic ALS. *Neurology.* 2005 Aug 23;65(4):586-90.

[184] Woolley SC, Jonathan SK. Cognitive and behavioral impairment in amyotrophic lateral sclerosis. *Phys. Med. Rehabil Clin. N Am.* 2008 Aug;19(3):607-17, xi.

[185] Grossman AB, Woolley-Levine S, Bradley WG, Miller RG. Detecting neurobehavioral changes in amyotrophic lateral sclerosis. *Amyotroph. Lateral Scler.* 2007 Feb;8(1):56-61.

[186] Neary D, Snowden JS, Gustafson L, Passant U, Stuss D, Black S, et al. Frontotemporal lobar degeneration: a consensus on clinical diagnostic criteria. *Neurology.* 1998 Dec;51(6):1546-54.

[187] Rosen HJ, Cummings J. A real reason for patients with pseudobulbar affect to smile. *Ann. Neurol.* 2007 Feb;61(2):92-6.

[188] Palmieri A, Abrahams S, Soraru G, Mattiuzzi L, D'Ascenzo C, Pegoraro E, et al. Emotional Lability in MND: Relationship to cognition and psychopathology and impact on caregivers. *J. Neurol. Sci.* 2009 Mar 15;278(1-2):16-20.

[189] Moore SR, Gresham LS, Bromberg MB, Kasarkis EJ, Smith RA. A self report measure of affective lability. *J. Neurol. Neurosurg Psychiatry.* 1997 Jul;63(1):89-93.

[190] Meininger V. Treatment of emotional lability in ALS. Lancet Neurol. 2005 Feb;4(2):70.

[191] Brooks BR, Thisted RA, Appel SH, Bradley WG, Olney RK, Berg JE, et al. Treatment of pseudobulbar affect in ALS with dextromethorphan/quinidine: a randomized trial. *Neurology.* 2004 Oct 26;63(8):1364-70.

[192] Kurt A, Nijboer F, Matuz T, Kubler A. Depression and anxiety in individuals with amyotrophic lateral sclerosis: epidemiology and management. *CNS Drugs.* 2007;21(4):279-91.

[193] Rabkin JG, Albert SM, Del Bene ML, O'Sullivan I, Tider T, Rowland LP, et al. Prevalence of depressive disorders and change over time in late-stage ALS. *Neurology.* 2005 Jul 12;65(1):62-7.

[194] Goldstein LH, Atkins L, Landau S, Brown RG, Leigh PN. Longitudinal predictors of psychological distress and self-esteem in people with ALS. *Neurology.* 2006 Nov 14;67(9):1652-8.

[195] Simmons Z, Bremer BA, Robbins RA, Walsh SM, Fischer S. Quality of life in ALS depends on factors other than strength and physical function. *Neurology.* 2000 Aug 8;55(3):388-92.

[196] Rabkin JG, Albert SM, Rowland LP, Mitsumoto H. How common is depression among ALS caregivers? A longitudinal study. *Amyotroph. Lateral Scler.* 2009 Oct-Dec;10(5-6):448-55.

[197] Goldstein LH, Atkins L, Landau S, Brown R, Leigh PN. Predictors of psychological distress in carers of people with amyotrophic lateral sclerosis: a longitudinal study. *Psychol. Med.* 2006 Jun;36(6):865-75.

[198] Ray RA, Street AF. Caregiver bodywork: family members' experiences of caring for a person with motor neurone disease. *J. Adv. Nurs.* 2006 Oct;56(1):35-43.

[199] Matuz T, Birbaumer N, Hautzinger M, Kubler A. Coping with amyotrophic lateral sclerosis: an integrative view. *J. Neurol. Neurosurg Psychiatry.* 2010 Aug;81(8):893-8.

[200] De Groot IJ, Post MW, van Heuveln T, Van den Berg LH, Lindeman E. Cross-sectional and longitudinal correlations between disease progression and different health-related quality of life domains in persons with amyotrophic lateral sclerosis. *Amyotroph. Lateral Scler.* 2007 Dec;8(6):356-61.

[201] Mitsumoto H, Bromberg M, Johnston W, Tandan R, Byock I, Lyon M, et al. Promoting excellence in end-of-life care in ALS. *Amyotroph. Lateral Scler Other Motor Neuron Disord.* 2005 Sep;6(3):145-54.

[202] McCluskey L. Amyotrophic Lateral Sclerosis: ethical issues from diagnosis to end of life. *NeuroRehabilitation.* 2007;22(6):463-72.

[203] Oliver D. Palliative care. In: Kiernan M, editor. *The motor neurone disease handbook.* Prymont: Australasian Medical Publishing Company Limited; 2007. p. 186-95.

[204] Albert SM, Wasner M, Tider T, Drory VE, Borasio GD. Cross-cultural variation in mental health at end of life in patients with ALS. *Neurology.* 2007 Mar 27;68(13):1058-61.

[205] Skyes NP. End of life care. In: Oliver D, Borasio GD, Walsh D, editors. *Palliative care in amyotrophic lateral sclerosis - from diagnosis to bereavement.* Oxford: Oxford University Press; 2006.

In: Motor Neuron Diseases
Editors: Bradley J. Turner and Julie B. Atkin

ISBN: 978-1-61470-101-9
© 2012 Nova Science Publishers, Inc.

Chapter II

MEMBRANE TRAFFICKING DEFECTS AS DETERMINANTS OF MOTOR NEURON SUSCEPTIBILITY AND DEGENERATION IN ALS

*Bradley J. Turner[*1] and Julie D. Atkin[*1,2]*
[1]Florey Neuroscience Institutes and Centre for Neuroscience,
University of Melbourne, Parkville, Victoria, Australia
[2]Department of Biochemistry, La Trobe Institute for Molecular Science,
La Trobe University, Bundoora, Victoria, Australia

ABSTRACT

Amyotrophic lateral sclerosis (ALS) is characterised by motor neuron death and accumulation of ubiquitinated protein inclusions. Motor neurons are large-calibre and long distance projection excitatory cells with unusually high energetic, synthetic and transport demands required for maintenance and survival. These neurons are therefore likely to be uniquely susceptible to intracellular transport abnormalities in cell bodies and distal axons. Here, we review increasing evidence that motor neuron vulnerability in ALS may be conferred by defects in intracellular trafficking pathways specialised for these cells. Firstly, many of the genes implicated in familial forms of ALS encode molecular machinery or enzymes directly mediating intracellular transport. Secondly, these ALS gene products and additional constituents of trafficking pathways form core components of pathology in familial and sporadic disease. Lastly, defective membrane, vesicle, protein and mRNA transport features prominently and early in motor neuron degeneration in ALS models. We provide a systematic summary of ALS-linked proteins including ALS2, CHMP2B, FIG4, FUS, OPTN, p150[Glued], SOD1, TDP-43, VAPB and VCP with respect to their localisation, function and dysfunction in intracellular

* Correspondence: B. Turner: Tel: +61 3 8344 1867, email: bradley.turner@florey.edu.au and J. Atkin: Tel: +61 3 9479 5480, email: j.atkin@latrobe.edu.au

trafficking pathways, such as anterograde and retrograde axonal transport, endoplasmic-Golgi, endosome-lysosome and nuclear transport. The role of molecular motor-linked proteins such as kinesin, dynein and neurofilaments in motor neurodegeneration will also be addressed. We propose that intracellular membrane trafficking defects affecting key neuronal functions, such as neurotransmission, extracellular signalling and synaptic activity, may be an early determinant of motor neuron loss and common denominator of potentially many ALS-linked proteins.

INTRODUCTION

Amyotrophic lateral sclerosis (ALS) is a rapidly progressing and fatal neurodegenerative disorder affecting motor neurons of the spinal cord, brainstem and frontal cortex. ALS has a consistent clinical pattern with striking similarities in cellular pathology, implying a common pathogenic process. Several proteins are linked to sporadic and familial forms of ALS, notably superoxide dismutase 1 (SOD1), TAR DNA binding protein 43 (TDP-43) and fused in sarcoma (FUS).

Approximately 20% of familial ALS cases are due to mutations in SOD1 and mutant SOD1 proteins have been extensively studied in cellular and animal models of disease. In spite of many studies into the possible molecular mechanisms underlying neurodegeneration, definition of the primary mechanism in ALS still remains elusive. In this review we describe the increasing evidence that defects in intracellular membrane trafficking pathways specifically target motor neurons and contribute to the pathophysiology of ALS. Efficient and reliable protein, vesicular and organelle trafficking during cellular transport is fundamental for the maintenance of neuronal homeostasis.

Motor neurons are uniquely vulnerable to transport defects because of their long axons, large cell bodies and high energetic requirements. Whilst axonal transport defects are most commonly reported, a long list of vesicle, endosome and intracellular transport proteins have now been linked to disorders of motor neurons, including classic ALS genes (Table 1.) and non-ALS genes such as atlastin, dynein, HspB1, KIF1Bβ, KIF5A, maspardin, NIPA1, protrudin, Rab7A, spartin and spastin.

Mechanisms of Intracellular Protein Trafficking

The general protein apparatus used by motor neurons is common to all intracellular transport processes in eukaryotic cells. Donor membranes are shaped into vesicles by cytoplasmic coats which then dissociate by the action of Rab small GTPases. The organelle or target membrane specificity of vesicles is also determined by Rab GTPases, of which over 40 members are currently known in mammals (Stenmark, 2009). Rabs switch between a GTP-bound active form catalysed by guanine nucleotide exchange factors (GEF) and GDP-bound inactive forms, resulting from GTP hydrolysis stimulated by a GTPase-activating protein (GAP) (Ali and Seabra, 2005). GTP hydrolysis drives vesicle budding while GTP-bound Rabs bind effector proteins, collectively mediating transport, docking and fusion with target compartments.

Table 1. Familial ALS genes and products

Type	Mode	Onset	Gene	Frequency	Protein	Localisation	Mislocalisation	Reference(s)
ALS1	AD	Adult	SOD1	2%	Superoxide dismutase 1	Ubiquitous	Cytoplasm	Rosen et al. (1993)
ALS2	AR	Juvenile	ALS2	rare	ALS2/Alsin	Early endosome	ND	Hadano et al. (2001); Yang et al. (2001)
ALS4	AD	Juvenile	SETX	very rare	Senataxin	Nucleus	ND	Chen et al. (2004)
ALS6	AD	Adult	FUS	0.5%	Fused in sarcoma	Nucleus	Cytoplasm	Kwiatkowski et al. (2009); Vance et al. (2009)
ALS8	AD	Adult	VAPB	very rare	Vesicle-associated protein B	ER	Cytoplasm	Nishimura et al. (2004)
ALS9	AD	Adult	ANG	rare	Angiogenin	Cytoplasm	ND	Greenway et al. (2006)
ALS10	AD	Adult	TARDBP	0.5%	TAR DNA binding protein 43	Nucleus	Cytoplasm	Sreedharan et al. (2008)
ALS11	AD	Adult	FIG4	very rare	Factor induced gene 4	Late endosome	ND	Chow et al. (2009)
ALS12	AD	Adult	OPTN	very rare	Optineurin	Golgi apparatus	Cytoplasm	Maruyama et al. (2010)
ALS	AD	Adult	DCTN1	rare	p150[Glued]	Cytoskeleton	Cytoplasm	Puls et al. (2003)
ALS	AD	Adult	CHMP2B	rare	Charged MVB protein 2B	MVB	Late endosome	Parkinson et al. (2006)
ALS	AD	Adult	VCP	0.2%	Valosin containing protein	ER-Golgi	ND	Johnson et al. (2010)

AD, autosomal dominant; AR, autosomal recessive; MVB, multivesicular body; ND, not described.

Intracellular Trafficking and Motor Neuron Diseases

A perplexing characteristic of ALS is why motor neurons are predominantly targeted by ubiquitously expressed proteins. Motor neurons are large, highly differentiated and polarized cells, with extremely long axons, up to 1 metre in length in an adult human. Hence, they have high synthetic and energy requirements, which therefore place heavy demands on cellular transport processes. Proteins, lipids, mRNAs and organelles need to rapidly move from the cell body over large distances along the axon to the synaptic terminals or neuromuscular junctions, where they are required for axoplasmic membrane remodeling, energy production, neurotransmission and local protein synthesis. Axonal transport is also required to collect neurotrophins, survival factors or potentially toxic factors from distal axons, peripheral synapses or muscle cells back to the soma. The complexity and fine regulation of this system is highly sensitive to perturbation, and minor alterations of cellular and vesicular transport processes may result in motor neuron dysfunctions (Sau et al., 2011). Here, we review the mechanisms underpinning four major transport pathways within motor neurons and the evidence implicating their dysfunction in ALS and other motor neuron disorders as determinants of neuronal susceptibility and degeneration.

1. Axonal Transport

Axonal transport is a key cellular trafficking process in motor neurons due to their high calibre and large projection axons. Axonal transport cargoes are actively transported either downstream to the synaptic terminal (anterograde transport) or upstream to the soma (retrograde transport). Transport occurs along cytoskeletal filaments (microtubules, actin or intermediate filaments), which provide structural support for these movements. In axons microtubules have unipolar orientation that provides stability and polarity, with the fast growing 'plus' end directed towards the synapse, and the 'minus' end directed towards the cell body. In contrast, dendrites have mixed microtubule polarity (Chevalier-Larsen and Holzbaur, 2006). Neurofilaments or intermediate filaments are the most abundant component in the neuronal cytoskeleton, and they assemble from three subunit polypeptides, light chain (NF-L), medium chain (NF-M) and heavy chain (NF-H). NFs are much more stable than actin or microtubules and they primarily provide structural stabilization to neurons. In axons and dendrites, microtubules and neurofilaments are the major cytoskeletal filaments, whereas in the synaptic regions, such as presynaptic terminals and postsynaptic spines, actin filaments predominate the cytoskeletal architecture. Actin filaments are composed of monomers which can extend and grow at very rapid rates during neurite extension (Sau et al., 2011).

Historically and functionally, axonal transport is divided into 'fast' transport, characterized by high speeds (up to 1 mm/s) and occurring in both anterograde and retrograde directions, and 'slow' transport, typically anterograde and less efficient, with low speeds (approx. 1 mm/day) (De Vos et al., 2008). Mitochondria, polyribosomes, membrane-bound organelles and synaptic vesicles typically use fast axonal transport, whereas cytoskeleton components and cytosolic enzymes generally rely on slow axonal transport. Cargoes are transported specifically along cytoskeletal structures by motor proteins which drive movement by intrinsic ATPase activity. Both fast and axonal transport processes involve the same molecular motor proteins (Roy et al., 2000). Transport along axons is powered by microtubule-based motor proteins dynein and kinesin, whereas transport at the synapse is driven by the motor molecule myosin, which transports the cargo along actin filaments.

Microtubule Motor Proteins, Kinesin and Dynein

Kinesin superfamily proteins transport cargoes in the anterograde direction and dyneins move cargoes in a retrograde direction, although a few kinesins also power retrograde transport (Brady, 1985; Vale et al., 1985; Paschal et al., 1987). The kinesin superfamily comprises at least 45 members in humans (Miki et al., 2005), whereas the cytoplasmic dynein family is much smaller, and only two members have been described: cytoplasmic dyneins and axonemal (or cilary) dyneins (Kamal and Goldstein, 2002). The direction of axonal transport depends on microtubule orientation and motor protein specificity.

Kinesins are heterotetramers composed of two heavy and two light chains, containing an ATPase motor domain (head domain), microtubule-binding regions and a cargo-binding domain (tail domain) (Morfini et al., 2009). Kinesins are classified into 14 families based on head domain homology (Hirokawa et al., 2009). The N-kinesin (kinesins 1−12) family members have an N-terminal motor domain and generally move towards microtubule plus ends. The M-kinesin (kinesin 13) family members possess a centrally located motor domain and are involved in microtubule depolymerization without actively moving along them. C-kinesin (kinesin 14) family members have a C-terminal motor domain and move retrogradely towards the microtubule minus end.

Cytoplasmic dynein is a large complex (approx. 2 MDa) formed by two dynein heavy chains, two dynein intermediate chains, four dynein light intermediate chains and several dynein light chains. Dynein functions strictly depend on an associated protein complex, dynactin, which acts as an adaptor protein between the molecular motor and its cargoes, and regulates dynein by increasing its binding to cargoes. Dynactin is composed of 11 different subunits including p62, dynamitin, and a coiled-coil domain, known as p150^{Glued}, which connects dynein to microtubules. There are many isoforms of each component and this facilitates the transport of multiple cargoes despite there being only one isoform of dynein (Hirokawa et al., 2010). Cytoplasmic dynein conveys cargoes retrogradely both in the axon and distal dendrites, whilst in the proximal dendrites it transports cargoes to both the periphery and cell body due to the mixed polarity of microtubules in this location. In dendrites, cytoplasmic dynein conveys cargos involving glycine receptor vesicles, mRNAs within protein complexes, and Rab5-positive endosomes. In contrast to the divergence of kinesins, there is only one species of dynein heavy chain involved in transport. Hence, dynein regulates cargo binding through light chains, the light intermediate chain, and the dynactin complex.

Dyneins and kinesins function in an inter-dependent manner, and the disruption of movement in one direction can affect movement in the opposite direction (Waterman-Storer et al., 1997). Moreover, the dynein intermediate chain directly interacts with and kinesin light chains 1 and 2 (Ligon et al., 2004) and the p150^{Glued} subunit of dynactin interacts with kinesin (Deacon et al., 2003). Molecular motors can also participate in signaling processes by transporting signaling molecules from one location to another within a neuron, from where they can modulate cellular behaviours (Hirokawa et al., 2010). Hence, regulation of axonal transport is a complex process.

Pre- and Post-Synaptic Transport Is Powered by Myosin

Myosin superfamily motor proteins move along actin filaments and are classified into 18 different groups (Foth et al., 2006). They play significant roles in cell movement, muscle contraction, cytokinesis, membrane trafficking, and signal transduction. Most myosins form a dimer and consist of a motor domain, a neck region, and a tail region.

Motor Neuron Diseases and Axonal Transport

There is now substantial evidence for the involvement of axonal transport defects in the pathogenesis of neurodegenerative disorders, including diseases of motor neurons (Sau et al., 2011). Direct evidence has come from the identification of disease-causative mutations in proteins involved in axonal transport, (Gunawardena and Goldstein, 2004) and indirect evidence comes from morphological abnormalities described in motor neuron diseases (MNDs), such as axonal swelling, cytoskeletal abnormalities and axonal accumulation of organelles or ubiquitinated proteins. Abnormalities in kinesin-mediated anterograde transport could lead to either synaptic defects or axonal die-back due to inadequate supply of new proteins and lipids from the cell body to the distal synapse. In contrast, defects in dynein-mediated retrograde transport could lead to a lack of neurotrophin support or the accumulation of cellular components at the synapse and distal axon. Alternatively, recent study suggested that retrograde transport defects trigger neurodegeneration by a change in the type of protein cargoes that are transported, from survival-promoting to death-promoting signaling molecules (Perlson et al., 2009).

Slowing of both fast and slow axonal transport is an early event in animal ALS disease models, detectable long before neuronal death (Coleman, 2005) , implying that disruption to axonal transport is a primary event in pathogenesis. Pathological intracellular protein inclusions are found in almost all MNDs linked to protein misfolding (Piccioni et al., 2002; Poletti, 2004) and these aggregates may sequester proteins essential for transport, perturbing transport protein function or by exacerbation of existing damage. Dynein, kinesin, NFs, α-internexin, peripherin, 14-3-3 protein, TDP-43 and FUS have all been found in ALS aggregates (Strong, 2010) which may perturb the axon and synapse of mitochondria, RNA granules or key proteins (Piccioni et al., 2002; De Vos et al., 2007). However these interactions appear late in disease course and thus do not explain the observed inhibition of transport (Perlson et al., 2009).

Kinesins

Anterograde axonal transport is essential for synapse generation and for maintaining synaptic transmission, and multiple roles have been described for kinesin motors in neurons. Human genetic pedigrees and reverse and forward genetic studies in animal models have highlighted the importance of kinesin in MNDs, particularly kinesin heavy chain genes, KIF5A and KIF1Bβ, which transport mitochondria, synaptic vesicles and macromolecular complexes, (Hirokawa et al., 2009). Postnatal disruption of KIF5A induces a reduction in slow anterograde axonal transport, resulting in accumulation of neurofilaments in dorsal root ganglion cell bodies, a reduction in axonal calibre and degeneration of sensory neurons (Xia et al., 2003). Similarly, the expression of KIF1Bβ mutants in mice induces slowing of anterograde transport of synaptic vesicle precursors, resulting in a late-onset axonopathy (Zhao et al., 2001). These pathological effects closely resemble those observed in two familial human MNDs caused by mutant kinesin family genes: KIF5A (Ebbing et al., 2008) in hereditary spastic paraplegia (SPG10) and KIF1β (Zhao et al., 2001) in Charcot-Marie Tooth type 2A (CMT2A) disease. Notably, not only mutations, but lower expression of wild-type kinesin proteins are implicated in MNDs (Pantelidou et al., 2007). For example, KIF1Bβ and KIF3Aβ mRNA and protein are downregulated in motor cortex specimens of ALS patients (Pantelidou et al., 2007), and KIFAP3, kinesin-associated protein 3, a subunit of kinesin-2 complexes, has been identified as a susceptibility gene in sporadic ALS (Landers et al., 2009). Furthermore, the sequestering of KAP3 by mutant SOD1 was suggested to cause reduced transport of ChAT (a known KAP3-kinesin-2 cargo) in an ALS model (Tateno et al., 2009). However, in comparison to dynein, relatively few degenerative diseases have been directly linked to mutations in kinesin, possibly due to functional redundancy in the large kinesin superfamily.

Dynein

Dynein is very highly expressed in neurons (Melloni et al., 1995) and neurons are particularly sensitive to defects in dynein/dynactin function (de Vos et al., 2008). There is now a wealth of evidence linking dynein/dynactin abnormalities and retrograde axonal transport failure to motor neuron degeneration. Mutations in the dynactin 1 gene (DCTN1), encoding the p150^{Glued} subunit of dynactin, cause human distal hereditary motor neuropathy (HMN7B) (Puls et al., 2003; Munch et al., 2005). Knock-in and transgenic mice expressing these mutations subsequently develop motor neuron degeneration (Lai et al., 2007; Laird et al., 2008). Over-expression of dynactin subunit dynamitin in mice leads to impairment of dynein-dynactin interaction and a late-onset progressive disease reminiscent of ALS (LaMonte et al., 2002). Mutation of the dynein heavy chain 1 gene causes motor neuron degeneration and inhibition of axonal transport (Hafezparast et al., 2003). *Loa* (legs at odd angles) and *Cra1* (Cramping1) mice which carry separate *N*-ethyl-*N*-nitrosourea-induced mutations of the dynein cytoplasmic heavy chain 1 gene, show selective impairment of axonal retrograde transport as well as progressive locomotor disorders associated with spinal motor neuron degeneration (Hafezparast et al., 2003). A third mouse model (*Swl*) with another dynein heavy chain gene mutation displays an early-onset sensory neuropathy with muscle spindle deficiency (Chen et al., 2007). These mice have severely compromised proprioceptive sensory neurons in lumbar dorsal root ganglia, but unaffected motor neurons. Defects in axonal transport are also well documented as an early event in pathology in motor neurons of transgenic mutant SOD1^{G93A} mice (Williamson and Cleveland, 1999; Bisland et al., 2010), the most widely used animal model of ALS (Murakami et al., 2001; Kieran et al.,

2005). Surprisingly, crossing these animals with *Loa* or *Cra1* (but not *Swl*) mice delays disease progression and significantly increases lifespan (Kieran et al., 2005). This correlates with a complete recovery of the axonal transport deficits in motor neurons of these mice (Kieran et al., 2005; Teuchert et al., 2006). However, this observation was partially explained recently by a proteomics study which revealed that the SOD1 mutation augments retrograde transport of stress factors (p-JNK, caspase-8 and p75[NTR] cleavage fragment) and simultaneously impairs retrograde transport of survival factors (p-Trk and p-Erk1/2) (Perlson et al., 2009).

In addition to a direct involvement of dynein in disease, defects in other proteins could also perturb dynein functions and lead to motor neuron degeneration. Notably, cytoplasmic dynein is sequestered into SOD1 aggregates (Ligon et al., 2005) through HDAC6 (histone deacetylase 6), a dynein interacting protein that poly-ubiquitinates misfolded proteins (Kawaguchi et al., 2003). The sequestration of dynein could perturb retrograde axonal transport and other dynein-mediated processes. Dynein is involved in the autophagic clearance of misfolded proteins (Komatsu et al., 2007 and removal of damaged organelles and proteins from the axonal compartment (Strom et al., 2008). Dynein also plays a role in the transport of nerve injury signals, phosphorylated Erk (Perlson et al., 2005), and phosphorylated JNK (Cavalli et al., 2005). Impairment of these functions would also contribute to a worsening neurological status. The transport of secretory proteins between the endoplasmic reticulum (ER) and Golgi apparatus is also a dynein mediated process, and is also implicated in diseases of motor neurons, suggesting a link between these two processes (LaMonte et al., 2002). Also, another well-established consequence of dynein dysfunction is fragmentation of the Golgi apparatus (Gonatas et al., 2006), which occurs in spinal and cortical motor neurons in ALS, cell lines over-expressing mutant SOD1 (Turner and Atkin, 2006) and is one of the first pathological events in SOD1[G93A] mice (Mourelatos et al., 1996), further linking axonal transport with ER-Golgi abnormalities. Alternatively the types of protein cargoes transported by dynein is implicated in ALS (Perlson et al., 2009). Impaired retrograde transport of activated neurotrophin receptors by direct association of the dynein light chain with Trk neurotrophin receptors may also trigger neurodegeneration (Heerssen et al., 2004; Yano et al., 2001). Whilst there is clear evidence that axonal transport abnormalities lead to motor neuron loss, the biological meaning of all these highly variable genotype/phenotype correlations remain largely obscure. It is also unclear why mutations in molecular motor genes affect primarily only a specific subset of motor neuron populations. For example, KIF5A mutations lead to upper motor neuron death in the cortex, whereas spinal cord motor neurons are spared. Conversely, DCTN1 mutations affect primarily the lower spinal cord motor neurons without significant alterations in the upper cortical motor neurons.

Regulation of Axonal Functions Are Also Linked to ALS

Axonal transport is a tightly regulated process, and deregulation or misregulation of axonal transport is also associated with neurodegeneration. Regulation of axonal transport involves cargo-specific membrane-bound Rab adaptor proteins that actively recruit motors to organelles. Mutant forms of Rab7 cause CMT2B and exhibit aberrant GTP hydrolysis

(Spinosa et al., 2008). As well as specific mutations perturbations in the regulatory environment of the cell also may significantly disrupt transport.

Cytoskeletal Abnormalities in Motor Neuron Diseases

Cytoskeletal integrity is absolutely essential for maintaining neuronal function, and perturbations within the cytoskeleton represent another level of regulation of axonal transport and motor neuronal dysfunction. Among the three main neuronal cytoskeleton structures, NFs are particularly important because they control axonal calibre and provide structural stabilization to neurons (Perrot and Eyer, 2009). Moreover, NF accumulations and inclusions are a common feature of motor neuron disorders. Furthermore, NF-L is mutated in CMT2E and CMT1F, and these mutations disrupt the transport of wild-type NFs and mitochondria (Perez-Olle et al., 2005). Modifications of proteins involved in cytoskeleton assemblage, dynamics or quality control is another potential source of axonal transport defects. Mutations of heat shock protein 27 kDa protein 1 (HspB1) disrupt NF assembly and organelle transport (Evgrafov et al., 2004), and lead to CMT2F. Also, mutations in the spastin gene (SPG4) gene, which lead to hereditary spastic paraplegia, induce neurite swellings and focal impairment of retrograde transport at the growth cone (Tarrade et al., 2006). Furthermore, atlastin and REEP1, two proteins which normally interact with spastin and play a role in microtubule assembly, are mutated in two hereditary spastic paraplegia forms. Notably, these three proteins not only interact in a single complex, but their mutations give rise to very similar hereditary spastic paraplegia phenotypes. Alterations of microtubule modification also disrupt axonal transport, such as acetylation or tyrosination of tubulin subunits. Microtubule associated proteins, which compete with motor proteins in binding to the microtubule surface, have also been demonstrated to perturb transport (Perlson et al., 2010).

Mutant SOD1 can also affect axonal transport by damaging cargoes such as NFs, inhibiting their transport or promoting their release from motors (Hirokawa et al., 2010). These effects depend on p38 mitogen-activated protein kinase activation, resulting in an aberrant hyperphosphorylation of NF-M/NF-H domains (Zhang et al., 2007). Furthermore, p38-dependent hyperphosphorylation promotes NF release from molecular motors, slowing NF transport (Shea et al., 2004; Jung et al., 2005). Mutant SOD1 can trigger axonal dysfunction and degeneration via NO-induced up-regulation of CRMP4a (collapsin response mediator protein 4a) via the death receptor Fas/CD95 (Duplan et al., 2010) . TDP-43 is altered in response to axotomy in normal mice, and axonal ligation induces nuclear exclusion and peripheral axonal accumulation of TDP-43 in hypoglossal neurons (Sato et al., 2009). This is accompanied by a concomitant decrease in active autophagosomes, possibly due to defective axonal autophagy. Moreover, in presymptomatic NF-L-knockout mice, cytosolic TDP-43 expression is up-regulated, suggesting that TDP-43 is involved in NF mRNA metabolism and transport (Moisse et al., 2009). Together, these results clearly indicate that several different axonal pathways could be targeted by disease-associated mutant proteins.

Alterations of Axonal Transport of Mitochondria, Vesicles and Other Cargoes

Axonal transport defects can also affect motor neuron viability by reducing the axon and synapse content of essential components such as mitochondria. Mitochondria play a fundamental role both in the cell body and in the synaptic terminal, where high Ca^{2+} buffering and strong energetics are required. Hence efficient mechanisms of transporting mitochondria to the synapse are necessary. Mitochondria also need to be transported from the synapse and distal axon to the lysosome when they are targeted for destruction. Hence, both anterograde and retrograde axonal transport of mitochondria are crucial for motor neuron metabolism and survival. Moreover, mitochondrial dysfunction is well documented in diseases of motor neurons (Pasinelli and Brown, 2006; Nagley et al., 2010). Three kinesins involved in mitochondrial transport are also implicated in diseases of motor neurons: KIF1B (responsible for CMT2A), KIF5B (SPG10) and kinesin light chain (Magrane and Manfredi, 2009). Damaged mitochondria are degraded through an autophagic process known as mitophagy. This is a finely regulated mechanism dependent on mitochondrial dynamic properties, and mitophagy dysregulation leads to perturbation of axonal mitochondrial content. Mitophagy requires active mitochondrial transport along microtubules, which is mediated by kinesins and dyneins (Hollenbeck, 2005).Slow movements over relatively short distances are driven by myosin and occur on actin filaments (Ligon and Steward, 2000).

2. ENDOPLASMIC RETICULUM AND GOLGI APPARATUS TRANSPORT

The endoplasmic reticulum (ER) and Golgi apparatus together exert a fundamental regulatory role in neurons, and there is now substantial evidence for ER and Golgi abnormalities in diseases involving motor neurons (Zhao et al., 2005; Ito and Suzuki 2007; Senderek et al., 2005). In particular, ER stress is emerging as important cellular pathway to motor neuron death in ALS. The ER is primarily responsible for the sorting, post-translational modification and trafficking of transmembrane and secretory proteins (Schroder, 2008). Proteins destined for secretion or for transport to distal sites within the cell are folded and packed into small vesicles which bud from the ER (Routledge et al., 2010) encased in the coat protein complex II (COPII). Vesicles containing the secretory protein cargo are then transported to the Golgi along microtubules by a dynein-dependent process (Figure 1). The dynein complex therefore an important motor driving both bidirectional transport between the ER and Golgi and retrograde axonal transport. Vesicles from the ER fuse with the *cis*-Golgi network and subsequently progress to the *trans*-Golgi network, from where they are dispatched to further cell locations. The Golgi apparatus is integral in modifying, sorting, and packaging secretory molecules. Secretion of proteins via the classical ER-Golgi pathway is a vital cellular function and approximately a third of all cellular proteins transit via this route. Hence, inhibition of ER-Golgi function and transport could severely impact on cellular function.

A high rate of protein folding is required within the ER and prevention of protein misfolding is vital to maintain cellular function. A proportion of proteins misfold as part of normal cellular physiology, but in some instances the burden of misfolded or unfolded proteins within the ER increases. This results in ER stress, which triggers signaling pathways collectively known as the unfolded protein response (UPR). Activation of the UPR results in a decrease in general protein translation, a specific up-regulation of UPR target genes such as those encoding protein chaperones, and an expansion of ER volume via increased lipid production (Ron and Walter, 2007). ER stress also induces ER-associated degradation (ERAD), a process by which constituent and transient proteins are removed from the ER and retrotranslocated to the cytosol, where they are degraded by the 26S proteasome. These initial UPR response mechanisms aim to restore homeostasis and alone are often sufficient to overcome a short-term insult. However, if homeostasis is not restored, cell death is triggered via apoptotic signaling mechanisms. Cellular insults which lead to increased protein misfolding in the ER include changes in intracellular calcium concentration, alterations in the redox state of the ER, nutrient deprivation, the failure of post-translational modifications and increases in secretory protein synthesis (Rutkowski et al., 2008). Disturbances of the Golgi, endosomal and vesicular transport pathways and mitochondrial-associated apoptosis, can also elicit ER stress (Short et al., 2007; Jonikas et al., 2009).

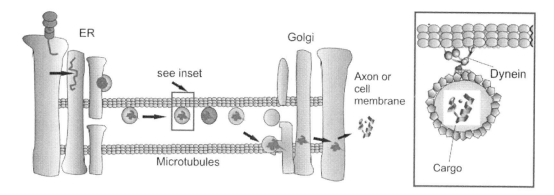

Figure 1. Trafficking of secretory proteins from the ER to Golgi. Newly synthesised proteins destined for secretion or transport to distal sites within the cell are folded and packed into small vesicles which bud from the ER. Vesicles containing protein cargoes are transported to the Golgi where they are then dispatched to further cell locations. The dynein complex (inset) is the important molecular motor which drives bidirectional transport between ER-Golgi and retrograde axonal transport.

ER-Golgi and Diseases of Motor Neurons

We were amongst the first groups to demonstrate that ER stress is present in the SOD1^{G93A} animal disease model (Atkin et al., 2006), prior to appearance of clinical signs (Atkin et al., 2008). Subsequently, it was shown that ER stress appears very early and selectively in those motor neurons which are targeted first in these animals (Saxena et al., 2009). Multiple *in vivo* studies have now demonstrated a key role for ER stress in disease in SOD1^{G93A} mice (Wootz et al., 2006a; Kieran et al., 2007; Nishitoh et al., 2008; Hetz et al., 2009). Disease progression in this animal model can also be altered by pharmacological agents that modulate ER stress (Saxena et al., 2009). Furthermore, ER stress is triggered in humans with sporadic ALS (Atkin et al., 2008), implicating the UPR in the pathophysiology of all ALS, not just SOD1-linked familial forms. Increasing evidence also implicates the ER-Golgi in disease induced by TDP-43 and FUS in ALS. Recently, TDP-43 was detected in the rough ER in spinal cord motor neurons of sporadic ALS patients (Sasaki, 2010), suggesting that TDP-43 could be redistributed to the ER in disease. Furthermore, TDP-43 has been detected in mouse brainstem microsomes which contain ER and other vesicles (Sato et al., 2009), and pharmacological induction of ER stress increases the accumulation of TDP-43 in cell culture (Suzuki et al., 2011). Similarly, FUS has also been linked to the ER: electron microscopy of spinal motor neurons of patients with juvenile ALS demonstrated FUS-positive inclusions associated with disorganised rough ER (Huang et al., 2010). A key UPR protein, BiP, is also found in FUS-immunoreactive inclusions in ALS patient tissue, providing further evidence that ER stress could be involved in mutant FUS-linked ALS (Tateishi et al., 2009).

An important question raised by these findings is how ER stress is induced in ALS and other motor neuron diseases? Protein misfolding within the ER lumen has been previously regarded as necessary for induction of the UPR. However most proteins linked to ALS are not normally located in the ER. Previous reports describing an ER presence for SOD1 were subsequently shown to be artifactual (Nishitoh et al., 2008).UPR induction has been attributed to the interaction of cytoplasmic mutant SOD1 with Derlin-1, a key protein involved in ERAD (Nishitoh et al., 2008), but this interaction was only detected after the onset of symptoms in transgenic SOD1 mice, suggesting that this mechanism is not the primary trigger of ER stress. However, it is now recognised that other cellular processes can cause secondary ER stress, such as disturbances of the ER, Golgi, endosomal and vesicular transport systems (Short et al., 2007; Preston et al., 2009; Jonikas et al., 2009) Similarly, cross-talk between ER stress, autophagy and the ubiquitin proteasome system indicates that aggregation of proteins within the cytoplasm can also lead to ER stress. Hence, a range of cellular mechanisms can trigger ER stress can be within or independent of the ER.

Fragmentation of the Golgi Apparatus

Golgi fragmentation, a well-established consequence of both ER stress and dynein dysfunction (Gonatas et al., 2006; Nakagomi et al., 2008), occurs in spinal and cortical motor neurons in ALS, in cell lines over-expressing mutant SOD1 (Turner and Atkin, 2006) and is one of the first pathological events in SOD1^{G93A} mice (Mourelatos et al., 1996; Nakagomi et al., 2008). Golgi fragmentation is not downstream of apoptosis or rough ER morphological disturbance, since it can occur in neurons with intact rough ER that are not undergoing apoptosis (Gonatas et al., 2006). Blockage of ER to Golgi trafficking also causes dispersal of the Golgi apparatus (Zaal et al., 1999).

ER-Golgi Vesicle Trafficking Defects

As well as ER stress, perturbation of vesicle trafficking within the ER-Golgi compartments is linked to diseases of motor neurons. Several spontaneous mouse mutants with motor phenotypes have been linked to defects in intracellular trafficking, such as the progressive motor neuronopathy (pmn) mouse, which accumulates the mutant tubulin-specific chaperone TBCE in the cis-Golgi compartment (Schaefer et al., 2007). Similarly, neurodegeneration in another spontaneous mutant, the wobbler mouse, is due to mutations in vacuolar-vesicular protein sorting factor Vps54, which is involved in Golgi-associated vesicular trafficking (Schmitt-John et al., 2005). Importantly, vesicle trafficking defects have also been linked to human motor neuron diseases. Two proteins implicated in endocytosis and vesicular transport (Wishart and Dixon, 2002) MTMR2 (myotubularin-related protein 2) and MTMR13 (myotubularin 13)/SBF2, are mutated in CMT4B1 and CMT4B2 respectively (Bolino et al., 2000; Azzedine et al., 2003). Both MTMR2 and MTMR13/SBF2 are phosphatases, and a loss of phosphatase activity results in impaired interaction with binding partners and vesicular traffic defects. Another vesicular traffic regulator, dynamin 2, is associated with dominant intermediate CMT type B (DICMTB) (Zuchner et al., 2005). Dynamin 2 modulates the actin cytoskeleton, interacts with actin-binding proteins such as profiling and Abp1 (Orth and McNiven, 2003), and is involved in the fusion and fission of vesicles and other membranous organelles (McNiven, 2005). Furthermore, atlastin 1 (SPG3A) and REEP1 mutations (SPG31) also result in marked ER morphological defects and altered synaptic vesicle recycling. Several familial forms of ALS are also linked to genes encoding proteins involved in the regulation and control of vesicle transport: VAPB, VCP and ALS2 (please see section 3 below) (Yang et al., 2001; Otomo et al., 2003; Johnson et al., 2010).

Vesicle-Associated Membrane Protein-Associated Protein B (VAPB)

Missense mutations of VAPB, a widely expressed ER transmembrane protein (Teuling et al., 2007), cause autosomal dominant typical ALS, slowly progressing atypical ALS or late-onset spinal muscular atrophy (SMA). VAPB belongs to a class of VAPs [VAMP (vesicle associated membrane protein)-associated proteins]; highly conserved proteins which are localized in the ER and associated with microtubules (Skehel et al., 2000). The human VAP family proteins were initially identified as homologues of vesicle-associated membrane protein (VAMP)-associated protein (VAP) with a size of 33 kDa in *Aplysia californica* (aVAP33) (Nishimura et al., 1999), which is involved in exocytosis of neurotransmitters. Several reports have suggested that VAPB is important in structural regulation of the ER and in, both ER and Golgi maintenance (Teuling et al., 2007; Peretti et al., 2008; Fasana et al., 2010). Importantly, VAPB is involved in the regulation of ER−Golgi vesicle transport (Foster et al., 2000) and in modulating ER stress (Kanekura et al., 2006). It also has other roles in protein transport, phospholipid metabolism, and also viral infection (Kagiwada et al., 1998).

The two VAPB mutations described in ALS, P56S and T46I, perturb ER and Golgi trafficking (Nishimura et al., 2004) and cause morphological disruption to the ER (Tsuda et al., 2008; Chen et al., 2010; Fasana et al., 2010). These mutations also appear to increase motor neuron vulnerability to ER stress-induced death, by sequestering wild-type VAPB (Suzuki et al., 2009). Mutant VAPB also induces the co-aggregation of wild-type VAPB (Kanekura et al., 2006; Chen et al., 2010), suggesting a dominant-negative mode of pathogenesis. Mutant P56S VAPB inclusions are ER derived (Teuling et al., 2007; Fasana et al., 2010), and co-locate with a subset of ER proteins (Tsuda et al., 2008). VAP proteins are usually cleaved releasing an N-terminal MSP (major sperm protein) domain, which acts as a diffusible hormone on Eph (Ephrin) receptors. Eph receptors are present on the growth cone of neurons and are involved in axonal guidance (Flanagan and Vanderhaeghen, 1998), suggesting that axonal dysfunctions related to loss-of-function of the MSP domain contribute to ALS (Tsuda et al., 2008).

Optineurin (OPTN)

Mutations in optineurin, a Golgi-localised protein involved in membrane and vesicle trafficking, have also been discovered in ALS pedigrees (Maruyama et al 2010). Optineurin mutations are also found in glaucoma, another neurodegenerative condition, from which its name is derived: "optic neuropathy inducing" protein optineurin (Rezaie et al., 2002). Optineurin plays an important role in the maintenance of the Golgi complex, in membrane trafficking, and in exocytosis via its interactions with Rab8 (Park et al., 2006) (Sahlender et al., 2005), huntingtin (Hattula and Peranen, 2000), and myosin VI (Park et al., 2006; Sahlender et al., 2005). Targeting of optineurin to the Golgi complex is also mediated via myosin VI (Park et al., 2006; Sahlender et al., 2005). siRNA studies have also suggested a role of optineurin in the exocytosis of vesicular-stomatitis-virus G protein (Sahlender et al., 2005).

Valosin Containing Protein (VCP)

Recently, ALS-causative mutations in the gene encoding valosin containing protein (VCP/p97) were identified in familial ALS patients (Johnson et al., 2010). VCP is a hexameric type II ATPase of the AAA family that mediates disparate cellular functions, including ERAD via the ubiquitin proteasome system (UPS) (Woodman, 2003; Dreveny et al., 2004; Halawani and Latterich, 2006) and the fusion of ER and Golgi membranes (Latterich et al., 1995; Patel and Latterich, 1998). VCP is required for normal ER function, and it interacts with at least 30 different cellular proteins, which may differentially mediate its functions. RNA interference (RNAi) of VCP in HeLa cells results in the formation of large intracellular vacuoles derived from the ER (Wojcik et al., 2004), and reduced levels of cellular VCP induce ER stress, perhaps as consequence of reduced constitutive ERAD and/or by disturbing the fusion of ER membranes (Nowis et al., 2006; Wojcik et al., 2006). Motor neurons of an ALS patient with a VCP mutation were recently found to contain TDP-43-positive inclusions (Johnson et al., 2010), similar to another VCP mutation linked to frontotemporal lobar dementia (FTLD) (Gitcho et al., 2009), similar to ALS. The FTLD VCP mutation was also found to induce ER stress and cell death in cell culture (Gitcho et al., 2009). Interestingly, VCP is involved in ERAD by binding to the ER transmembrane protein Derlin-1 (Rabinovich et al., 2002; Ye et al., 2004). The association of Derlin-1 with activation of the UPR in mutant SOD1 cellular and mouse models of ALS (Nishitoh et al., 2008) suggests overlap in the pathogenic disease mechanisms triggered by VCP, TDP-43 and SOD1 related to ER stress and ERAD.

A Link between ER-Golgi and Axonal Transport?

The relationship between cellular transport events within the cell body and along the axon is poorly understood. However, there is evidence of a functional link between the two systems. An essential prerequisite for axonal transport is efficient ER to Golgi trafficking: proteins which are transported along the axon require intact ER-Golgi transport in order to reach their correct destination (Reiterer et al., 2008). COPII also plays a role in the growth of axons during development (Aridor et al., 1998), indicating involvement of this system in neuritic transport. Furthermore, all newly synthesised proteins destined for fast axonal transport first transit through the Golgi apparatus before being transported in the axon (Hammerschlag et al., 1982).

Perturbations of both the ER-Golgi system and axonal transport mechanisms are also well documented in ALS, and both events are mediated by the dynein molecular motor . Furthermore, both ER-Golgi and axonal transport are linked to ER stress and Golgi fragmentation, suggesting that these apparently disparate systems may be linked into a single mechanism in diseases of MNDs.

3. ENDOSOME-LYSOSOME TRANSPORT

The endosome-lysosome system (ELS) represents a network of organelles that mediate vesicular uptake of extracellular, plasma membrane or cytoplasmic proteins destined for recycling, degradation, signalling or secretion (Figure 2). Cell surface receptor recycling and degradation is a well characterised example while pinocytosis of fluid-phase molecules is another, but not the subject of this chapter. Ligand-bound receptors for transferrin or EGF for instance are internalised by clathrin-coated pits to primary endocytic vesicles which fuse into early or sorting endosomes (Raiborg and Stenmark 2009). Clathrin-mediated endocytosis is largely driven by two factors: Rab5 GTPases localised on the periphery of early endosomes for correct targeting and dynamin GTPases at the cell membrane which recruit adaptor proteins that interact with the actin cytoskeleton to invaginate the plasma membrane (Kim and Chang 2006). Receptors are returned to the cell surface by fission of early endosomes into recycling endosomes. The rate of recycling is determined by Rab4 (slow) and Rab11 (fast)-mediated transport from early and recycling endosomes, respectively (Stenmark 2009). Early endosomes mature into late endosomes by transition of Rab5 to Rab7 expression. At this point, endocytosed cargoes are incorporated into intraluminal vesicles (ILVs) within late endosomes, which precludes their recycling, which in turn progress into multivesicular bodies (MVBs).

The primary role of MVBs is to deliver cargoes to lysosomes for destruction by a process known as autophagy. This is achieved by fusing MVBs with phagosomes or autophagosomes mediated by Rab7. Lysosomal-resident cathepsins A, B and D are serine, cysteine and aspartate proteases, respectively, and mediate clearance of proteins. The ELS does not exist in isolation, but rather intersects and creates a number of pathways, most prominently late endosome-*trans*-Golgi anterograde transport driven by Rab9 which supplies enzymes to lysosomes via mannose-6-phosphate receptors (M6PR), and retrieval of such receptors by retrograde transport (Stenmark 2009).

Exosomes and Neurodegeneration

The second fate of MVBs is to fuse with the plasma membrane and discharge ILVs known as exosomes. Exosomes are small secretory microvesicles, 50-100 nm in diameter, shed into conditioned medium in culture and biological fluids such as plasma, lymph, urine, saliva (Vella et al., 2008a) and most recently cerebrospinal fluid (CSF) *in vivo* (Vella et al., 2008b). They contain discrete sets of proteins, mRNA and miRNA termed exosomal shuttle RNA (Valadi et al., 2007) from donor cells, and thus function in cell-cell transmission, signalling and pathogen transfer in the immune system (Thery et al., 2009). Using an RNAi approach, it was recently determined that Rab27a is a central mediator of exosome secretion (Ostrowski et al., 2010). Exosomes were previously regarded as a mechanism of purging obsolete proteins from cell, however they are now regarded as potential important players in neurodegeneration (Vella et al., 2008a). Exosomal secretion of α-synuclein (Emmanouilidou et al., 2010), β-amyloid (Rajendran et al., 2006), β-amyloid protein precursor C-terminal fragments (Sharples et al., 2009), cellular prion protein (Fevrier et al., 2004) and scrapie prion protein (Vella et al., 2007), suggesting relevance of exosomal transmission of misfolded pathogenic proteins to disease propagation in Parkinson's, Alzheimer's and Creutzfeldt-Jacob diseases.

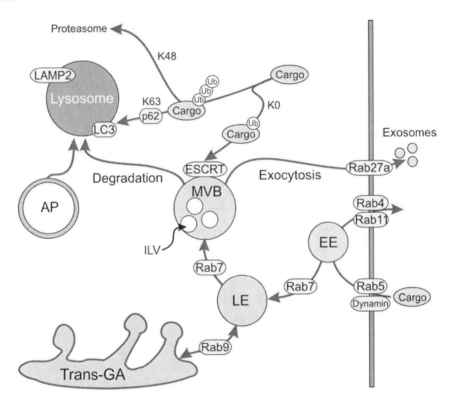

Figure 2. Endosome-lysosome system transport. (1) Extracellular cargoes are endocytosed by action of dynamin and Rab5 leading to their incorporation into early endosomes (EEs). Receptors are returned to the cell surface by recycling endosomes via Rab4 and Rab11. Endocytosed cargoes progress to late endosomes (LEs) by action of Rab7. LEs also receive contents from the ER-GA by action of Rab9. Cargoes are captured into intraluminal vesicles (ILVs) of multivesicular bodies (MVBs) which mature from LEs. Cargoes then have two major fates: they are degraded by lysosomes which result from fusion of MVBs with autophagosomes (APs) or they are secreted by externalised ILVs now termed exosomes by Rab27a activity. (2) Intracellular proteins may also enter the MVB pathway by their monoubiquitination (Ub) and capture by the endosomal sorting complex required for transport (ESCRT). Alternatively, polyubiquitination of cargoes signals their trafficking to the proteasome (K48) or lysosome (K63), in the latter case via recognition by p62 which binds to lysosomal LC3.

Exosomes and ALS

We first reported secretion of normal and ALS-linked mutant SOD1 in motor neurons and into CSF (Turner et al., 2005). Extracellular accumulation of mutant SOD1 was reduced, suggesting that low level secretion may be sufficient for propagating its cell-cell transfer and/or reflecting a more fundamental disturbance of the secretory pathway linked to neurodegeneration. In support of the first proposal, others demonstrated that secreted SOD1 mutants mediated non-cell autonomous killing of motor neurons by activation of proinflammatory microglia (Urushitani et al., 2006). This killing effect was subsequently linked to extracellular mutant SOD1 activation of TLR2/4 and CD14 pathway signalling in microglia (Zhao et al., 2010). One caveat to this proposal is that the level of interstitial SOD1 in nature and ALS is about 1000-fold lower than doses necessary to stimulate microglia and harm motor neurons *in vitro* (Zetterstrom et al., 2011). More recently, extracellular mutant SOD1 was shown to very effectively penetrate cells and propagate intraneuronal protein misfolding and infect neighbouring cells (Munch et al., 2011). The mode(s) of physiological and pathological SOD1 secretion however, is not clear from these studies. A role for ER-Golgi secretion of SOD1 has been recently disputed (Nishitoh et al., 2008), pointing to non-classical pathways. SOD1 transcript and protein, however, were reported in exosomes, compatible with exosomal secretion (Valadi et al., 2007; Gomes et al., 2007).

Confirming this result with SOD1, we have also discovered that other major ALS-linked proteins are present in exosomes which is surprising given their intracellular localisation outside the cytoplasm (Turner et al., unpublished). Furthermore exosomal accumulation of SOD1 was reduced, implying disruption of endosomal trafficking in ALS models. In support of this, endocytic Rab5 and Rab7 abnormalities were shown in SALS patients and SOD1^{G93A} mice (Matej et al., 2010; Palmisano et al., 2011), and were especially pronounced in Wobbler mice (Palmisano et al., 2011), implying defective ELS transport in many forms of ALS.

Ubiquitin-Dependent Signalling in the ELS

One question raised by this section is how then are proteins marked for degradative or exocytotic MBVs? The key machinery responsible involves ubiquitinating enzymes. Ubiquitin is a 76 residue protein consisting of 7 lysines and a C-terminal glycine (Tan et al., 2008). Attachment of ubiquitin via its C-terminus to target proteins via their lysines, referred to as ubiquitination, signals cargoes for intracellular sorting. However, true specificity of trafficking is conferred by self-association of ubiquitin into multimers on protein substrates.

Ubiquitin crosslinkage at lysine-48 (K48), typically tetraubiquitin, is recognised by the proteasome for targeting and clearance (Kirkin et al., 2009). Polyubiquitination at K63 is known to direct substrates to lysosomes, whereas monoubiquitination (K0) signals uptake by MVBs (Figure 2). K0-tagged proteins are captured by the endosomal sorting complex required for transport (ESCRT) on MVBs. This occurs in four steps: ESCRT0 selects cargoes via its ubiquitin binding domain, ESCRTI interacts with and passages cargoes, ESCRTII binds cargoes and recruits endosomal membrane, and ESCRTIII mediates inward budding of MVB lumen to generate ILVs loaded with cargoes (Raiborg and Stenmark 2009). Interestingly, forced K63-ubiquitination of mutant SOD1 triggers inclusion formation, suggesting that enhanced autophagy contributes to aggregation (Tan et al., 2008).

Autophagy and ALS

Autophagy is a routine homeostatic mechanism for turnover of cellular constituents (Nagley et al., 2010). Lysosomes clear substrates via three distinct mechanisms. (1) Macroautophagy, often just autophagy, is the process whereby K63-polyubiquitinated proteins, ribosomes or organelles are recognised by the ubiquitin receptors p62/sequestersome 1, NBR1 or NDP52, which in turn are captured by lysosomal microtubule-associated light chain 3 (LC3) on the surface of autophagosomes (Clague and Urbe 2010). This triggers lipidation of LC3 and conversion to $LC3_{II}$, facilitating fusion to form mature lysosomes. (2) Chaperone-mediated autophagy (CMA) is when cytoplasmic Hsp72 recognises misfolded proteins and binds lysosomal-associated membrane protein 2 (LAMP2), promoting their translocation into lysosomes. (3) Microautophagy involves direct engulfment of cytoplasm by lysosomes which is less well characterised (Nagley et al., 2010).

Autophagy is strongly implicated in progression of ALS. Spinal motor neuron expression and activation of cathepsins was increased in MND (Kikuchi et al., 2003) and spinal cords of presymptomatic $SOD1^{G93A}$ mice (Wootz et al., 2006b). p62 accumulates in neuronal inclusions of MND patients (Mizuno et al., 2006) and mutant SOD1 mice (Gal et al., 2007), although autophagosome formation and $LC3_{II}$ processing was only evident in mice with advanced disease (Li et al., 2008), suggesting that autophagy is probably a late player in pathogenesis. Treatment of $SOD1^{G93A}$ mice with rapamycin, an inhibitor of mTOR, to promote autophagy surprisingly worsened paralysis and neurodegeneration (Zhang et al., 2011). Although counter-intuitive, these findings are in line with cell culture data showing that K63- polyubiquitination of SOD1 aggravates inclusion formation propensity (Tan et al., 2008).

The most compelling evidence backing a role for ELS transport and autophagy defects in ALS is evident from mutations in genes encoding machinery mediating these membrane trafficking pathways which are discussed below.

Alsin (ALS2)

Inactivating mutations in *ALS2* encoding a novel multifunctional protein were identified in rare juvenile forms of ALS, primary lateral sclerosis and infantile ascending spastic paraparesis (Hadano et al., 2001; Yang et al., 2001). ALS2/Alsin localises to peripheral membranes of early endosomes where it activates Rab5 via its GEF domain (Otomo et al., 2003). Later studies showed widespread presence of ALS2/Alsin throughout the ELS including pinosomes, autophagosomes and amphisomes, a type of autophagic vacuole (Otomo et al. 2011). ALS2/Alsin has been linked to regulation of Rac1-dependent macropinocytosis (Kunita et al., 2007), endosomal-lysosomal fusion (Hadano et al., 2010) and trafficking of calcium impermeable GluR2 AMPA receptors in motor neurons (Lai et al., 2006), functions presumed to be disrupted by mutations in ALS. Some of these effects were recapitulated in mice deficient for ALS/Alsin where impaired cargo-specific endocytosis affecting neurotrophic factors was reported in neurons (Devon et al., 2006; Hadano et al., 2006). However, these animals did not reveal a gross disease phenotype, most likely due to the redundancy of the corticospinal tract in rodents which bears the brunt of damage in human ALS2 disease.

Charged Multivesicular Body Protein 2B (CHMP2B)

Mutations in *CHMP2B* were first reported in a Danish kindred with FTLD (Skibinski et al., 2006) and later confirmed in Belgian families (van der Zee et al., 2008). *CHMP2B* encodes a subunit of ESCRTIII which is the sorting step prior to MVB loading with ILVs (Williams and Urbe, 2007). Mutant CHMP2B was sequestered to abnormally enlarged endosomes in neuronal culture, suggesting impaired late endosome progression to MVBs (van der Zee et al., 2008). Abnormal endosomes were also a feature of CHMP2B-linked FTLD patient brains and cell lines (Urwin et al., 2010). In cells depleted of endogenous CHMP2B, p62- and ubiquitin-positive inclusions accumulated, providing evidence that efficient autophagic clearance of proteins relies on functional MVBs (Filimonenko et al., 2007). Curiously, TDP-43 pathology was not characteristic of CHMP2B mutation or depletion (Filimonenko et al., 2007; Holm et al., 2007), suggesting a distinct disease mechanism for CHMP2B-induced pathogenesis. *CHMP2B* mutations have been reported in ALS and associated with p62 and $LC3_{II}$ induction (Parkinson et al., 2006; Cox et al., 2010), again linking defective autophagic activation to the pathogenic mechanism of motor neuron loss.

FIG1 (Factor-Induced Gene 4)

FIG4 encodes a lipid phosphatase that associates with early and late endosomes. FIG4 forms a complex with the kinase PIP5K3 and scaffold protein VAC14 to regulate levels of $PI(3,5)P_2$, a phospholipid essential for late endosome to trans-Golgi retrograde traffic (Rutherford et al., 2004). In the spontaneous mouse mutant "pale tremor", *FIG4* mutation leads to widespread neuronal loss and vacuolation due to enlarged late endosomes, and multisystem depigmentation resulting from impaired melanosome formation (Chow et al., 2007). Interestingly, mutation of *VAC14* is responsible for the spontaneous neurological mouse mutant "infantile gliosis" characterised by spongiform brain degeneration (Jin et al., 2008). Recessive *FIG4* mutations were subsequently identified in CMT4J patients (Chow et al., 2007) and a gene candidate screen in ALS revealed possible pathogenic variants consistent with a loss-of-function mechanism (Chow et al., 2009). In mice lacking FIG4, the autophagic markers p62 and $LC3_{II}$ accumulate in brain and spinal cord, in addition to ubiquitinated inclusions which are TDP-43 negative (Ferguson et al., 2009). However, autophagic pathway beclin and mTOR were not recruited in these mice, suggesting that $PI(3,5)P_2$ deficiency incurred by FIG4 or VAC14 mutation blocks rather than activates autophagy (Ferguson et al., 2009), providing further evidence that impaired autophagy may contribute to ALS and other neurodegenerative disorders.

4. NUCLEAR TRANSPORT

Motor neurons rely on efficient nucleocytoplasmic transport which involves the relocation of cargo molecules through the nuclear envelope (Figure 3). For instance, import of transcription factors and histones, and export of RNA and RNA-binding proteins. This is achieved through nuclear pore complexes (NPCs), large MDa assemblies comprising around 30 structural proteins called nucleoporins which are phenylalanine-glycine (FG) domain rich (McLane and Corbett 2009). Of these, nucleoporins-88 and -358 orient towards the cytoplasm, nucleoporin-62 lines the inner channel and nucleoporin-153 is situated facing the nucleoplasm (Ben-Efrain and Gerace, 2001). Small molecules can passively diffuse through the NPC, however proteins >40 kDa require active and regulated transport across the nuclear membrane. A large family of cytoplasmic soluble transport receptors known as importins or karyopherins mediate nuclear import of cargoes. Importins bind Ran GTPases which are essential for nuclear transport. Proteins containing a nuclear localisation sequence (NLS) which are lysine and arginine-rich first bind to the adaptor protein importin-α which is recognised by importin-β (McLane and Corbett 2009). This ternary complex migrates through the pore due to importin affinity to FG-rich nucleoporins and Ran-GTP hydrolysis. Conversely, outbound cargoes requires a nuclear export sequence (NES) to interact with soluble nuclear exportins.

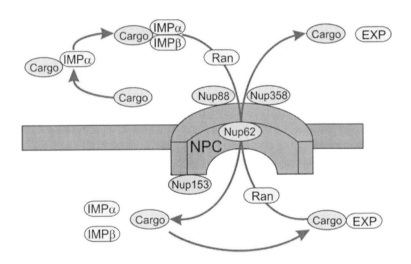

Figure 3. Nuclear-cytoplasmic transport. (1) Cytoplasmic cargoes bind to the karyopherins importin-α and importin-β. This ternary complex is imported via the nuclear pore complex (NPC) into the nucleoplasm via energy derived from Ran. Once imported, the karyopherins dissociate from cargoes. (2) Nuclear cargoes are exported by binding exportins which facilitate passage through the NPC powered by Ran. Both importins and exportins interact with nucleoporins (Nuc) embedded throughout the NPC structure.

There is increasing recognition for a central role of nuclear transport defects in neurodegeneration, most strikingly in the case of motor neurons in sporadic ALS. Disruption of nuclear envelope integrity and depletion of nucleoporin-62 and importin-β was reported in ALS tissue, supported by presymptomatic downregulation of nucleoporin-62 in motor neurons of SOD1^{G93A} mice (Kinoshita et al., 2009), contending for a causal role of nuclear transport defects in disease. More importantly, several nuclear resident proteins mislocalise in ALS and are detailed below.

TAR DNA Binding Protein 43 (TDP-43)

Cytoplasmic mislocalisation of nuclear TDP-43 is a signature pathological hallmark of affected neurons in ALS and FTLD (Neumann et al., 2006). TDP-43 is a DNA and RNA binding protein housed primarily in the nucleus with putative roles in transcription, mRNA splicing and shuttling. Redistribution of TDP-43 to neuronal cytoplasm provokes inclusions and biochemical abnormalities ranging from its hyperphosphorylation, ubiquitination and fragmentation into TDP-35 and TDP-25 species. While *TARDBP* mutations may account for these abnormalities in about 0.5% of ALS patients (Sreedharan et al., 2008), the mechanisms underlying TDP-43 pathology in all sporadic cases, but not SOD1, FUS, CHMP2B and FIG4-linked familial forms, remain puzzling. Recent studies have shown that axonal transection or ligation transiently mislocalises TDP-43 to the cytoplasm, suggesting an adaptive and stress-inducible response to injury (Moisse et al., 2009; Sato et al., 2009), presumably through global translational arrest and selective transcription of repair factors. Another possibility is that TDP-43 pathology arises from defective nuclear transport. RNAi-mediated knockdown of importin-β or cellular apoptosis susceptibility (CAS) protein triggered TDP-43 redistribution in culture (Sato et al., 2009; Nishimura et al., 2010), strengthening a causal role for nuclear transporter defects in TDP-43 pathology.

Fused in Sarcoma (FUS)

Mutations in the TDP-43 homolog FUS are causative in a form of familial ALS (Vance et al., 2009; Kwiatkowski et al., 2009). Expression of FUS mutants leads to drastic cytoplasmic mislocalisation in culture, suggesting a nuclear transport defect mechanism in common with TDP-43. Abnormal FUS redistribution was also reported in sporadic ALS (Deng et al., 2010), but not SOD1 cases, in accordance with a potentially wider disturbance of nuclear transport. Again, the mechanism of FUS mislocalisation is unresolved. Mutation of residues, oxidative stress and heat shock all promote FUS recruitment into cytoplasmic stress granules (Bosco et al., 2010). RNAi-mediated knockdown of nuclear import receptors also resulted in FUS migration to stress granules (Dormann et al., 2010), suggesting overlapping causal mechanisms with pathological TDP-43.

CONCLUSIONS

The studies reported above collectively suggest that, in highly polarized motor neurons, even subtle alterations of dynamics and transport mechanisms of intracellular organelles and compartments, such as the axoplasm, ER-Golgi system, ELS and nucleus can have dramatic impacts on proximal and distal cellular functions, which are fundamental for the survival of these cells. The close association of the ER with the Golgi/microtubule networks involved in somal and axonal transport processes provides a possible explanation for the involvement of each of these systems in ALS. Other intracellular organelles and membranous systems can be involved in the molecular mechanisms triggering neurodegeneration via an alteration of cellular transport processes and can be affected by cellular toxic insults.

ACKNOWLEDGMENTS

This work was supported by the Australian National Health and Medical Research Council (NHMRC) Project Grants 1008910 (B.J.T.), 1006141 (J.D.A.), Motor Neuron Disease Research Institute of Australia, Mick Rodger Benalla MND Research Grant (B.J.T), zo-ee MND Research Grant (J.D.A.) and Bethlehem Griffiths Research Foundation.

REFERENCES

Ali BR, Seabra MC (2005) Targeting of Rab GTPases to cellular membranes. *Biochem. Soc. Trans* 33:652-656.

Aridor M, Weissman J, Bannykh S, Nuoffer C, Balch WE (1998) Cargo selection by the COPII budding machinery during export from the ER. *J. Cell Biol.* 141:61-70.

Atkin JD, Farg MA, Walker AK, McLean C, Tomas D, Horne MK (2008) Endoplasmic reticulum stress and induction of the unfolded protein response in human sporadic amyotrophic lateral sclerosis. *Neurobiol. Dis.* 30:400-407.

Azzedine H, Bolino A, Taieb T, Birouk N, Di Duca M, Bouhouche A, Benamou S, Mrabet A, Hammadouche T, Chkili T, Gouider R, Ravazzolo R, Brice A, Laporte J, LeGuern E (2003) Mutations in MTMR13, a new pseudophosphatase homologue of MTMR2 and Sbf1, in two families with an autosomal recessive demyelinating form of Charcot-Marie-Tooth disease associated with early-onset glaucoma. *Am. J. Hum. Gen.* 72:1141-1153.

Ben-Efraim I, Gerace L (2001) Gradient of increasing affinity of importin beta for nucleoporins along the pathway of nuclear import. *J. Cell. Biol.* 152:411-7.

Bilsland LG, Sahai E, Kelly G, Golding M, Greensmith L, Schiavo G (2010) Deficits in axonal transport precede ALS symptoms in vivo. *Proc. Natl. Acad. Sci.USA* 107:20523-8.

Bolino A, Muglia M, Conforti FL, LeGuern E, Salih MA, Georgiou DM, Christodoulou K, Hausmanowa-Petrusewicz I, Mandich P, Schenone A, Gambardella A, Bono F, Quattrone A, Devoto M, Monaco AP (2000) Charcot-Marie-Tooth type 4B is caused by mutations in the gene encoding myotubularin-related protein-2. *Nat. Genet* 25:17-19.

Bosco DA, Lemay N, Ko HK, Zhou H, Burke C, Kwiatkowski TJ Jr, Sapp P, McKenna-Yasek D, Brown RH Jr, Hayward LJ (2010) Mutant FUS proteins that cause amyotrophic lateral sclerosis incorporate into stress granules. *Hum. Mol. Genet.* 19:4160-75.

Brady ST (1985) A novel brain ATPase with properties expected for the fast axonal transport motor. *Nature* 317:73-75.

Cavalli V, Kujala P, Klumperman J, Goldstein LS (2005) Sunday Driver links axonal transport to damage signaling. *J. Cell Biol.* 2005 168:775-87.

Chen HJ, Anagnostou G, Chai A, Withers J, Morris A, Adhikaree J, Pennetta G, de Belleroche JS (2010) Characterization of the properties of a novel mutation in VAPB in familial amyotrophic lateral sclerosis. *J. Biol. Chem.* 285:40266-40281.

Chen XJ, Levedakou EN, Millen KJ, Wollmann RL, Soliven B, Popko B (2007) Proprioceptive sensory neuropathy in mice with a mutation in the cytoplasmic Dynein heavy chain 1 gene. *J. Neurosci.* 27:14515-14524.

Chen YZ, Bennett CL, Huynh HM, Blair IP, Puls I, Irobi J, Dierick I, Abel A, Kennerson ML, Rabin BA, Nicholson GA, Auer-Grumbach M, Wagner K, De Jonghe P, Griffin JW, Fischbeck KH, Timmerman V, Cornblath DR, Chance PF (2004) DNA/RNA helicase gene mutations in a form of juvenile amyotrophic lateral sclerosis (ALS4). *Am. J. Hum. Genet.* 74:1128-35.

Chevalier-Larsen E, Holzbaur EL (2006) Axonal transport and neurodegenerative disease. *Biochim. Biophys. Acta* 1762:1094-1108.

Chow CY, Zhang Y, Dowling JJ, Jin N, Adamska M, Shiga K, Szigeti K, Shy ME, Li J, Zhang X, Lupski JR, Weisman LS, Meisler MH (2007) Mutation of FIG4 causes neurodegeneration in the pale tremor mouse and patients with CMT4J. *Nature* 448:68-72.

Chow CY, Landers JE, Bergren SK, Sapp PC, Grant AE, Jones JM, Everett L, Lenk GM, McKenna-Yasek DM, Weisman LS, Figlewicz D, Brown RH, Meisler MH (2009) Deleterious variants of FIG4, a phosphoinositide phosphatase, in patients with ALS. *Am. J. Hum. Genet.* 84(1):85-8.

Clague MJ, Urbe S (2010) Ubiquitin: same molecule, different degradation pathways. *Cell* 143:682-5.

Coleman M (2005) Axon degeneration mechanisms: commonality amid diversity. Nature reviews. *Neuroscience* 6:889-898.

Cox LE, Ferraiuolo L, Goodall EF, Heath PR, Higginbottom A, Mortiboys H, Hollinger HC, Hartley JA, Brockington A, Burness CE, Morrison KE, Wharton SB, Grierson AJ, Ince PG, Kirby J, Shaw PJ (2010) Mutations in CHMP2B in lower motor neuron predominant amyotrophic lateral sclerosis (ALS). *PLoS ONE* 5:e9872.

De Vos KJ, Grierson AJ, Ackerley S, Miller CC (2008) Role of axonal transport in neurodegenerative diseases. *Annu. Rev. Neurosci.* 31:151-173.

De Vos KJ, Chapman AL, Tennant ME, Manser C, Tudor EL, Lau KF, Brownlees J, Ackerley S, Shaw PJ, McLoughlin DM, Shaw CE, Leigh PN, Miller CC, Grierson AJ (2007) Familial amyotrophic lateral sclerosis-linked SOD1 mutants perturb fast axonal transport to reduce axonal mitochondria content. *Hum. Mol. Genet.* 16:2720-2728.

Deacon SW, Serpinskaya AS, Vaughan PS, Lopez Fanarraga M, Vernos I, Vaughan KT, Gelfand VI (2003) Dynactin is required for bidirectional organelle transport. *J. Cell Biol.* 160:297-301.

Deng HX, Zhai H, Bigio EH, Yan J, Fecto F, Ajroud K, Mishra M, Ajroud-Driss S, Heller S, Sufit R, Siddique N, Mugnaini E, Siddique T (2010) FUS-immunoreactive inclusions are a common feature in sporadic and non-SOD1 familial amyotrophic lateral sclerosis. *Ann Neurol.* 67:739-48.

Devon RS, Orban PC, Gerrow K, Barbieri MA, Schwab C, Cao LP, Helm JR, Bissada N, Cruz-Aguado R, Davidson TL, Witmer J, Metzler M, Lam CK, Tetzlaff W, Simpson EM, McCaffery JM, El-Husseini AE, Leavitt BR, Hayden MR (2006) Als2-deficient mice exhibit disturbances in endosome trafficking associated with motor behavioral abnormalities. *Proc. Natl. Acad. Sci. USA* 103:9595-9600.

Dormann D, Rodde R, Edbauer D, Bentmann E, Fischer I, Hruscha A, Than ME, Mackenzie IR, Capell A, Schmid B, Neumann M, Haass C (2010) ALS-associated fused in sarcoma (FUS) mutations disrupt Transportin-mediated nuclear import. *EMBO J.* 29:2841-57.

Dreveny I, Pye VE, Beuron F, Briggs LC, Isaacson RL, Matthews SJ, McKeown C, Yuan X, Zhang X, Freemont PS (2004) p97 and close encounters of every kind: a brief review. *Biochem. Soc Trans* 32:715-720.

Duplan L, Bernard N, Casseron W, Dudley K, Thouvenot E, Honnorat J, Rogemond V, De Bovis B, Aebischer P, Marin P, Raoul C, Henderson CE, Pettmann B (2010) Collapsin response mediator protein 4a (CRMP4a) is upregulated in motoneurons of mutant SOD1 mice and can trigger motoneuron axonal degeneration and cell death. *J. Neurosci.* 30:785-796.

Ebbing B, Mann K, Starosta A, Jaud J, Schols L, Schule R, Woehlke G (2008) Effect of spastic paraplegia mutations in KIF5A kinesin on transport activity. *Hum. Mol. Genet* 17:1245-1252.

Emmanouilidou E, Melachroinou K, Roumeliotis T, Garbis SD, Ntzouni M, Margaritis LH, Stefanis L, Vekrellis K (2010) Cell-produced alpha-synuclein is secreted in a calcium-dependent manner by exosomes and impacts neuronal survival. *J. Neurosci.* 30:6838-51.

Evgrafov OV, Mersiyanova I, Irobi J, Van Den Bosch L, Dierick I, Leung CL, Schagina O, Verpoorten N, Van Impe K, Fedotov V, Dadali E, Auer-Grumbach M, Windpassinger C, Wagner K, Mitrovic Z, Hilton-Jones D, Talbot K, Martin JJ, Vasserman N, Tverskaya S, Polyakov A, Liem RK, Gettemans J, Robberecht W, De Jonghe P, Timmerman V (2004) Mutant small heat-shock protein 27 causes axonal Charcot-Marie-Tooth disease and distal hereditary motor neuropathy. *Nat. Genet.* 36:602-6.

Fasana E, Fossati M, Ruggiano A, Brambillasca S, Hoogenraad CC, Navone F, Francolini M, Borgese N (2010) A VAPB mutant linked to amyotrophic lateral sclerosis generates a novel form of organized smooth endoplasmic reticulum. *FASEB J.* 24:1419-1430.

Fevrier B, Vilette D, Archer F, Loew D, Faigle W, Vidal M, Laude H, Raposo G (2004) Cells release prions in association with exosomes. *Proc. Natl. Acad. Sci. USA* 101:9683-8.

Flanagan JG, Vanderhaeghen P (1998) The ephrins and Eph receptors in neural development. *Annu. Rev. Neurosci* 21:309-345.

Foster LJ, Weir ML, Lim DY, Liu Z, Trimble WS, Klip A (2000) A functional role for VAP-33 in insulin-stimulated GLUT4 traffic. *Traffic* 1:512-521.

Foth BJ, Goedecke MC, Soldati D (2006) New insights into myosin evolution and classification. *Proc. Natl. Acad. Sci. USA* 103:3681-3686.

Ferguson CJ, Lenk GM, Meisler MH (2009) Defective autophagy in neurons and astrocytes from mice deficient in PI(3,5)P2. *Hum. Mol. Genet* 18:4868-78.

Filimonenko M, Stuffers S, Raiborg C, Yamamoto A, Malerød L, Fisher EM, Isaacs A, Brech A, Stenmark H, Simonsen A (2007) Functional multivesicular bodies are required for autophagic clearance of protein aggregates associated with neurodegenerative disease. *J. Cell Biol.* 179:485-500.

Gal J, Ström AL, Kilty R, Zhang F, Zhu H (2007) p62 accumulates and enhances aggregate formation in model systems of familial amyotrophic lateral sclerosis. *J. Biol. Chem.* 82:11068-11077.

Gitcho MA, Strider J, Carter D, Taylor-Reinwald L, Forman MS, Goate AM, Cairns NJ (2009) VCP mutations causing frontotemporal lobar degeneration disrupt localization of TDP-43 and induce cell death. *J. Biol. Chem.* 284:12384-12398.

Gomes C, Keller S, Altevogt P, Costa J (2007) Evidence for secretion of Cu,Zn superoxide dismutase via exosomes from a cell model of amyotrophic lateral sclerosis. *Neurosci. Lett.* 428:43-6.

Gonatas NK, Stieber A, Gonatas JO (2006) Fragmentation of the Golgi apparatus in neurodegenerative diseases and cell death. *J. Neurol. Sci.* 246:21-30.

Greenway MJ, Andersen PM, Russ C, Ennis S, Cashman S, Donaghy C, Patterson V, Swingler R, Kieran D, Prehn J, Morrison KE, Green A, Acharya KR, Brown RH Jr, Hardiman O (2006) ANG mutations segregate with familial and 'sporadic' amyotrophic lateral sclerosis. *Nat. Genet.* 38:411-3.

Gunawardena S, Goldstein LS (2004) Cargo-carrying motor vehicles on the neuronal highway: transport pathways and neurodegenerative disease. *J. Neurobiol.* 58:258-271.

Hadano S, Hand CK, Osuga H, Yanagisawa Y, Otomo A, Devon RS, Miyamoto N, Showguchi-Miyata J, Okada Y, Singaraja R, Figlewicz DA, Kwiatkowski T, Hosler BA, Sagie T, Skaug J, Nasir J, Brown RH Jr, Scherer SW, Rouleau GA, Hayden MR, Ikeda JE (2001) A gene encoding a putative GTPase regulator is mutated in familial amyotrophic lateral sclerosis 2. *Nat. Genet* 29:166-73.

Hadano S, Benn SC, Kakuta S, Otomo A, Sudo K, Kunita R, Suzuki-Utsunomiya K, Mizumura H, Shefner JM, Cox GA, Iwakura Y, Brown RH Jr, Ikeda JE (2006) Mice deficient in the Rab5 guanine nucleotide exchange factor ALS2/alsin exhibit age-dependent neurological deficits and altered endosome trafficking. *Hum. Mol. Genet* 15:233-250.

Hadano S, Otomo A, Kunita R, Suzuki-Utsunomiya K, Akatsuka A, Koike M, Aoki M, Uchiyama Y, Itoyama Y, Ikeda JE (2010) Loss of ALS2/Alsin exacerbates motor dysfunction in a SOD1-expressing mouse ALS model by disturbing endolysosomal trafficking. *PLoS One* 5:e9805.

Hafezparast M, Klocke R, Ruhrberg C, Marquardt A, Ahmad-Annuar A, Bowen S, Lalli G, Witherden AS, Hummerich H, Nicholson S, Morgan PJ, Oozageer R, Priestley JV, Averill S, King VR, Ball S, Peters J, Toda T, Yamamoto A, Hiraoka Y, Augustin M, Korthaus D, Wattler S, Wabnitz P, Dickneite C, Lampel S, Boehme F, Peraus G, Popp A, Rudelius M, Schlegel J, Fuchs H, Hrabe de Angelis M, Schiavo G, Shima DT, Russ AP, Stumm G, Martin JE, Fisher EM (2003) Mutations in dynein link motor neuron degeneration to defects in retrograde transport. *Science* 300:808-812.

Halawani D, Latterich M (2006) p97: The cell's molecular purgatory? *Mol Cell* 22:713-717.

Hammerschlag R, Stone GC, Bolen FA, Lindsey JD, Ellisman MH (1982) Evidence that all newly synthesized proteins destined for fast axonal transport pass through the Golgi apparatus. *J. Cell Biol.* 93:568-575.

Hattula K, Peranen J (2000) FIP-2, a coiled-coil protein, links Huntingtin to Rab8 and modulates cellular morphogenesis. *Curr. Biol.* 10:1603-1606.

Heerssen HM, Pazyra MF, Segal RA (2004) Dynein motors transport activated Trks to promote survival of target-dependent neurons. *Nat. Neurosci.* 7:596-604.

Hetz C, Thielen P, Matus S, Nassif M, Court F, Kiffin R, Martinez G, Cuervo AM, Brown RH, Glimcher LH (2009) XBP-1 deficiency in the nervous system protects against amyotrophic lateral sclerosis by increasing autophagy. *Genes Dev.* 23:2294-2306.

Hirokawa N, Nitta R, Okada Y (2009) The mechanisms of kinesin motor motility: lessons from the monomeric motor KIF1A. Nature reviews Mol. *Cell Biol.* 10:877-884.

Hirokawa N, Niwa S, Tanaka Y (2010) Molecular motors in neurons: transport mechanisms and roles in brain function, development, and disease. *Neuron* 68:610-638.

Hollenbeck PJ (2005) Mitochondria and neurotransmission: evacuating the synapse. *Neuron.* 47:331-3.

Holm IE, Englund E, Mackenzie IR, Johannsen P, Isaacs AM (2007) A reassessment of the neuropathology of frontotemporal dementia linked to chromosome 3. *J. Neuropathol Exp. Neurol.* 66:884-891.

Huang EJ, Zhang J, Geser F, Trojanowski JQ, Strober JB, Dickson DW, Brown RH Jr, Shapiro BE, Lomen-Hoerth C (2010) Extensive FUS-immunoreactive pathology in juvenile amyotrophic lateral sclerosis with basophilic inclusions. *Brain Pathol* 20:1069-76.

Jin N, Chow CY, Liu L, Zolov SN, Bronson R, Davisson M, Petersen JL, Zhang Y, Park S, Duex JE, Goldowitz D, Meisler MH, Weisman LS (2008) VAC14 nucleates a protein complex essential for the acute interconversion of PI3P and PI(3,5)P(2) in yeast and mouse. *EMBO J.* 27:3221-34.

Johnson JO, Mandrioli J, Benatar M, Abramzon Y, Van Deerlin VM, Trojanowski JQ, Gibbs JR, Brunetti M, Gronka S, Wuu J, Ding J, McCluskey L, Martinez-Lage M, Falcone D, Hernandez DG, Arepalli S, Chong S, Schymick JC, Rothstein J, Landi F, Wang YD, Calvo A, Mora G, Sabatelli M, Monsurro MR, Battistini S, Salvi F, Spataro R, Sola P, Borghero G, Galassi G, Scholz SW, Taylor JP, Restagno G, Chio A, Traynor BJ (2010) Exome sequencing reveals VCP mutations as a cause of familial ALS. *Neuron* 68:857-864.

Jonikas MC, Collins SR, Denic V, Oh E, Quan EM, Schmid V, Weibezahn J, Schwappach B, Walter P, Weissman JS, Schuldiner M (2009) Comprehensive characterization of genes required for protein folding in the endoplasmic reticulum. *Science* 323:1693-1697.

Jung C, Lee S, Ortiz D, Zhu Q, Julien JP, Shea TB (2005) The high and middle molecular weight neurofilament subunits regulate the association of neurofilaments with kinesin: inhibition by phosphorylation of the high molecular weight subunit. *Brain Res. Mol. Brain Res.* 141:151-155.

Kagiwada S, Hosaka K, Murata M, Nikawa J, Takatsuki A (1998) The Saccharomyces cerevisiae SCS2 gene product, a homolog of a synaptobrevin-associated protein, is an integral membrane protein of the endoplasmic reticulum and is required for inositol metabolism. *J. Bacteriol.* 180:1700-1708.

Kamal A, Goldstein LS (2002) Principles of cargo attachment to cytoplasmic motor proteins. *Curr. Opin. Cell Biol.* 14:63-68.

Kanekura K, Nishimoto I, Aiso S, Matsuoka M (2006) Characterization of amyotrophic lateral sclerosis-linked P56S mutation of vesicle-associated membrane protein-associated protein B (VAPB/ALS8). *J. Biol. Chem.* 281:30223-30233.

Kawaguchi Y, Kovacs JJ, McLaurin A, Vance JM, Ito A, Yao TP (2003) The deacetylase HDAC6 regulates aggresome formation and cell viability in response to misfolded protein stress. *Cell* 115:727-738.

Kikuchi H, Yamada T, Furuya H, Doh-ura K, Ohyagi Y, Iwaki T, Kira J (2003) Involvement of cathepsin B in the motor neuron degeneration of amyotrophic lateral sclerosis. *Acta Neuropathol.* 105:462-8.

Kieran D, Woods I, Villunger A, Strasser A, Prehn JH (2007) Deletion of the BH3-only protein puma protects motoneurons from ER stress-induced apoptosis and delays motoneuron loss in ALS mice. *Proc. Natl. Acad. Sci. USA* 104:20606-20611.

Kieran D, Hafezparast M, Bohnert S, Dick JR, Martin J, Schiavo G, Fisher EM, Greensmith L (2005) A mutation in dynein rescues axonal transport defects and extends the life span of ALS mice. *J. Cell Biol.* 169:561-567.

Kim Y, Chang S (2006) Ever-expanding network of dynamin-interacting proteins. *Mol. Neurobiol.* 34:129-36.

Kinoshita Y, Ito H, Hirano A, Fujita K, Wate R, Nakamura M, Kaneko S, Nakano S, Kusaka H (2009) Nuclear contour irregularity and abnormal transporter protein distribution in anterior horn cells in amyotrophic lateral sclerosis. *J. Neuropathol. Exp. Neurol.* 68:1184-1192.

Kirkin V, McEwan DG, Novak I, Dikic I (2009) A role for ubiquitin in selective autophagy. *Mol Cell* 34:259-69.

Komatsu M, Waguri S, Koike M, Sou YS, Ueno T, Hara T, Mizushima N, Iwata J, Ezaki J, Murata S, Hamazaki J, Nishito Y, Iemura S, Natsume T, Yanagawa T, Uwayama J, Warabi E, Yoshida H, Ishii T, Kobayashi A, Yamamoto M, Yue Z, Uchiyama Y, Kominami E, Tanaka K (2007) Homeostatic levels of p62 control cytoplasmic inclusion body formation in autophagy-deficient mice. *Cell* 131:1149-1163.

Kunita R, Otomo A, Mizumura H, Suzuki-Utsunomiya K, Hadano S, Ikeda JE (2007) The Rab5 activator ALS2/alsin acts as a novel Rac1 effector through Rac1-activated endocytosis. *J. Biol. Chem.* 282:16599-16611.

Kwiatkowski TJ Jr, Bosco DA, Leclerc AL, Tamrazian E, Vanderburg CR, Russ C, Davis A, Gilchrist J, Kasarskis EJ, Munsat T, Valdmanis P, Rouleau GA, Hosler BA, Cortelli P, de Jong PJ, Yoshinaga Y, Haines JL, Pericak-Vance MA, Yan J, Ticozzi N, Siddique T, McKenna-Yasek D, Sapp PC, Horvitz HR, Landers JE, Brown RH Jr (2009) Mutations in the FUS/TLS gene on chromosome 16 cause familial amyotrophic lateral sclerosis. *Science* 323:1205-8.

Lai C, Lin X, Chandran J, Shim H, Yang WJ, Cai H (2007) The G59S mutation in p150(glued) causes dysfunction of dynactin in mice. *J. Neurosci.* 27:13982-13990.

Lai C, Xie C, McCormack SG, Chiang HC, Michalak MK, Lin X, Chandran J, Shim H, Shimoji M, Cookson MR, Huganir RL, Rothstein JD, Price DL, Wong PC, Martin LJ, Zhu JJ, Cai H (2006) Amyotrophic lateral sclerosis 2-deficiency leads to neuronal degeneration in amyotrophic lateral sclerosis through altered AMPA receptor trafficking. *J. Neurosci.* 26:11798-11806.

Laird FM, Farah MH, Ackerley S, Hoke A, Maragakis N, Rothstein JD, Griffin J, Price DL, Martin LJ, Wong PC (2008) Motor neuron disease occurring in a mutant dynactin mouse model is characterized by defects in vesicular trafficking. *J. Neurosci.* 28:1997-2005.

LaMonte BH, Wallace KE, Holloway BA, Shelly SS, Ascano J, Tokito M, Van Winkle T, Howland DS, Holzbaur EL (2002) Disruption of dynein/dynactin inhibits axonal transport in motor neurons causing late-onset progressive degeneration. *Neuron* 34:715-727.

Landers JE, Melki J, Meininger V, Glass JD, van den Berg LH, van Es MA, Sapp PC, van Vught PW, McKenna-Yasek DM, Blauw HM, Cho TJ, Polak M, Shi L, Wills AM, Broom WJ, Ticozzi N, Silani V, Ozoguz A, Rodriguez-Leyva I, Veldink JH, Ivinson AJ, Saris CG, Hosler BA, Barnes-Nessa A, Couture N, Wokke JH, Kwiatkowski TJ, Jr., Ophoff RA, Cronin S, Hardiman O, Diekstra FP, Leigh PN, Shaw CE, Simpson CL, Hansen VK, Powell JF, Corcia P, Salachas F, Heath S, Galan P, Georges F, Horvitz HR, Lathrop M, Purcell S, Al-Chalabi A, Brown RH, Jr. (2009) Reduced expression of the Kinesin-Associated Protein 3 (KIFAP3) gene increases survival in sporadic amyotrophic lateral sclerosis. *Proc. Natl. Acad. Sci. USA* 106:9004-9009.

Latterich M, Frohlich KU, Schekman R (1995) Membrane fusion and the cell cycle: Cdc48p participates in the fusion of ER membranes. *Cell* 82:885-893.

Li L, Zhang X, Le W (2008) Altered macroautophagy in the spinal cord of SOD1 mutant mice. *Autophagy* 4:290-3.

Ligon LA, Steward O (2000) Role of microtubules and actin filaments in the movement of mitochondria in the axons and dendrites of cultured hippocampal neurons. *J. Comp. Neurol.* 427:351-361.

Ligon LA, Tokito M, Finklestein JM, Grossman FE, Holzbaur EL (2004) A direct interaction between cytoplasmic dynein and kinesin I may coordinate motor activity. *J. Biol. Chem.* 279:19201-19208.

Ligon LA, LaMonte BH, Wallace KE, Weber N, Kalb RG, Holzbaur EL (2005) Mutant superoxide dismutase disrupts cytoplasmic dynein in motor neurons. *Neuroreport* 16:533-536.

Magrane J, Manfredi G (2009) Mitochondrial function, morphology, and axonal transport in amyotrophic lateral sclerosis. *Antioxid Redox Signal* 11:1615-1626.

Maruyama H, Morino H, Ito H, Izumi Y, Kato H, Watanabe Y, Kinoshita Y, Kamada M, Nodera H, Suzuki H, Komure O, Matsuura S, Kobatake K, Morimoto N, Abe K, Suzuki N, Aoki M, Kawata A, Hirai T, Kato T, Ogasawara K, Hirano A, Takumi T, Kusaka H, Hagiwara K, Kaji R, Kawakami H (2010) Mutations of optineurin in amyotrophic lateral sclerosis. *Nature* 465:223-6.

Matej R, Botond G, László L, Kopitar-Jerala N, Rusina R, Budka H, Kovacs GG (2010) Increased neuronal Rab5 immunoreactive endosomes do not colocalize with TDP-43 in motor neuron disease. *Exp. Neurol.* 225:133-9.

McLane LM, Corbett AH (2009) Nuclear localization signals and human disease. *IUBMB Life* 61:697-706.

McNiven MA (2005) Dynamin in disease. *Nat. Genet.* 37:215-216.

Melloni RH, Jr., Tokito MK, Holzbaur EL (1995) Expression of the p150Glued component of the dynactin complex in developing and adult rat brain. *J. Comp. Neurol.* 357:15-24.

Miki H, Okada Y, Hirokawa N (2005) Analysis of the kinesin superfamily: insights into structure and function. *Trends Cell Biol.* 15:467-476.

Mizuno Y, Amari M, Takatama M, Aizawa H, Mihara B, Okamoto K (2006) Immunoreactivities of p62, an ubiqutin-binding protein, in the spinal anterior horn cells of patients with amyotrophic lateral sclerosis. *J. Neurol. Sci.* 249:13-8.

Moisse K, Mepham J, Volkening K, Welch I, Hill T, Strong MJ (2009) Cytosolic TDP-43 expression following axotomy is associated with caspase 3 activation in NFL-/- mice: support for a role for TDP-43 in the physiological response to neuronal injury. *Brain Res.* 1296:176-186.

Morfini GA, Burns M, Binder LI, Kanaan NM, LaPointe N, Bosco DA, Brown RH, Jr., Brown H, Tiwari A, Hayward L, Edgar J, Nave KA, Garberrn J, Atagi Y, Song Y, Pigino G, Brady ST (2009) Axonal transport defects in neurodegenerative diseases. *J. Neurosci.* 29:12776-12786.

Mourelatos Z, Gonatas NK, Stieber A, Gurney ME, Dal Canto MC (1996) The Golgi apparatus of spinal cord motor neurons in transgenic mice expressing mutant Cu,Zn superoxide dismutase becomes fragmented in early, preclinical stages of the disease. *Proc. Natl. Acad. Sci. USA* 93:5472-5477.

Munch C, Prechter F, Xu R, Linke P, Prudlo J, Kuzma M, Kwiecinski H, Ludolph AC, Meyer T (2005) Frequency of a tau genotype in amyotrophic lateral sclerosis. *J. Neurol. Sci.* 236:13-16.

Munch C, O'Brien J, Bertolotti A (2011) Prion-like propagation of mutant superoxide dismutase-1 misfolding in neuronal cells. *Proc. Natl. Acad. Sci. USA* 108:3548-53.

Murakami T, Warita H, Hayashi T, Sato K, Manabe Y, Mizuno S, Yamane K, Abe K (2001) A novel SOD1 gene mutation in familial ALS with low penetrance in females. *J. Neurol. Sci.* 189:45-47.

Nagley P, Higgins GC, Atkin JD, Beart PM (2010) Multifaceted deaths orchestrated by mitochondria in neurones. *Biochim. Biophys Acta* 1802:167-185.

Nakagomi S, Barsoum MJ, Bossy-Wetzel E, Sutterlin C, Malhotra V, Lipton SA (2008) A Golgi fragmentation pathway in neurodegeneration. *Neurobiol. Dis.* 29:221-231.

Neumann M, Sampathu DM, Kwong LK, Truax AC, Micsenyi MC, Chou TT, Bruce J, Schuck T, Grossman M, Clark CM, McCluskey LF, Miller BL, Masliah E, Mackenzie IR, Feldman H, Feiden W, Kretzschmar HA, Trojanowski JQ, Lee VM (2006) Ubiquitinated TDP-43 in frontotemporal lobar degeneration and amyotrophic lateral sclerosis. *Science* 314:130-3.

Nishimura AL, Mitne-Neto M, Silva HC, Richieri-Costa A, Middleton S, Cascio D, Kok F, Oliveira JR, Gillingwater T, Webb J, Skehel P, Zatz M (2004) A mutation in the vesicle-trafficking protein VAPB causes late-onset spinal muscular atrophy and amyotrophic lateral sclerosis. Am J Hum Genet 75:822-831.

Nishimura Y, Hayashi M, Inada H, Tanaka T (1999) Molecular cloning and characterization of mammalian homologues of vesicle-associated membrane protein-associated (VAMP-associated) proteins. *Biochem. Biophys. Res. Comm.* 254:21-26.

Nishimura AL, Zupunski V, Troakes C, Kathe C, Fratta P, Howell M, Gallo JM, Hortobágyi T, Shaw CE, Rogelj B (2010) Nuclear import impairment causes cytoplasmic trans-activation response DNA-binding protein accumulation and is associated with frontotemporal lobar degeneration. *Brain* 133:1763-71.

Nishitoh H, Kadowaki H, Nagai A, Maruyama T, Yokota T, Fukutomi H, Noguchi T, Matsuzawa A, Takeda K, Ichijo H (2008) ALS-linked mutant SOD1 induces ER stress- and ASK1-dependent motor neuron death by targeting Derlin-1. *Genes Dev* 22:1451-1464.

Nowis D, McConnell E, Wojcik C (2006) Destabilization of the VCP-Ufd1-Npl4 complex is associated with decreased levels of ERAD substrates. *Exp. Cell Res.* 312:2921-2932.

Orth JD, McNiven MA (2003) Dynamin at the actin-membrane interface. *Curr. Opin. Cell Biology* 15:31-39.

Ostrowski M, Carmo NB, Krumeich S, Fanget I, Raposo G, Savina A, Moita CF, Schauer K, Hume AN, Freitas RP, Goud B, Benaroch P, Hacohen N, Fukuda M, Desnos C, Seabra MC, Darchen F, Amigorena S, Moita LF, Thery C (2010) Rab27a and Rab27b control different steps of the exosome secretion pathway. *Nat. Cell. Biol.* 12:19-30.

Otomo A, Hadano S, Okada T, Mizumura H, Kunita R, Nishijima H, Showguchi-Miyata J, Yanagisawa Y, Kohiki E, Suga E, Yasuda M, Osuga H, Nishimoto T, Narumiya S, Ikeda JE (2003) ALS2, a novel guanine nucleotide exchange factor for the small GTPase Rab5, is implicated in endosomal dynamics. *Hum. Mol. Genet.* 12:1671-1687.

Otomo A, Kunita R, Suzuki-Utsunomiya K, Ikeda JE, Hadano S (2011) Defective relocalization of ALS2/alsin missense mutants to Rac1-induced macropinosomes accounts for loss of their cellular function and leads to disturbed amphisome formation. *FEBS Lett* 585:730-6.

Palmisano R, Golfi P, Heimann P, Shaw C, Troakes C, Schmitt-John T, Bartsch JW (2011) Endosomal accumulation of APP in wobbler motor neurons reflects impaired vesicle trafficking: Implications for human motor neuron disease. *BMC Neurosci* 12:24.

Pantelidou M, Zographos SE, Lederer CW, Kyriakides T, Pfaffl MW, Santama N (2007) Differential expression of molecular motors in the motor cortex of sporadic ALS. *Neurobiol. Dis.* 26:577-589.

Park BC, Shen X, Samaraweera M, Yue BY (2006) Studies of optineurin, a glaucoma gene: Golgi fragmentation and cell death from overexpression of wild-type and mutant optineurin in two ocular cell types. *Am. J. Pathol.* 169:1976-1989.

Parkinson N, Ince PG, Smith MO, Highley R, Skibinski G, Andersen PM, Morrison KE, Pall HS, Hardiman O, Collinge J, Shaw PJ, Fisher EM; MRC Proteomics in ALS Study; FReJA Consortium (2006) ALS phenotypes with mutations in CHMP2B (charged multivesicular body protein 2B). *Neurology* 67:1074-1077.

Paschal BM, King SM, Moss AG, Collins CA, Vallee RB, Witman GB (1987) Isolated flagellar outer arm dynein translocates brain microtubules in vitro. *Nature* 330:672-674.

Pasinelli P, Brown RH (2006) Molecular biology of amyotrophic lateral sclerosis: insights from genetics. *Nat. Rev. Neurosci.* 7:710-723.

Patel S, Latterich M (1998) The AAA team: related ATPases with diverse functions. *Trends Cell Biol.* 8:65-71.

Patel SK, Indig FE, Olivieri N, Levine ND, Latterich M (1998) Organelle membrane fusion: a novel function for the syntaxin homolog Ufe1p in ER membrane fusion. *Cell* 92:611-620.

Peretti D, Dahan N, Shimoni E, Hirschberg K, Lev S (2008) Coordinated lipid transfer between the endoplasmic reticulum and the Golgi complex requires the VAP proteins and is essential for Golgi-mediated transport. *Mol. Biol Cell* 19:3871-3884.

Pérez-Ollé R, López-Toledano MA, Goryunov D, Cabrera-Poch N, Stefanis L, Brown K, Liem RK (2005) Mutations in the neurofilament light gene linked to Charcot-Marie-Tooth disease cause defects in transport. *J. Neurochem.* 93:861-74.

Perlson E, Hanz S, Ben-Yaakov K, Segal-Ruder Y, Seger R, Fainzilber M (2005) Vimentin-dependent spatial translocation of an activated MAP kinase in injured nerve. *Neuron* 45:715-26.

Perlson E, Jeong GB, Ross JL, Dixit R, Wallace KE, Kalb RG, Holzbaur EL (2009) A switch in retrograde signaling from survival to stress in rapid-onset neurodegeneration. *J. Neurosci.* 29:9903-9917.

Perrot R, Eyer J (2009) Neuronal intermediate filaments and neurodegenerative disorders. *Brain Res. Bull* 80:282-95.

Piccioni F, Pinton P, Simeoni S, Pozzi P, Fascio U, Vismara G, Martini L, Rizzuto R, Poletti A (2002) Androgen receptor with elongated polyglutamine tract forms aggregates that alter axonal trafficking and mitochondrial distribution in motor neuronal processes. *FASEB J.* 16:1418-1420.

Poletti A (2004) The polyglutamine tract of androgen receptor: from functions to dysfunctions in motor neurons. *Front Neuroendocrinol* 25:1-26.

Preston AM, Gurisik E, Bartley C, Laybutt DR, Biden TJ (2009) Reduced endoplasmic reticulum (ER)-to-Golgi protein trafficking contributes to ER stress in lipotoxic mouse beta cells by promoting protein overload. *Diabetologia* 52:2369-2373.

Puls I, Jonnakuty C, LaMonte BH, Holzbaur EL, Tokito M, Mann E, Floeter MK, Bidus K, Drayna D, Oh SJ, Brown RH, Jr., Ludlow CL, Fischbeck KH (2003) Mutant dynactin in motor neuron disease. *Nat. Genet.* 33:455-456.

Rabinovich E, Kerem A, Frohlich KU, Diamant N, Bar-Nun S (2002) AAA-ATPase p97/Cdc48p, a cytosolic chaperone required for endoplasmic reticulum-associated protein degradation. *Mol. Cell Biol.* 22:626-634.

Raiborg C, Stenmark H (2009) The ESCRT machinery in endosomal sorting of ubiquitylated membrane proteins. *Nature.* 458:445-52.

Rajendran L, Honsho M, Zahn TR, Keller P, Geiger KD, Verkade P, Simons K (2006) Alzheimer's disease beta-amyloid peptides are released in association with exosomes. *Proc. Natl. Acad. Sci .USA* 103:11172-7.

Reiterer V, Maier S, Sitte HH, Kriz A, Ruegg MA, Hauri HP, Freissmuth M, Farhan H (2008) Sec24- and ARFGAP1-dependent trafficking of GABA transporter-1 is a prerequisite for correct axonal targeting. *J. Neurosci.* 28:12453-12464.

Rezaie T, Child A, Hitchings R, Brice G, Miller L, Coca-Prados M, Heon E, Krupin T, Ritch R, Kreutzer D, Crick RP, Sarfarazi M (2002) Adult-onset primary open-angle glaucoma caused by mutations in optineurin. *Science* 295:1077-1079.

Ron D, Walter P (2007) Signal integration in the endoplasmic reticulum unfolded protein response. *Nat. Rev. Mol Cell Biol.* 8:519-529.

Rosen DR, Siddique T, Patterson D, Figlewicz DA, Sapp P, Hentati A, Donaldson D, Goto J, O'Regan JP, Deng HX, Rahmani Z, Krizus A, McKenna-Yasek D, Cayabyab A, Gaston SM, Berger R, Tanzi RE, Halperin JJ, Hertzfeldt B, Van den Bergh R, Hung WY, Bird T, Deng G, Mulder DW, Smyth C, Laing NG, Soriano E, Pericak-Vance MA, Haines J, Rouleau GA, Gusella JS, Horvitz HR, Brown RH (1993) Mutations in Cu/Zn superoxide dismutase gene are associated with familial amyotrophic lateral sclerosis. *Nature* 362:59-62.

Routledge KE, Gupta V, Balch WE (2010) Emergent properties of proteostasis-COPII coupled systems in human health and disease. *Mol. Membrane Biol.* 27:385-397.

Roy S, Coffee P, Smith G, Liem RK, Brady ST, Black MM (2000) Neurofilaments are transported rapidly but intermittently in axons: implications for slow axonal transport. *J. Neuroscience* 20:6849-6861.

Rutkowski DT, Wu J, Back SH, Callaghan MU, Ferris SP, Iqbal J, Clark R, Miao H, Hassler JR, Fornek J, Katze MG, Hussain MM, Song B, Swathirajan J, Wang J, Yau GD, Kaufman RJ (2008) UPR pathways combine to prevent hepatic steatosis caused by ER stress-mediated suppression of transcriptional master regulators. *Dev Cell* 15:829-840.

Rutherford AC, Traer C, Wassmer T, Pattni K, Bujny MV, Carlton JG, Stenmark H, Cullen PJ (2006) The mammalian phosphatidylinositol 3-phosphate 5-kinase (PIKfyve) regulates endosome-to-TGN retrograde transport. *J. Cell Sci.* 119:3944-57.

Sahlender DA, Roberts RC, Arden SD, Spudich G, Taylor MJ, Luzio JP, Kendrick-Jones J, Buss F (2005) Optineurin links myosin VI to the Golgi complex and is involved in Golgi organization and exocytosis. *J. Cell Biol.* 169:285-295.

Sasaki S (2010) Endoplasmic reticulum stress in motor neurons of the spinal cord in sporadic amyotrophic lateral sclerosis. *J. Neuropathol. Exp. Neurol.* 69:346-355.

Sato T, Takeuchi S, Saito A, Ding W, Bamba H, Matsuura H, Hisa Y, Tooyama I, Urushitani M (2009) Axonal ligation induces transient redistribution of TDP-43 in brainstem motor neurons. *Neuroscience* 164:1565-1578.

Sau D, Rusmini P, Crippa V, Onesto E, Bolzoni E, Ratti A, Poletti A (2011) Dysregulation of axonal transport and motorneuron diseases. *Biol. Cell* 103:87-107.

Saxena S, Cabuy E, Caroni P (2009) A role for motoneuron subtype-selective ER stress in disease manifestations of FALS mice. *Nat. Neurosci.* 12:627-636.

Schaefer MK, Schmalbruch H, Buhler E, Lopez C, Martin N, Guenet JL, Haase G (2007) Progressive motor neuronopathy: a critical role of the tubulin chaperone TBCE in axonal tubulin routing from the Golgi apparatus. *J. Neurosci.* 27:8779-8789.

Schmitt-John T, Drepper C, Mussmann A, Hahn P, Kuhlmann M, Thiel C, Hafner M, Lengeling A, Heimann P, Jones JM, Meisler MH, Jockusch H (2005) Mutation of Vps54 causes motor neuron disease and defective spermiogenesis in the wobbler mouse. *Nat Genet.* 37:1213-1215.

Schroder M (2008) Endoplasmic reticulum stress responses. *Cell Mol Life Sci.* 65:862-894.

Sharples RA, Vella LJ, Nisbet RM, Naylor R, Perez K, Barnham KJ, Masters CL, Hill AF (2008) Inhibition of gamma-secretase causes increased secretion of amyloid precursor protein C-terminal fragments in association with exosomes. *FASEB J.* 22:1469-78.

Shea TB, Yabe JT, Ortiz D, Pimenta A, Loomis P, Goldman RD, Amin N, Pant HC (2004) Cdk5 regulates axonal transport and phosphorylation of neurofilaments in cultured neurons. *J. Cell Sci.* 117:933-941.

Short DM, Heron ID, Birse-Archbold JL, Kerr LE, Sharkey J, McCulloch J (2007) Apoptosis induced by staurosporine alters chaperone and endoplasmic reticulum proteins: Identification by quantitative proteomics. *Proteomics* 7:3085-3096.

Skehel PA, Fabian-Fine R, Kandel ER (2000) Mouse VAP33 is associated with the endoplasmic reticulum and microtubules. *Proc. Natl. Acad. Sci. USA* 97:1101-1106.

Skibinski G, Parkinson NJ, Brown JM, Chakrabarti L, Lloyd SL, Hummerich H, Nielsen JE, Hodges JR, Spillantini MG, Thusgaard T, Brandner S, Brun A, Rossor MN, Gade A, Johannsen P, Sorensen SA, Gydesen S, Fisher EM, Collinge J (2005) Mutations in the endosomal ESCRTIII-complex subunit CHMP2B in frontotemporal dementia. *Nat. Genet.* 37:806-8.

Spinosa MR, Progida C, De Luca A, Colucci AM, Alifano P, Bucci C (2008) Functional characterization of Rab7 mutant proteins associated with Charcot-Marie-Tooth type 2B disease. *J. Neurosci.* 28:1640-8.

Sreedharan J, Blair IP, Tripathi VB, Hu X, Vance C, Rogelj B, Ackerley S, Durnall JC, Williams KL, Buratti E, Baralle F, de Belleroche J, Mitchell JD, Leigh PN, Al-Chalabi A, Miller CC, Nicholson G, Shaw CE (2008) TDP-43 mutations in familial and sporadic amyotrophic lateral sclerosis. *Science* 319:1668-72.

Stenmark H (2009) Rab GTPases as co-ordinators of vesicle traffic. *Nat. Rev. Mol. Cell Biol.* 10:513-525.

Strom AL, Shi P, Zhang F, Gal J, Kilty R, Hayward LJ, Zhu H (2008) Interaction of amyotrophic lateral sclerosis (ALS)-related mutant copper-zinc superoxide dismutase with the dynein-dynactin complex contributes to inclusion formation. *J. Biol. Chem.* 283:22795-22805.

Strong MJ (2010) The evidence for altered RNA metabolism in amyotrophic lateral sclerosis (ALS). *J. Neurol. Sci.* 288:1-12.

Suzuki H, Lee K, Matsuoka M (2011) TDP-43-induced death is associated with altered regulation of BIM and BCL-XL and attenuated by caspase-mediated TDP-43 cleavage. *J. Biol. Chem.* 286:13171-13183.

Suzuki H, Kanekura K, Levine TP, Kohno K, Olkkonen VM, Aiso S, Matsuoka M (2009) ALS-linked P56S-VAPB, an aggregated loss-of-function mutant of VAPB, predisposes motor neurons to ER stress-related death by inducing aggregation of co-expressed wild-type VAPB. *J. Neurochem.* 108:973-985.

Tan JM, Wong ES, Kirkpatrick DS, Pletnikova O, Ko HS, Tay SP, Ho MW, Troncoso J, Gygi SP, Lee MK, Dawson VL, Dawson TM, Lim KL (2008) Lysine 63-linked ubiquitination promotes the formation and autophagic clearance of protein inclusions associated with neurodegenerative diseases. *Hum. Mol. Genet* 17:431-9.

Tateishi T, Hokonohara T, Yamasaki R, Miura S, Kikuchi H, Iwaki A, Tashiro H, Furuya H, Nagara Y, Ohyagi Y, Nukina N, Iwaki T, Fukumaki Y, Kira JI (2010) Multiple system degeneration with basophilic inclusions in Japanese ALS patients with FUS mutation. *Acta Neuropathol.* 119:355-364.

Tateno M, Kato S, Sakurai T, Nukina N, Takahashi R, Araki T (2009) Mutant SOD1 impairs axonal transport of choline acetyltransferase and acetylcholine release by sequestering KAP3. *Hum. Mol. Genet.* 18:942-55.

Teuchert M, Fischer D, Schwalenstoecker B, Habisch HJ, Bockers TM, Ludolph AC (2006) A dynein mutation attenuates motor neuron degeneration in SOD1(G93A) mice. *Exp. Neurol.* 198:271-274.

Teuling E, Ahmed S, Haasdijk E, Demmers J, Steinmetz MO, Akhmanova A, Jaarsma D, Hoogenraad CC (2007) Motor neuron disease-associated mutant vesicle-associated membrane protein-associated protein (VAP) B recruits wild-type VAPs into endoplasmic reticulum-derived tubular aggregates. *J. Neurosci.* 27:9801-9815.

Théry C, Ostrowski M, Segura E (2009) Membrane vesicles as conveyors of immune responses. *Nat.Rev. Immunol.* 9:581-93.

Tsuda H, Han SM, Yang Y, Tong C, Lin YQ, Mohan K, Haueter C, Zoghbi A, Harati Y, Kwan J, Miller MA, Bellen HJ (2008) The amyotrophic lateral sclerosis 8 protein VAPB is cleaved, secreted, and acts as a ligand for Eph receptors. *Cell* 133:963-977.

Turner BJ, Atkin JD (2006) ER Stress and UPR in Familial Amyotrophic Lateral Sclerosis. *Curr. Mol. Med.* 6:79-86.

Turner BJ, Atkin JD, Farg MA, Zang DW, Rembach A, Lopes EC, Patch JD, Hill AF, Cheema SS (2005) Impaired extracellular secretion of mutant superoxide dismutase 1 associates with neurotoxicity in familial amyotrophic lateral sclerosis. *J. Neurosci.* 25:108-17.

Urushitani M, Sik A, Sakurai T, Nukina N, Takahashi R, Julien JP (2006) Chromogranin-mediated secretion of mutant superoxide dismutase proteins linked to amyotrophic lateral sclerosis. *Nat. Neurosci.* 9:108-18.

Urwin H, Authier A, Nielsen JE, Metcalf D, Powell C, Froud K, Malcolm DS, Holm I, Johannsen P, Brown J, Fisher EM, van der Zee J, Bruyland M; FReJA Consortium, Van Broeckhoven C, Collinge J, Brandner S, Futter C, Isaacs AM (2010) Disruption of endocytic trafficking in frontotemporal dementia with CHMP2B mutations. *Hum. Mol. Genet* 19:2228-38.

Valadi H, Ekström K, Bossios A, Sjöstrand M, Lee JJ, Lötvall JO (2007) Exosome-mediated transfer of mRNAs and microRNAs is a novel mechanism of genetic exchange between cells. *Nat. Cell Biol.* 9:654-9.

Vale RD, Schnapp BJ, Reese TS, Sheetz MP (1985) Movement of organelles along filaments dissociated from the axoplasm of the squid giant axon. *Cell* 40:449-454.

van der Zee J, Urwin H, Engelborghs S, Bruyland M, Vandenberghe R, Dermaut B, De Pooter T, Peeters K, Santens P, De Deyn PP, Fisher EM, Collinge J, Isaacs AM, Van Broeckhoven C. (2008) CHMP2B C-truncating mutations in frontotemporal lobar degeneration are associated with an aberrant endosomal phenotype in vitro. *Hum. Mol. Genet.* 17:313-22.

Vance C, Rogelj B, Hortobágyi T, De Vos KJ, Nishimura AL, Sreedharan J, Hu X, Smith B, Ruddy D, Wright P, Ganesalingam J, Williams KL, Tripathi V, Al-Saraj S, Al-Chalabi A, Leigh PN, Blair IP, Nicholson G, de Belleroche J, Gallo JM, Miller CC, Shaw CE (2009) Mutations in FUS, an RNA processing protein, cause familial amyotrophic lateral sclerosis type 6. *Science* 323:1208-11.

Vella LJ, Sharples RA, Lawson VA, Masters CL, Cappai R, Hill AF (2007) Packaging of prions into exosomes is associated with a novel pathway of PrP processing. *J. Pathol.* 211:582-90.

Vella LJ, Sharples RA, Nisbet RM, Cappai R, Hill AF (2008a) The role of exosomes in the processing of proteins associated with neurodegenerative diseases. *Eur. Biophys J.* 37:323-32.

Vella LJ, Greenwood DL, Cappai R, Scheerlinck JP, Hill AF (2008b) Enrichment of prion protein in exosomes derived from ovine cerebral spinal fluid. *Vet. Immunol. Immunopathol.* 124:385-93.

Waterman-Storer CM, Karki SB, Kuznetsov SA, Tabb JS, Weiss DG, Langford GM, Holzbaur EL (1997) The interaction between cytoplasmic dynein and dynactin is required for fast axonal transport. *Proc. Natl. Acad. Sci. USA* 94:12180-12185.

Williams RL, Urbe S (2007) The emerging shape of the ESCRT machinery. *Nat. Rev. Mol. Cell Biol.* 8:355-68.

Williamson TL, Cleveland DW (1999) Slowing of axonal transport is a very early event in the toxicity of ALS-linked SOD1 mutants to motor neurons. *Nat. Neurosci.* 2:50-56.

Wishart MJ, Dixon JE (2002) PTEN and myotubularin phosphatases: from 3-phosphoinositide dephosphorylation to disease. *Trends Cell Biol.* 12:579-585.

Wojcik C, Yano M, DeMartino GN (2004) RNA interference of valosin-containing protein (VCP/p97) reveals multiple cellular roles linked to ubiquitin/proteasome-dependent proteolysis. *J. Cell Sci.* 117:281-292.

Wojcik C, Rowicka M, Kudlicki A, Nowis D, McConnell E, Kujawa M, DeMartino GN (2006) Valosin-containing protein (p97) is a regulator of endoplasmic reticulum stress and of the degradation of N-end rule and ubiquitin-fusion degradation pathway substrates in mammalian cells. *Mol. Biol. Cell* 17:4606-4618.

Woodman PG (2003) p97, a protein coping with multiple identities. *J. Cell Sci.* 116:4283-4290.

Wootz H, Hansson I, Korhonen L, Lindholm D (2006a) XIAP decreases caspase-12 cleavage and calpain activity in spinal cord of ALS transgenic mice. *Exp. Cell Res.* 312:1890-1898.

Wootz H, Weber E, Korhonen L, Lindholm D (2006b) Altered distribution and levels of cathepsinD and cystatins in amyotrophic lateral sclerosis transgenic mice: possible roles in motor neuron survival. *Neuroscience* 143:419-30.

Xia CH, Roberts EA, Her LS, Liu X, Williams DS, Cleveland DW, Goldstein LS (2003) Abnormal neurofilament transport caused by targeted disruption of neuronal kinesin heavy chain KIF5A. *J. Cell Biol.* 161:55-66.

Yang Y, Hentati A, Deng HX, Dabbagh O, Sasaki T, Hirano M, Hung WY, Ouahchi K, Yan J, Azim AC, Cole N, Gascon G, Yagmour A, Ben-Hamida M, Pericak-Vance M, Hentati F, Siddique T (2001) The gene encoding alsin, a protein with three guanine-nucleotide exchange factor domains, is mutated in a form of recessive amyotrophic lateral sclerosis. *Nat. Genet.* 29:160-165.

Yano H, Lee FS, Kong H, Chuang J, Arevalo J, Perez P, Sung C, Chao MV (2001) Association of Trk neurotrophin receptors with components of the cytoplasmic dynein motor. *J. Neurosci.* 21:RC125.

Ye Y, Shibata Y, Yun C, Ron D, Rapoport TA (2004) A membrane protein complex mediates retro-translocation from the ER lumen into the cytosol. *Nature* 429:841-847.

Zaal KJ, Smith CL, Polishchuk RS, Altan N, Cole NB, Ellenberg J, Hirschberg K, Presley JF, Roberts TH, Siggia E, Phair RD, Lippincott-Schwartz J (1999) Golgi membranes are absorbed into and reemerge from the ER during mitosis. *Cell* 99:589-601.

Zetterstrom P, Andersen PM, Brännström T, Marklund SL (2011) Misfolded superoxide dismutase-1 in CSF from amyotrophic lateral sclerosis patients. *J. Neurochem.* 117:91-9.

Zhang F, Strom AL, Fukada K, Lee S, Hayward LJ, Zhu H (2007) Interaction between familial amyotrophic lateral sclerosis (ALS)-linked SOD1 mutants and the dynein complex. *J. Biol. Chem.* 282:16691-16699.

Zhang X, Li L, Chen S, Yang D, Wang Y, Zhang X, Wang Z, Le W (2011) Rapamycin treatment augments motor neuron degeneration in SOD1 (G93A) mouse model of amyotrophic lateral sclerosis. *Autophagy* 7, in press.

Zhao C, Takita J, Tanaka Y, Setou M, Nakagawa T, Takeda S, Yang HW, Terada S, Nakata T, Takei Y, Saito M, Tsuji S, Hayashi Y, Hirokawa N (2001) Charcot-Marie-Tooth disease type 2A caused by mutation in a microtubule motor KIF1Bbeta. *Cell* 105:587-597.

Zhao W, Beers DR, Henkel JS, Zhang W, Urushitani M, Julien JP, Appel SH (2010) Extracellular mutant SOD1 induces microglial-mediated motoneuron injury. *Glia* 58:231-43.

Zuchner S, Noureddine M, Kennerson M, Verhoeven K, Claeys K, De Jonghe P, Merory J, Oliveira SA, Speer MC, Stenger JE, Walizada G, Zhu D, Pericak-Vance MA, Nicholson G, Timmerman V, Vance JM (2005) Mutations in the pleckstrin homology domain of dynamin 2 cause dominant intermediate Charcot-Marie-Tooth disease. *Nat. Genet.* 37:289-294.

In: Motor Neuron Diseases
Editors: Bradley J. Turner and Julie B. Atkin

ISBN 978-1-61470-101-9
© 2012 Nova Science Publishers, Inc.

Chapter III

MOTONEURON SPECIFIC CALCIUM DYSREGULATION AND PERTURBED CELLULAR CALCIUM HOMESTASIS IN AMYOTROPHIC LATERAL SCLEROSIS: RECENT ADVANCES GAINED FROM GENETICALLY MODIFIED ANIMALS AND CELL CULTURE MODELS

*Manoj Kumar Jaiswal**
McGovern Institute for Brain Research,
Massachusetts Institute of Technology, Cambridge, MA, U. S.

ABSTRACT

Amyotrophic lateral sclerosis (ALS) is a fatal neurodegenerative disorder characterized by the selective loss of defined subgroups of motoneuorn populations in the brainstem and spinal cord with signature hallmarks of mitochondrial Ca^{2+} overload, free radical damage, excitotoxicity and impaired axonal transport. Although intracellular disruptions of cytosolic and mitochondrial calcium and in particular low cytosolic calcium ($[Ca^{2+}]_i$) buffering and a strong interaction between metabolic mechanisms and $[Ca^{2+}]_i$ have been associated with selective motoneuron degeneration, the underlying mechanisms are not well understood. The present evidence supports a hypothesis that mitochondria are a primary target of mutant superoxide dismutase1 (mtSOD1)-mediated toxicity in ALS and intracellular alterations of cytosolic and mitochondria-ER microdomain calcium accumulation might aggravate the course of this neurodegenerative disease. Furthermore, chronic excitotoxicity mediated by Ca^{2+}- permeable AMPA and

* Corresponding author: Manoj Kumar Jaiswal, PhD, McGovern Institute for Brain Research, Massachusetts Institute of Technology, 77 Massachusetts Avenue, Cambridge, MA 02139, USA. Email: jaiswal@mit.edu
Present address: Center for Neuroscience and Regenerative Medicine and Department of Anatomy, Physiology and Genetics, USUHS, School of Medicine, 4301 Jones Bridge Road, Bethesda, MD 20814, USA.

NMDA receptors seems to initiate a vicious cycle of intracellular calcium dysregulation which leads to toxic Ca^{2+} overload and thereby selective neurodegeneration. Recent advancement in the experimental analysis of calcium signals at high spatiotemporal precision has allowed investigations of calcium regulation in different cell types, in particular selectively vulnerable/resistant cell types in different animal models of this motoneuron disease. This chapter provides an overview of recent advances in this field and discusses in detail what has been learned about Ca^{2+} homeostasis and the role of mitochondria in motoneurons in pathophysiological conditions such as ALS.

Keywords: Amyotrophic lateral sclerosis, Motoneuron, Calcium dysregulation, Mitochondria, Selective vulnerability, Calcium buffer.

ABBREVIATIONS

ALS	amyotrophic lateral sclerosis;
aCSF	artificial cerebrospinal fluid;
AMPA	alpha-amino-3-hydroxy-5-methyl-4-isoxazolepropionic acid;
$[Ca^{2+}]i$,	cytosolic calcium;
CB-D_{28K}	calbidin D_{28K};
CSF	cerebrospinal fluid;
EAAT2	excitatory amino acid transporter 2;
ER	endoplasmic reticulum;
fALS	familial amyotrophic lateral sclerosis;
FCCP	Carbonyl cyanide 4-(trifluoromethoxy) phenylhydrazone;
GluR	glutamate receptors;
GLT	glutamate transporter;
hALS	human amyotrophic lateral sclerosis;
ROS	reactive oxygen species;
SOD1	Cu/Zn superoxide dismutase 1;
mtSOD1	mutant superoxide dismutase1;
MNs	motoneurons;
NMDA	N-Methyl-D-aspartic acid;
PV	parvalbumin;
Tg	transgenic;
VEGF	vascular endothelial-cell growth factor;
WT	wild-type;
$\Delta\psi_m$,	mitochondrial membrane potential;
τ	decay time constant.

INTRODUCTION

Amyotrophic lateral sclerosis (ALS) is an incurable adult-onset fatal neurodegenerative disorder characterized by the selective loss of a defined motoneuron (MN) population in the brain stem and spinal cord leading to paralysis and death within 5 years [1]. The majority of

ALS cases are sporadic, but ~10% of ALS cases are familial ALS (fALS). About 20% of these familial cases are caused by dominantly inherited mutations in the gene encoding the enzyme Cu/Zn-superoxide dismutase (mtSOD1) [2]. Although the process of MN degeneration both in sporadic and familial forms is still little understood, it is generally agreed that there are cell-specific features, particulaly impaired uptake of Ca^{2+} into mitochondria and low content of Ca^{2+} binding proteins which modulate physiological as well as pathophysiological processes and may render MNs selectively vulnerable to degeneration [3, 4, 5, 6].

In fact, recent evidence suggests that abnormalities in cellular Ca^{2+} signaling are common features in the pathogenesis of a range of neurodegenerative disorders, including ALS [7]. It is well known that Ca^{2+} is one of the most relevant intracellular messengers, being essential in neuronal development, synaptic transmission and plasticity, as well as in the regulation of various metabolic pathways in the brain. In both subtypes, ALS associated with SOD1 mutation and in the sporadic disease, there have been several reports indicating that the involvement of mitochondria in the pathogenesis includes the generation of intracellular free radical species [8], ultrastructral changes in mitochondrial morphology [9, 10], swollen and vacuolar mitochondria [11] and increased activity of complex I, III and IV in frontal cortex and spinal cord [12, 13, 14]. Impaired spinal cord [15] and vulnerable individual spinal MNs [16] have also been reported. It has been proposed that these changes trigger the functional decline of MNs and the onset of pathology in ALS. The loss of mitochondrial membrane potential ($\Delta\Psi$m) [17], excitotoxic stimulation of AMPA/kainite receptors [18] and age related MN injury reported by many groups may also contribute to ALS pathogenesis [19, 20].

Further evidence for the involvement of impaired intracellular Ca^{2+} homeostasis arises from several studies of *in-vitro* and *in-vivo* models in which the absence of Ca^{2+} binding proteins such as calbidin D_{28K} (CB-D_{28K}) and parvalbumin (PV) is characteristics of MN populations that are lost early in ALS, e.g. hypoglossal, spinal, and lower cranial MNs [3]. These findings are in good agreement with a quantitative comparison of Ca^{2+} homeostasis, where low cytosolic Ca^{2+} buffering capacity acts as an important risk factor for MN degeneration and, in contrast, an increase in cytosolic Ca^{2+} buffering capacity could protect vulnerable MNs from degeneration, both *in-vitro* and *in-vivo* [21, 6]. Several lines of evidence could explain how altered Ca^{2+} homeostasis leads to MN degeneration in ALS, notably disturbance of glutamate neurotransmission and subsequent glutamate triggered Ca^{2+} entry [22, 23], increased extracellular glutamate levels probably due to reduced glial glutamate uptake caused by oxidative damage to excitatory amino acid transporter 2 (EAAT2) [24]. Studies of fALS in cell lines and mouse models where the potential mechanism for Ca^{2+} disruption is inhibition of glial glutamate transport by mtSOD1 similar to effects proposed in sALS [25]. In addition, in cell culture experiments, partial protection was also obtained by treatment with nifedipine, implicating Ca^{2+} entry through voltage-gated Ca^{2+} channels in mediating the toxicity of mSOD1^{G93A} in MNs [26]. Evidence also suggests that reactive oxygen species (ROS) generated in MNs can cross the plasma membrane and cause oxidative disruption of glutamate transporters in neighboring astrocytes [27, 23]. However, in ALS pathology, the nature of dysfunction has become highly controversial after recent findings where non-cell autonomous effects of glia on MNs in an embryonic stem cell-based ALS model and astrocytes expressing ALS-linked mtSOD1 that release factors selectively toxic to MNs was shown [28, 29, 30, 31].

The kinetics of calcium signals in MNs are shaped by multiple processes including Ca^{2+} influx, Ca^{2+} uptake and release phenomenon, MN specific Ca^{2+} buffering and extrusion across cellular membrane and microdomains in vicinity [32, 33]. Over the past decade, there has been an increased understanding of local interactions between Ca^{2+} and its target signaling pathways. In particular, an impaired interaction between calcium signaling and mitochondrial processes has been identified as one cellular factor contributing to neurodegenerative processes like those found in motoneuron diseases. In addition, previous studies also indicate the importance of calcium and mitochondria for normal physiological function of MNs [34, 35]. Under pathophysiological conditions, low cytosolic calcium buffering and a strong interaction between metabolic mechanisms and $[Ca^{2+}]i$ have been associated with selective and severe MN damage resulting from excitotoxic stress and disruptions of cellular homeostasis [36, 37]. Considering the prime participation of mitochondria not only in calcium homeostasis directly but also in the energy transduction (to operate other Ca^{2+} clearing mechanisms) and in enacting apoptosis, this aspect of cellular function is of immense importance.

Despite rigorous research, since description of ALS by Charcot more than 130 years ago, the molecular abnormalities which lead to damage of specific MNs are still dodging the scientific community. The aim of this review is to discuss and determine the role of mtSOD1 toxicity on cellular Ca^{2+} homeostasis and mitochondrial signaling pathways in selectively vulnerable MNs in ALS. This review will focus on what has been learned about motoneuron specific calcium dysregulation and perturbed cellular calcium homestasis in ALS from genetically modified animals and cell culture models. Taken together, this review proposes an intregative view, describing mechanisms and critical elements of the pathology of SOD1-mediated motoneuron degeneration in ALS.

DISEASE MECHANISM IN AMYOTROPHIC LATERAL SCLEROSIS

Many pathophysiological mechanisms have been suggested to play a role in the etiology of ALS. Corresponding to the clinical feature, ALS is characterized by a progressive loss of cortical, spinal and brain stem MNs. MN damage as a result of oxidative stress and excitotoxicity is a key hypothesis in ALS etiology. The present evidence supports the hypothesis of mitochondrial dysfunction acting with oxidative stress to cause neurodegeneration via an apoptotic mechanism. Oxidative stress is also linked with other proposed disease mechanisms such as excitotoxicity causing an increase in intracellular calcium, which in turn leads to increased nitric oxide formation. Peroxynitrite, generated by the reaction of superoxide anions and nitric oxide, can subsequently lead to oxidative damage [23]. Glutamate excitotoxicity is another mechanism implicated in ALS pathogenesis through disruption of intracellular calcium homeostasis and free radical production [22]. For example in human ALS (hALS), overexpression of glutamatergic synapses and excess calcium influx have been associated with MN damage [38]. The oxidative stress evident in ALS might also promote increased excitotoxicity, as glutamate transporters are particularly susceptible to disruption by oxidants, and oxidative modifications to the transporters have been reported in ALS and the mtSOD1 mouse model [23]. Moreover, in geneticallty determined forms of

ALS, mutations in axonal neurofilaments (NFL) trigger MN degeneration [39]. Role of individual cellular domains at organelles level have suggested that high calcium buffering enhances MNs vulnerability [40]. In summery, ALS involves the interplay of several mechanisms from initiation and spread of MN cell death by mitochondrial dysfunction and/or by enhanced MN excitability by intracellular calcium overload. Therefore the etiology of the disease is most likely to be multifactorial [41, 34, 42]. This article will focus on and further discuss the hypotheses and key mechanism that have been most influential in the present and past decade of ALS research.

DISRUPTED CALCIUM HOMEOSTASIS IN AMYOTROPHIC LATERAL SCLEROSIS

Several groups have reported that independent of the cellular and molecular mechanisms, disruption of intracellular Ca^{2+} homeostasis plays a prominent role in the etiology of ALS. The involvement of Ca^{2+} as a risk factor was suggested by the observation that Ca^{2+}-binding proteins such as CB-D_{28k} and PV were absent in MN populations lost early in ALS, whereas MNs less prone to damage expressed markedly higher levels of CB-D_{28k} and/or PV [43, 3]. This observation identified a low cytosolic Ca^{2+} buffering capacity as an important risk factor for MN degeneration. Data from different groups shows that vulnerable populations of MNs display low endogenous calcium buffering capacity [44]. The ability of MNs to buffer increases in intracellular Ca^{2+} is impaired due to low expression levels of Ca^{2+}-buffering proteins. This low Ca^{2+}-buffering capacity could be essential under physiological conditions as it allows rapid relaxation times of Ca^{2+} transients in MNs during high frequency rhythmic activity. However, these characteristics make MNs more susceptible to an excessive influx of Ca^{2+} ions by evoking large amplitudes of intracellular free Ca^{2+} concentrations and thus increasing the risk for activation of excitotoxic second messenger cascades and related cellular disturbances [43]. Another argument in favor of this hypothesis is that high concentrations of mobile buffers accelerate the dispersion of local Ca^{2+} gradients by a process commonly known as buffering diffusion (Figure 1a, b). According to this concept, under pathophysiological conditions, differential buffering reflects a basic diversity in the spatio-temporal organization of Ca^{2+} signaling rather than a singular difference in one cellular parameter [45, 46, 47]. Likewise, an increase in cytosolic Ca^{2+} buffering capacity could protect vulnerable MNs from degeneration both *in vitro* and *in-vivo* [48, 6].

The observation of high buffering capacity in selectively resistant MNs is consistent with earlier immunocytochemical studies of endogenous calcium buffering proteins. Moreover, *in-vitro* cell culture models have shown that elevated cytosolic buffer concentration reduces ALS related MN damage providing further support in favor of the idea that increased buffer concentrations create beneficial protection [49]. The low Ca^{2+} buffering properties, together with a high AMPA/kainate current density, could explain the particular vulnerability of MNs to increased stimulation by glutamate and concomitant Ca^{2+} influx [50]. Another proposed factor for calcium disregulation could be an ALS-related immune reaction targeted at voltage-dependent calcium channels, where a disruption of homeostasis results from impaired voltage-dependent calcium influx [51]. Furthermore, synaptic glutamate transport is also thought to be involved in other forms of ALS-related neurodegeneration.

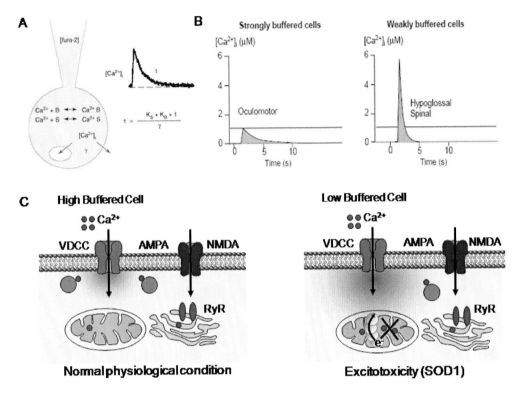

Figure 1. Ca^{2+} homeostasis and its correlation with weakly and strongly buffered motoneurons under physiological and pathophysiological conditions. (A) The Ca^{2+} buffering capacity (K$_S$) of a cell, reflecting relative fraction of bound versus free Ca^{2+}, can be calculated by using the 'added buffer' approach by linear one-compartment model. The recovery time of cytosolic [Ca^{2+}]$_i$ elevations (τ) depends on the amount of endogenous buffer (S; denotes Ca^{2+}-binding proteins), the amount of exogenous buffer (B; i.e. Fura-2) and the transport rate (γ) of Ca^{2+} across cellular membranes. Gradual introduction of exogenous buffer via the patch pipette enables the cytosolic K$_S$ to be determined. K$_B$ indicates the buffer capacity of the exogenous buffer (i.e. Fura-2). (B) Ca^{2+} homeostasis in weakly and strongly buffered MNs. Low cytosolic Ca^{2+}-buffering capacity has several implications for spatial and temporal Ca^{2+} signaling. The amplitude of Ca^{2+} transients is several times larger in weakly buffered cells (e.g. hypoglossal and spinal MNs) than in strongly buffered cells (e.g. oculomotor neurons), and the recovery time is significantly accelerated (τ). (C) Low Ca^{2+} buffering in ALS-vulnerable HMNs exposes mitochondria to higher Ca^{2+} loads compared to high buffered cells. Under normal physiological conditions the neurotransmitter opens glutamate, NMDA and AMPA receptor channels along with voltage-dependent Ca^{2+} channels (VDCC) with high glutamate release and reuptake by EAAT1 and EAAT2. This results in a small rise in intracellular calcium that can be buffered by the cell. In ALS disorder, the glutamate receptor channels possess high calcium conductivity and thereby high Ca^{2+} loads; increase the risk for mitochondrial damage. This triggers mitochondrial production of reactive oxygen species (ROS), which then inhibit glial EAAT2 function. This leads to further increase in glutamate concentrations in the synapse and further rises in postsynaptic calcium levels which contributes to the selective vulnerability of MNs in ALS. Low cytosolic Ca^{2+} buffering capacity promotes Ca^{2+} accumulation and formation of subcellular domains around influx sites (red), and thus facilitates the interaction of elevated calcium levels with intracellular organelles such as mitochondria (modified after Neher and Augustine, 1992; Vanselow and Keller, 2000; Von Lewinski and Keller, 2005; Jaiswal et al., 2009).

In a cell-culture study, partial protection was obtained by treatment with nifedipine, implicating Ca^{2+} entry through voltage-gated Ca^{2+} channels, in addition to glutamate receptors, in mediating the toxicity of mtSOD1 in MNs. Recently, the crucial role of Ca^{2+}-permeable AMPA receptors was further underlined by cross-breeding of transgenic SOD1 mice with mice that showed markedly reduced Ca^{2+} permeability of AMPA/kainate receptors, due to GluR2 overexpression [52]. Finally, impaired mitochondrial calcium transport capacity in mtSOD1 mice may play an important role. Firstly, it links mitochondrial dysfunction to glutamate excitotoxicity and secondly, elevation of cytosolic calcium levels in neurons compromises mitochondrial integrity and function by inducing enhanced production of free radicals from mitochondria [53] (Figure 1C).

OXIDATIVE STRESS AND MITOCHONDRIAL DYSFUNCTION

Oxidative stress and mitochondrial dysfunction is implicated in the pathogenesis of both normal aging and neurodegenerative diseases. Motoneuron damage as a consequence of oxidative stress is supposed to be the key premise in ALS. A number of studies have established the presence of elevated oxidative metabolism in ALS, such as the detection of increased biochemical markers of oxidative injury in post-mortem samples from patients. Free radical scavenging proteins like SOD1, mitochondrial manganese SOD (SOD2), catalase, and cytochrome c can neutralize free radicals but can not prevent cellular damage by ROS [54, 41]. Increased ˙OH generation may occur as a consequence of either enhanced peroxidase activity or decreased Cu-binding affinity of mtSOD1. mtSOD1 transgenic (Tg) mice show elevated levels of protein and lipid oxidation at both pre- and post-symptomatic stages [55]. Oxidative stress is also associated with other proposed disease mechanisms such as excitotoxicity and axonal transport defects. Studies suggest that ROS generated in motoneurons can cross the plasma membrane and cause oxidative disruption of glutamate transporters in neighboring astrocytes by excitotoxic stimulation of AMPA/kainate receptors followed by local excitotoxicity and initiation of a vicious cycle of motoneuron overactivation and damage [18, 27].

Morphological and ultrastructural abnormalities observed in mitochondria of both, sporadic and familial forms of ALS point towards a crucial involvement of mitochondria in ALS [56]. There are now several observations suggest that mitochondria play a crucial role in disturbing energy metabolism by predisposing calcium-mediated excitotxicity leading to ROS generation and initiation of apoptotic pathway, thereby jeopardizing cell function and normal cellular metabolism [57, 58, 16].

Abnormalities in mitochondrial function have been found in fALS and some sALS patients. Initial clues were provided by histological observations of mitochondrial abnormalities such as swelling and vacuolization, as some of the earliest signs of pathology in ALS mouse models and in human ALS [11, 9, 12, 59, 20] (Figure 2A). Morphological abnormalities were not only confined to CNS but were also found in skeletal muscles, intramuscular nerve fibers and proximal horns of the spinal cord [60, 61, 62]. Recently, in a SOD1-transfected cell culture model of MN disease, our laboratory has shown impairement of mitochondrial calcium handling and impaired cross-talk between mitochondria-ER microdomains [63] (Figure 2B -D).

Many other studies have recently focused on mitochondrial dysfunction, in particular on altered activity of the mitochondrial respiratory chain necessary for ATP synthesis and on increased production of ROS.

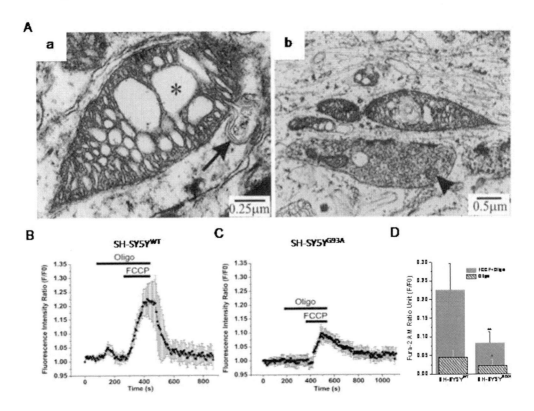

Figure 2. Mitochondrial structure of motor neurons in mutant SOD1 transgenic mice and calcium load in microdomains in a cell culture model of motoneuron disease. (A) a, Shows abnormalities like dilated cristae (asterisk) and leaking outer membrane (indicated with arrow) in mitochondrion. (A) b, Swollen dendritic mitochondria with dilated and disorganized cristae (adapted from Kong and Xu, 1998). (B) The quantitative kinetic profile of the oligomycin (mitochondrial ATP synthase inhibitor) and FCCP (mitochondrial uncoupler)-evoked [Ca^{2+}]i release in WT transfected SH-SY5Y cells. (C) The corresponding quantitative kinetic profile of the oligo and FCCP-evoked [Ca^{2+}]i release in the G93A transfected SH-SY5Y cells. The trace is representative of mean of 4-6 cells in focus stimulated with 5 μg/ml oligo and 2μM FCCP. (D) A bar diagram of oligo and FCCP plus oligo-induced Ca^{2+} release in the WT and G93A transfected SH-SY5Y neuroblastoma cells. Gray bars represent oligo plus FCCP-induced Ca^{2+} release in WT and G93A transfected SH-SY5Y cells. Striped bars represent oligo-induced Ca^{2+} release in WT and G93A transfected cells. Values represent means ± SD, *$p<0.01$, **$p<0.001$ (significanct level of SOD1^{G93A} compare to WT^{G93A} transfected SHSY-5Ycells; adapted from Jaiswal et al., 2009).

Lack of supply of requisite energy can result in the loss of integrity of neuronal cell membranes, leaving them permeable to ions and water which can cause damage. Deficits in the activities of complex I [64] and complex IV [65], as a result of mutations in mitochondrial DNA, have been identified in the skeletal muscles and spinal cord of sALS patients [14].

The question of whether alterations in the mitochondrial genome can lead to alterations in cell function has been addressed by transferring mitochondrial DNA from ALS subjects to mitochondrial DNA-depleted human neuroblastoma cells. This resulted in abnormal electron transport chain function, increase in activity of free radical scavenging enzymes, disturbed Ca^{2+} homeostasis and altered mitochondrial ultrastructure, suggesting a pathological role for mitochondrial DNA mutations in some forms of ALS [66]. A striking recent set of publications provides evidence that mtSOD1 might disrupt association of complex IV (cytochrome c) with the inner mitochondrial membrane, and by this mechanism interfere with mitochondrial respiration. Cultured MNs expressing mtSOD1 and MNs in brain slices where complex IV was inhibited by cyanide also show mitochondrial involvement [67, 68, 69].

Although these results are intriguing, they do not resolve the question of whether mitochondrial abnormalities are causally involved in the disease process or merely a byproduct of neuronal degeneration. However, pathological features like the presence of membrane-bound vacuoles in MNs in Tg mice expressing SOD1 mutants G93A or G37R suggest that mitochondrial alterations represent an early event triggering the onset of the disease, rather than simply a byproduct of cell degeneration [70, 71]. Further detailed studies using markers for different mitochondrial compartments demonstrated unequivocally that mitochondrial vacuolization develops from a progressive detachment of the outer membrane from the inner membrane and expansion of the intermembrane space. Once the outer membrane expands to form the mature vacuoles, the inner membrane collapses or disintegrates and becomes inner membrane remnants inside the vacuoles [72, 73]. A recent publication demonstrates the localization of a significant fraction of SOD1 in intermitochondrial space thereby causing toxicity. Inhibition of mitochondrial respiratory metabolism is reported in Tg ALS mice models [74]. Independent of the cause of mitochondrial damage, various other studies indicate that chronic mitochondrial inhibition (chemical hypoxia) induced by inhibitors like sodium cyanide and azide leads to selective motoneuron death, which can be counteracted by free-radical scavengers and AMPA receptor blockers [75]. In tune with these observations, ALS-like symptoms can be induced in mice by a targeted deletion of vascular endothelial-cell growth factor (VEGF) that eliminates the ability to respond to tissue hypoxia. Cross-breeding these mice with the mtSOD1 severely enhanced MN degeneration, while treatment of SOD1-Tg mice with VEGF delayed progression of symptoms and prolonged survival [76, 77, 78, 79, 80].

GLUTAMATE TRANSMISSION AND EXCITOTOXICITY

Glutamate is known as the predominant excitatory neurotransmitter in the CNS acting at both ionotropic and metabotropic receptors. It is synthesized and stored in synaptic nerve components and released in response to depolarization of the neuron. Excessive glutamate exposure is toxic to neurons via glutamate-triggered Ca^{2+} influx [81, 42]. Several lines of evidence implicate the disturbance of glutamate neurotransmission and subsequent glutamate-triggered Ca^{2+} entry as important factors in ALS. Increased extracellular glutamate levels presumably result from reduced glial glutamate uptake, which can be caused by oxidative damage to the excitatory amino acid transporter 2 (EAAT2) or by aberrant RNA processing. Increased glutamate levels in the cerebrospinal fluid (CSF) in a subset of ALS patients were shown earlier by many groups. Elevation of this glutamate level may be attributed to deficient glutamate transporter capacity (loss of EAAT2 function), as low levels of the transport protein have been found in some post mortem ALS brains [42, 82, 36, 22]. Furthermore, inhibitors of glutamate uptake cause selective motoneuron damage in organotypic slices [36] and in dissociated spinal cord culture models [83], suggesting that reduction of glutamate transport could contribute to the motoneuron damage seen in the disease. The most important argument for a role of glutamate excitotoxicity in ALS is the efficacy of riluzole, the only drug which proved effective against disease progression in patients and has anti-excitotoxic properties. It was shown that this drug inhibits the release of glutamate via the inactivation of voltage-dependent Na^+ channels on glutamatergic nerve terminals as well as to activate a G-protein-dependent signal transduction process.

In-vivo evidence for a possible role of GluR1-4 (AMPA receptor subunits) in ALS comes from several studies. Transgenic mice lacking GluR2 (GluR2 subunit is a component in the AMPA receptor complex, which renders them particularly impermeable to calcium) do not suffer from MN disease. This suggests that a low GluR2 level is a modifier of motoneuron degeneration rather than being sufficient to cause ALS [84]. Furthermore, glutamate excitotoxicity in sALS is caused by a selective loss of astrocytic glutamate transporter-1(GLT-1) and is reproduced in mice by knockout of GLT-1, a homologue of EAAT-2 [85]. Oral administration of glutamate inhibitors prolonged the life of $SOD1^{G93A}$ mice [86]. Further studies have pointed to the significance of GluR2 in neuronal survival where phenotypes of transgenic mice in which the extent of RNA edition at the Q/R site leads to generation of a lethal phenotype involving seizure and acute neurodegeneration [87]. Recent studies have provided clues that Glu2-N overexpression induces a progressive decline in the functions of spinal cord as well as long-onset degeneration of spinal motoneurons [88].

MISFOLDED PROTEIN STRESS

Abnormal protein aggregates are an inevitable byproduct of protein synthesis and degradation. Several illnesses, including most neurodegenerative disorders, are characterized by the presence of insoluble aggregates of proteins that are deposited in intracellular inclusions or extracellular plaques and are typical for the diseases. Unfolded proteins including Bunina bodies, ubiquitinated inclusions and neurofilament rich hyaline in ALS [89], amyloid and tau in Alzheimer's disease, α-synuclein in Parkinson's disease and huntingtin in Huntington's disease are pathological hallmarks. Potentially dangerous misfolded proteins also arise through oxidation, isomerization or glycation and by transcriptional or translational errors. Such proteins engage in non-native interactions and aggregate to form oligomeric complexes that are insoluble and metabolically stable and ultimately harmful to the cell [90, 91]. Cells have "quality control" machinery that consists of 1) molecular chaperones that assist in protein folding or refolding 2) the ubiquitin proteasome proteolytic pathway that recognizes and degrades misfolded proteins, to prevent damage from unfolded and aggregated protein, and 3) aggresome-autophagosome pathway that degrades aggregated proteins. The rate of misfolded protein production can increase markedly upon exposure of cells to oxidative or thermal stress, or as a result of mutations, and under these conditions the rate of misfolded protein production may exceed the capacity of the protein quality control machinery, disturbing cell function and inducing cell death [92].

A number of other studies point to a contribution of misfolded protein, consisting of irregular, loosely arranged bundles or spherical inclusions, to the pathogenesis of ALS. In

SOD1-linked ALS patients inclusions contain mtSOD1, but in sALS patients SOD1 usually is not present in ubiquitinated structures [93]. Ubiquitinated and non-ubiquitinated aggregates of SOD1 are a constant feature prior to the death and disappearance of MNs in Tg mtSOD1 mice. However, the presence of ubiquitinated structures in mtSOD1 mice as well as studies in chimeric mice has shown that MNs that do not express mtSOD1 may become strongly immunoreactive for ubiquitin [94]. There is ongoing debate whether this aggregate accumulation contributes to the death of MNs or whether it represents the cell's protective response in ALS pathology. Impairment of the function of intracellular organelles like mitochondria by SOD1-containing inclusions through accumulation within or on the organelles is also suggested [95].

CYTOSKELETAL DISORGANISATION AND NEUROFILAMENT DEFECTS

Neurofilaments are intermediate cytoskeletal fibrils composed of the neuron specific heavy (NFH), middle (NFM) and light (NFL) triplet proteins. The accumulation of Phosphorylated neurofilaments in chromatolytic neurons and swollen axons followed by impaired axonal transport is observed in patients suffering from sporadic or SOD1 mutant fALS, as well as in SOD1-knockout mice. Abnormalities in neurofilaments could be either casual or a by-product of neuronal degeneration [96, 97]. The direct involvement of neurofilaments in pathogenesis was suggested by the finding that overexpression of the WT NFL subunit in mice causes progressive motor neuropathy without MN loss, similar to those seen in patients with ALS [98]. On the other hand, knock-out of the endogenous WT NFL subunit in G85R mice delays the onset of MN disease [99]. Peripherin and internexin are two other intermediate-filament proteins that co-localise with neurofilaments and form part of the axonal inclusion bodies in patients with sALS and mice with SOD1 mutations. Overexpression of peripherin or internexin in Tg mice induces selective degeneration of motor axons [100]. Peripherin is encoded by a single gene and has splice variants of 56, 58 and 61 kDa. Peripherin (61 kDa) is toxic to primary motor neuron cultures, even at very low levels, and has been detected in the spinal cord of sALS patients [101].

In the past decade, studies on mtSOD1^{G93A} mice spinal MNs have shown that there is an increase of neurofilaments and mitochondria in the axon hillock and initial segment of these MN. This abnormality continues with aging in Tg mice compared to WT mice [102]. The reason for this distribution remains unclear but two theories for its effect on MNs have been proposed. First, the accumulated neurofilament protein might provide a buffer from other deleterious processes such as increases in intracellular calcium from excitotoxicity or aberrant protein modification caused by oxidative stress. Second, trapping neurofilament protein in the cell body might reduce the burden on axonal transport [99].

ABNORMALITIES IN INTRACELLULAR AXONAL TRANSPORT

The transport of molecules and organelles is a fundamental cellular process that is important for the development, function and survival of neurons. The molecular motors for anterograde and retrograde transport are kinesin and dynein-dynactin complex respectively. Several findings indicate that defects in axonal transport might contribute to the demise of MNs in ALS. One of the characteristics of ALS is a reduced activity of axonal transport, described initially in patients with ALS [9] and more recently in Tg mouse model of ALS [102]. The mtSOD1 mouse shows axonal transport defects as one of the earliest pathological features, and recent reports suggest this may even occur during development in embryonic neurons [103].

It is important to note that abnormalities in anterograde transport do not lead to MN death but cause diseases of the axon and usually affect both sensory and motor neurons. In contrast, several lines of evidence have linked impaired dynein-dynactin dependent (i.e. retrograde) trafficking to ALS. The dynein–dynactin complex is involved in fast retrograde transport. Mutations in the p150 subunit of dynactin have been reported in a family with an unusual Lumber MN disorder that begins with vocal cord paralysis [104]. Mutations in dynein and impaired retrograde axonal transport leads to MN disease in two lines of induced mouse mutants [105]. Furthermore, mice overexpressing the p50 subunit of dynactin have reduced axonal transport and develop progressive MN degeneration [106]. More interestingly, crossing mice overexpressing p50 with mtSOD1 mice results in amelioration of the disease and increased survival [104]. Finally, aberrant neurofilament aggregation, a common pathological hallmark in ALS MNs, has been linked to abnormal dynein trafficking [95]. The question still perplexing scientists is why impairment of dynein trafficking selectively afflicts MNs. A possible explanation is that MNs, more than other cell types, depend on retrograde trophic signaling [107, 108].

MECHANISM UNDERLYING MITOCHONDRIA-ER Ca^{2+} STORES COUPLING

Different intracellular pools participate in generating Ca^{2+} signals in neuronal cells and in shaping their spatio-temporal patterns as well as cell fate. Kinetic and "hot spot" hypothesis of mitochondria,different classes of channels with distinct properties and highly defined expression patterns on ER have been implicated in the regulation of $[Ca^{2+}]_i$ in many systems [109, 110].

In an attempt to understand more about the Ca^{2+} metabolism of hypogloosal motoneuorns MNs, Jaiswal et al. studied the role of ER in Ca^{2+} handling where it was shown that ER in MNs retained a comparatively lower quantity of calcium than mitochondria after $[Ca^{2+}]_i$ elevation, indicating its low efficiency to sequester Ca^{2+} in the MNs of SOD1^{G93A} mice compare to WT. These results indicate that the conventional Ca^{2+} storing function of mitochondria is dominating over ER Ca^{2+} accumulation in these MNs. These results are in good agreement with the "hotspot" hypothesis that proposes that mitochondria preferentially accumulate Ca^{2+} at microdomains of elevated Ca^{2+}concentration ($[Ca^{2+}]i$) that exist near ER

Ca^{2+} release sites and other Ca^{2+} channels. Accordingly, mitochondria may affect both Ca^{2+} release from the ER and capacitative Ca^{2+} entry across the plasma membrane, thereby shaping the size and duration of the intracellular Ca^{2+} signal in MNs of WT and SOD1^{G93A} mice and recruitment of these signals for selective MN degeneration. These events depend upon the Ca^{2+} sensitivity of the Ca^{2+} channels of the ER (allowing, for different Ca^{2+} concentrations and channel isoforms, positive or negative modulation of the Ca^{2+} release process) and the capacity of mitochondria to remove Ca^{2+} from the microdomain at the mouth of the channel. This effect has been confirmed *in-vitro*, but the situation appears distinctly different in various cell models [111, 112]. This indicates that various modulatory mechanisms exist, many of which still await molecular clarification at cellular and molecular level. As discussed above, overwhelming evidence supports the idea that the measured high rate of Ca^{2+} accumulation of MNs mitochondria *in situ* largely depends on the proximity of mitochondria to the channels through which Ca^{2+} enters the cytosol. A key, but still unanswered, question is whether this proximity is random and occurs only because some of these very abundant organelles, which are present throughout the cytosol, happen to be close to these channels, or whether there is a specific mechanism to ensure that mitochondria are located close to sites of Ca^{2+} influx and release (stochastic versus specific localization). The molecular mechanisms that define the organization of mitochondria in MNs of mice with regard to the ER and other Ca^{2+} sources, and the extent to which mitochondrial function varies among different cell types, are open questions of great importance.

ROLE OF CROSS-TALK BETWEEN MOTONEURONS AND GLIA IN ALS VULNERABILITY AND PATHOGENESIS

The role of glia contribution to the pathophysiology of ALS, particularly through dysfunction of their glutamate transporters, which results in reduced glutamate uptake, increased extracellular glutamate levels, and excitotoxic damage to MNs has been described earlier in great detail by Rothstein and colleagues. Reduced clearance of extracellular glutamate was disease- and region-specific, particularly in the brain stem and spinal cord [113, 36]. It is unclear whether dysfunction of the glial glutamate transporter is causative of ALS or whether this dysfunction follows from oxidative damage that is initiated in MNs. One suggestion is that activation of AMPA receptors might lead to the release of ROS from spinal cord and brain stem MNs, which results in oxidation and local decrease of glutamate uptake in neighboring astrocytes. Accordingly, a pathological type of MN-glia interaction that might contribute to the initiation of ALS is defined by a sequence of events- initiation of Ca^{2+} entry through glutamate receptors, followed by mitochondrial Ca^{2+} overload and subsequent production of ROS that impair glial glutamate uptake, which results in extracellular accumulation of glutamate and eventually exacerbation of Ca^{2+} entry into MNs [27, 114]. Recent work suggests an alternative ALS pathogenic model suggesting that not only the proportion of mutant gene expressing cells but also the topographical relationship between affected MNs and healthy glial cells can influence the progression of the disease [115, 116].

Moreover, microglial cells have been long suspected as central components in neurodegenerative diseases where their role may include secretion of trophic or toxic molecules. The role of glia in neuronal degeneration during development is well established

[117]. In ALS, microglial activation has been described in the brain and spinal cord of the patients [118, 119] and in the spinal cord of mtSOD1 mouse models [120, 121]. The microglial reactivity is initiated before MN loss. Several groups have tried to treat motor neuron disease by using minocycline, shown to inhibit microglial activation. Minocycline is potent in increasing survival of ALS mice and reduces microglial activation. Since minocycline also exerts an anti-apoptotic property on neurons, it is unclear which cells the minocycline affected [121, 6, 122]. In addition, mtSOD1, which has now been reported to be released by motor neurons, is a potent activator of microglial cells [116], emphasizing the likely crosstalk between motor neurons, microglial cells, and potentially other non-neuronal cells that may interact to drive disease progression.

This new prospective has revived the question regarding the role of glia and its interaction with MNs in ALS. Correct functioning of glia and their partnership with neighboring MNs seems to be essential for normal brain function and study of their interaction in physiology and pathophysiology of ALS is of great importance. However, this wealth of findings raises further questions most importantly, what is the basis for cell-type specificity in ALS? Further investigation of this question will probably provide a more fundamental understanding of ALS, because cell selectivity is a hallmark of this deadly yet obscure disease.

CHARACTERISTICALLY LOW CA^{2+} BUFFERING CAPACITY OF MOTONEURONS AND ITS IMPACT ON SELECTIVE MOTONEURON VULNERABILITY

The existence and localization of calcium microdomains and the rapid Ca^{2+} uptake and release phenomenon are well established facts [123, 124, 125, 126]. How and to what concentrations Ca^{2+} in the mitochondrial matrix of MNs rises is a matter of great debate because of the widely varying results obtained with different probes and calibration procedures used by different groups. However, there is evidence that favors the hypothesis that resistant MNs have a fairly high concentration of calcium binding proteins, which control calcium transients and plasma membrane extrusion in these neurons, where mitochondria have little role in terms of calcium buffering. On the other hand, in the vulnerable neurons (e.g. Hypoglossal MNs and Facial MNs), rapid Ca^{2+} uptake to control the [Ca^{2+}]i during neuronal activity is made by mitochondria, coexisting with the reduced amount of calcium buffering proteins [47]. This may offer a precise localization of the mitochondria into the hotspots of Ca^{2+} entry or a wide spread distribution of these organelles in the low buffer cytoplasm of susceptible MNs. Supporting evidence also comes from results where Ca^{2+} involvement as a risk factor was indicated by the observation that Ca^{2+}-binding proteins such as CB-D$_{28k}$ and parvalbumin were absent in MN populations (hypoglossal MN and spinal MN) that are lost early in ALS [3]. In contrast, results from dorsal vagal neurons containing plenty of Ca^{2+} sequestering proteins [127], the delay in the decay time constant (τ) of Ca^{2+} transients (FCCP influx) was not caused by mitochondrial permeability.

In order to check whether CB-D$_{28k}$ protects cells from dysfunction and degeneration via buffering of [Ca^{2+}]i, our group performed Ca^{2+} imaging studies following a depolarization stimulus (60mM K^+) in primary neuronal cells obtained from mice cortex at E_{18} expressing low and high CB-D_{28k} (Data not shown). Results show that indeed CB-D_{28k} buffer $[Ca^{2+}]i$ where low CB-D_{28k} transfected neuronal cells display a significant (~2 times) reduction in the peak amplitude of the sustained $[Ca^{2+}]i$ increase compare to high CB-D_{28k} transfected neuronal cells. τ in CB-D_{28k} transfected cells is also slower (~60s) compared to non-transfected cells where baseline recovery time is ~30-35s while showing little differences in the area under the time - concentration curve (AUC). This observation is in good agreement with the "low buffering hypothesis" which states that low buffer capacity allows for rapid Ca^{2+} dynamics during physiological activity, but represents a significant risk factor during ALS-related MN disease [128]. In conclusion, we believe that two of the most important features for MNs in ALS are: (i) low buffer capacity generates exceptionally large Ca^{2+} domains, but not in case of serious end stage ALS like symptoms and (ii) in ALS vulnerable MNs buffering capacity critically depends upon the domain size of mitochondria and ER. Therefore, we proposed a model where a portion of MN mitochondria interacts with areas of high $[Ca^{2+}]$ around influx sites due to low buffering induced excitotoxicity shown in Figure 1C.

MITOCHONDRIAL DYSFUNCTION, Ca^{2+} HOMEOSTASIS AND ALS: A MULTIFACTORIAL DISEASE MECHANISM

Selective vulnerability of MNs in ALS-related disease and associated mouse models is closely linked to specific Ca^{2+} signaling mechanisms that are part of the physiological cell function, but seemingly also enhance the risk of disruption of Ca^{2+} homeostasis and mitochondrial dysfunction in vulnerable cells. Earlier studies have suggested that uncontrolled Ca^{2+} entry and inefficacy to sequester this calcium leads to formation of vacuoles derived from the degenerating mitochondria in the MNs of the mouse model of ALS [12, 10]. In contrast to most other neurons, MNs have a low Ca^{2+}-buffering capacity due to the low expression of Ca^{2+}-buffering proteins and a high number of Ca^{2+}-permeable AMPA receptors resulting from a low expression of the GluR2 subunit. The combination of these two properties seems to be specific to MNs and is most likely essential for their normal function. However, under pathological conditions, MNs could become over stimulated by glutamate and overwhelmed by Ca^{2+}, although whether downstream pathways activated by the intracellular Ca^{2+} increase are different in MNs compared to other neurons is not yet known.

Apparently, in the last few years, attention was drawn to the role of mitochondria as an efficient regulator of cytosolic calcium signals [129, 130]. Studies with mitochondria-targeted calcium probes indicate a rapid, dramatic increase in free intramitochondrial calcium upon stimulation. This uptake by mitochondria has an immense effect on the metabolic state of the cell as it can up-regulate the activity of the enzymes in oxidative metabolism [131, 132, 133]. Malformation in mitochondrial structure and massive vacuoles derived from degenerating mitochondria found in post mortem human ALS samples [9, 12] further strengthen this proposition. Although the exact molecular mechanism is still not known, we hypothesize that vulnerability to ALS is a consequence of specific physiological features, particularly highly specialized Ca^{2+} homeostasis, continuous activity-dependent Ca^{2+} cycling and the predominant role of mitochondria in buffering Ca^{2+} transients.

Vulnerable MNs are characterized by low cytosolic Ca^{2+} buffering, with mitochondria playing a major role for regulation of $[Ca^{2+}]_i$ transients by taking up more than 50% of Ca^{2+} even during small cytosolic Ca^{2+} increases. Low cytosolic Ca^{2+} buffering enhances the role of low-affinity organelle buffers such as mitochondria in the cell. For example, large and long-lasting Ca^{2+} domains around influx sites increase the risk of toxic Ca^{2+} accumulations and a subsequent activation of Ca^{2+} dependent neurodegenerative pathways under excitotoxic conditions. Indeed, a strong contribution of mitochondria and not ER Ca^{2+} uptake to buffer Ca^{2+} profiles has been demonstrated recently [68, 63, 134]. The prominent role of mitochondria in regulating moderate Ca^{2+} loads in MNs has important implications for pathological conditions such as in ALS. First, the amount of Ca^{2+} taken up by the mitochondria is probably higher in MNs than in many other cell types [18, 135]. These high Ca^{2+} loads enhance the risk for generation of ROS, which are suggested to play a major role in initiating a positive feedback loop resulting in MN degeneration [27]. Second, our experiments provide evidence that cytosolic Ca^{2+} critically depends on intact Ca^{2+} uptake into mitochondria. Thus, when mitochondrial Ca^{2+} uptake is disturbed as seen by low Ca^{2+} uptake in SOD1^{G93A} MNs compare to WT, MNs are directly put at risk to elevated Ca^{2+} levels during repetitive oscillations. Additionally, the decreased ability to limit Ca^{2+} transient amplitudes in the cytosol, in particular in local domains when mitochondria are depolarised, enhances the risk of initiating Ca^{2+} dependent neurodegenerative pathways leading to cell death.

Combining the lessons learned from multiple animal models as well as cell culture model used to determine pathogenic mechanisms in ALS, the central insight is that selective vulnerability of MNs likely arises from a combination of several mechanisms; two of them, mitochondrial dysfunction and Ca^{2+} homeostasis [136], are prominent. Considering the involvement and importance of mitochondrial dysfunction and Ca^{2+} homeostasis we hypothesize that MN possess large number of voltage and ligand gated Ca^{2+} channels that, when activated, cause rapid Ca^{2+} influx, which, in part because of relatively weak cytosolic Ca^{2+} buffering, results in mitochondrial Ca^{2+} overload and strong ROS generation. Furthermore, MN selective loss goes a long way explaining the oxidative damage, mitochondrial abnormalities and apoptotic contributions observed in ALS MNs. Chronic mitochondrial membrane depolarisation due to Ca^{2+} entry can cause the release of pro-apoptotic proteins and activate enzymes involved in apoptotic pathways [137, 138]. A summary of the mechanisms identified is given in Figure 3 where in vulnerable MNs, the calcium buffering machinery is signified by the predominance of mitochondria, while calcium binding proteins are more abundant in the non-vulnerable MNs.

DRUG TARGETS AND MULTIDRUG THERAPIES IN ALS: WHERE SHOULD WE AIM?

A decade of experimentation using mice and rodents made Tg for human mtSOD1 has yielded valuable information about the mechanisms that underlie ALS, and suggestions for therapy. However, the main reason for the failure to translate experimentation in animals to therapies for patients might be that ALS is not only a multifactorial disease but also a multisystemic disease, result of a complex neurotoxic cascade that involves molecular cross-talk between MNs, glia and astrocytes [95]. Preclinical tests suffer from the fact that data are usually collected in animals of the same age and with the same mutation expressed in a homogeneous genetic background. By contrast, the age of onset, the progression and the severity of ALS in patients are heterogeneous, indicating that many (only partially known) potential genetic risk factors and modifying factors exist for sALS and some drugs are effective only if given before onset [139].

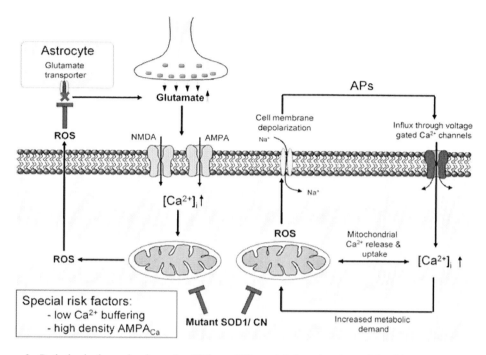

Figure 3. Pathological mechanisms in ALS, a differential functional model of interaction between mitochondria and high Ca^{2+}. Mitochondrial disturbance is predicted to be the key trigger to ALS etiology. The production of reactive oxygen species (ROS) by disturbed mitochondrial metabolism can be readily cytotoxic as ROS can destroy the membrane integrity by averting the specificity of membrane channels or triggering the opening of particular leak channels as well as by destroying the lipid components of the membrane. Furthermore, events following mitochondrial misfunction in MNs inhibits complex IV of the electron transport chain which leads to ROS generation. In addition, inhibition of the respiratory chain furthermore decreases the $\Delta\Psi m$ leading to reduced Ca^{2+} uptake into the mitochondrial matrix and potentially release of Ca^{2+}. The impact for the cell becomes more severe when mitochondria are placed cardinally to buffer the calcium and to control the subsequent metabolic pathways, since an uncontrolled elevation in the cytosolic Ca^{2+} can lead to immediate cell death. Mitochondrial inhibition additionally decreases cellular ATP levels, and this further enhances accumulation of intracellular Ca^{2+}. It is also hypothesised that ROS produced in motoneurons can escape to the extracellular environment and can damage the glutamate transporters on astrocytes. The observed changes provide a potential mechanism of how mitochondrial inhibition can lead to selective motoneuron degeneration (modified after Von Lewinski and Keller, 2005; Jaiswal et al., 2009; Jaiswal and Keller, 2009).

In view of recent findings of a non-cell-autonomous demise of MNs [28, 29, 30, 31], design of multi drug combination therapies should be targeted at the intersection of multiple aspects of this cascade, rather than a single-drug treatment. Until now animal studies have shown that multi-drug combination therapies and the method of delivery of a treatment is also often have synergistic effects in ALS, for example, riluzole administered with melatonin and vitamine E (inhibits Na+-current activation and the apoptotic cascade), minocycline administered with creatine (inhibits microglia activation and the apoptotic cascade), or treatment with IGF-1 or VEGF retrogradely transported in MNs through viral vectors [86, 140, 141, 79]. As an alternative to pharmacological treatments, the recent developments in stem-cell research might provide possibilities for neural implantation therapy in patients with ALS [142, 143]. The lessons learned from a decade of research using the mtSOD1 animal model might help researchers in finding cures for neurodegeneration where single-drug approaches have proven insufficient for effective treatment.

CONCLUSIONS

It is hypothesized that disrupted Ca^{2+} homeostasis and oxidative stress induced ROS have a vital role in propagating injury by increasing the excitability of MNs and by targeting neighboring glia. Perhaps as a consequence, excitotoxicty builds up with increased activity-dependent Ca^{2+} influx and associated mitochondrial Ca^{2+} cycling. Given the mitochondrial disturbances, Ca^{2+} buffering becomes inefficient and cytosolic Ca^{2+} levels rise. Protective options are to increase the resistance of MNs to high intracellular Ca^{2+} concentrations by inducing defense mechanism and/or to inhibit the downstream pathways activated by increased intracellular Ca^{2+} concentrations. However, severely impaired MNs are not amendable from taking functional advantage for neuronal protection in ALS. These include a more defined separation of spatial Ca^{2+} gradient signal cascades. Moreover, recent research data indicates that therapeutic options do not have to focus on MNs alone, as ALS seems to be a more intricate disease involving MNs, glia, astrocytes as well as muscle and in some cases inflammation and apoptosis. As a consequence, inhibiting microglial activation which prevents the release of toxic substances by these cells or stimulating astrocytes to increase glutamate uptake and/or secrete growth factors that modify the properties of the AMPA receptors present on the MNs could also be a viable option. In conclusion, it seems that ALS is a multifactorial disease where under physiological conditions diffusion-restricted and tightly controlled domains might indeed have several functional advantages. Accordingly, therapeutic measures aimed at protecting mitochondrial function could be useful in various forms of ALS.

Finally, a combined pharmacological interference with many facets of excitotoxicity both at the MNs and at the surrounding glial cells will be most likely essential to extend survival of ALS patients. It is conceivable that a combination of therapies addressing several intercellular targets in ALS could be successful at treating this once-obscure disease. At present however it is clear that more structural and functional studies are needed to identify other potential cytosolic pathways and barriers that could lead to MN degeneration in ALS. Forthcoming studies will hopefully add to the understanding of why these processes preferentially damage MNs and the role non-cell autonomous cell death (glia and astrocytes) might play.

ACKNOWLEDGMENTS

I would like to thank Drs. Bernhard U. Keller, Zygmunt Galdzicki and Fritz Lischka for their valuable discussions.

REFERENCES

[1]   Rowland LP and Shneider NA (2001). Amyotrophic Lateral Sclerosis. *N. Engl. J. Med.* 344: 1688-1700.

[2]   Rosen DR, Siddique T, Patterson D, Figlewicz DA, Sapp P, Hentati A, Donaldson D, Goto J, O'Regan JP, Deng HX, *et al*. (1993). Mutations in Cu/Zn superoxide dismutase gene are associated with familial amyotrophic lateral sclerosis. *Nature,* 362(6415): 59-62.

[3]   Alexianu ME, Ho, BK, Mohamed AH, La Bella V, Smith RG and Appel SH (1994). The role of calcium-binding proteins in selective motoneuron vulnerability in amyotrophic lateral sclerosis. *Ann. Neurol.* 36: 846-58.

[4]   Jaiswal MK and Keller BU (2009). Cu/Zn superoxide dismutase typical for familial amyotrophic lateral sclerosis increases the vulnerability of mitochondria and perturbs Ca^{2+} homeostasis in SOD1G93A mice. *Mol. Pharmacol.* 75: 478-489.

[5]   Lips MB and Keller BU (1998). Endogenous calcium buffering in motoneurones of the nucleus hypoglossus from mouse. *J. Physiol.* 511: 105–117.

[6]   Van Den Bosch L, Schwaller B, Vleminckx V, Meijers B, Stork S, Ruehlicke T, Van Houtte E, Klaassen H, Celio MR and Missiaen L (2002). Protective effect of parvalbumin on excitotoxic motor neuron death. *Exp. Neurol.* 174: 150-161.

[7]   Mattson MP, LaFerla FM, Chan SL, Leissring MA, Shepel PN and Geiger JD (2000). Calcium signaling in the ER: its role in neuronal plasticity and neurodegenerative disorders. *Trends Neurosci.* 23: 222-229.

[8]   Radi R, Rubbo H, Bush K and Freeman BA (1997). Xanthine Oxidase Binding to Glycosaminoglycans: Kinetics and Superoxide Dismutase Interactions of Immobilized Xanthine Oxidase-Heparin Complexes. *Arch. Biochem. Biophys* 339: 125-135.

[9]   Sasaki S and Iwata M (1996). Ultrastructural study of synapses in the anterior horn neurons of patients with amyotrophic lateral sclerosis. *Neurosci. Lett.* 204(1-2): 53-6.

[10]   Sasaki S, Warita H, Murakami T, Abe K and Iwata M (2004). Ultrastructural study of mitochondria in the spinal cord of transgenic mice with a G93A mutant SOD1 gene. *Acta Neuropathol.* 107: 461-74.

[11]   Wong PC, Pardo CA, Borchelt DR, Lee MK, Copeland NG, Jenkins NA, Sisodia SS, Cleveland DW and Price DL (1995). An adverse property of a familial ALS-linked SOD1 mutation causes motor neuron disease characterized by vacuolar degeneration of mitochondria. *Neuron* 14: 1105-16.

[12]   Kong J and Xu Z (1998). Massive mitochondrial degeneration in motor neurons triggers the onset of amyotrophic lateral sclerosis in mice expressing a mutant SOD1. *J. Neurosci.* 18: 3241-50.

[13]   Mattiazzi M, D'Aurelio M, Gajewski CD, Martushova K, Kiaei M, Beal MF and Manfredi G (2002). Mutated human SOD1 causes dysfunction of oxidative phosphorylation in mitochondria of transgenic mice. *J. Biol. Chem.* 277: 29626-33.

[14]   Wiedemann FR, Manfredi G, Mawrin C, Beal MF and Schon EA (2002). Mitochondrial DNA and respiratory chain function in spinal cords of ALS patients. *J. Neurochem.* 80: 616-625.

[15]   Fujita K, Yamauchi M, Shibayama K, Ando M, Honda M and Nagata Y (1996). Decreased cytochrome c oxidase activity but unchanged superoxide dismutase and

glutathione peroxidase activities in the spinal cords of patients with amyotrophic lateral sclerosis. *J. Neurosci. Res.* 45: 276-81.

[16] Borthwick GM, Johnson MA, Ince PG, Shaw PJ and Turnbull DM (1999). Mitochondrial enzyme activity in amyotrophic lateral sclerosis: implications for the role of mitochondria in neuronal cell death. *Ann. Neurol.* 46: 787-90.

[17] Carri MT, Ferri A, Battistoni A, Famhy L, Gabbianelli R, Poccia F and Rotilio G (1997). Expression of a Cu, Zn superoxide dismutase typical of familial amyotrophic lateral sclerosis induces mitochondrial alteration and increase of cytosolic Ca^{2+} concentration in transfected neuroblastoma SH-SY5Y cells. *FEBS Lett.* 414: 365-8.

[18] Carriedo SG, Sensi SL, Yin HZ and Weiss JH (2000). AMPA exposures induce mitochondrial Ca^{2+} overload and ROS generation in spinal motor neurons in vitro. *J. Neurosci* 20: 240-50.

[19] Beal MF (2002). Oxidatively modified proteins in aging and disease. *In Free Radic. Biol. Med.* pp. 797-803.

[20] Menzies FM, Cookson MR, Taylor RW, Turnbull DM, Chrzanowska-Lightowlers ZM, Dong L, Figlewicz DA and Shaw PJ (2002). Mitochondrial dysfunction in a cell culture model of familial amyotrophic lateral sclerosis. *Brain* 125: 1522–1533.

[21] Beers DR, Ho, BK, Siklos L, Alexianu ME, Mosier DR, Habib Mohamed A, Otsuka Y, Kozovska ME, Smith RE, McAlhany RG and Appel SH (2001). Parvalbumin overexpression alters immune-mediated increases in intracellular calcium, and delays disease onset in a transgenic model of familial amyotrophic lateral sclerosis. *J. Neurochem.* 79: 499-509.

[22] Heath PR and Shaw PJ (2002). Update on the glutamatergic neurotransmitter system and the role of excitotoxicity in amyotrophic lateral sclerosis. *Muscle Nerve* 26(4):438-58.

[23] Rao SD and Weiss JH (2004). Excitotoxic and oxidative cross-talk between motor neurons and glia in ALS pathogenesis. *Trends Neurosci.* 27: 17-23.

[24] Maragakis NJ and Rothstein JD (2001). Glutamate transporters in neurologic disease. *Arch. Neurol.* 58(3): 365-70.

[25] Trotti D, Rolfs A, Danbolt NC, Brown RH and Hediger MA (1999). SOD1 mutants linked to amyotrophic lateral sclerosis selectively inactivate a glial glutamate transporter. *Nat. Neurosci.* 2: 427-433.

[26] Tateno M, Sadakata H, Tanaka M, Itohara S, Shin RM, Miura M, Masuda M, Aosaki T, Urushitani M, Misawa H and Takahashi R (2004). Calcium-permeable AMPA receptors promote misfolding of mutant SOD1 protein and development of amyotrophic lateral sclerosis in a transgenic mouse model. *Hum. Mol. Genet* 13: 2183-2196.

[27] Rao SD, Yin HZ and Weiss JH (2003). Disruption of glial glutamate transport by reactive oxygen species produced in motor neurons. *J. Neurosci.* 23: 2627-2633.

[28] Di Giorgio FP, Carrasco MA, Siao MC, Maniatis T and Eggan K (2007). Non-cell autonomous effect of glia on motor neurons in an embryonic stem cell-based ALS model. *Nat. Neurosci.* 10(5): 608-614.

[29] Holden C (2007). NEUROSCIENCE: Astrocytes secrete substance that kills motor neurons in ALS. *Science* 316: 353a.

[30] Julien JP (2007). ALS: astrocytes move in as deadly neighbors. *Nat. Neurosci.* 10(5):535-537.

[31] Nagai M, Re DB, Nagata T, Chalazonitis A, Jessell TM, Wichterle H and Przedborski S (2007). Astrocytes expressing ALS-linked mutated SOD1 release factors selectively toxic to motor neurons. *Nat. Neurosci.* 10: 615-622.

[32] Neher E (1995). The use of fura-2 for estimating Ca^{2+} buffers and Ca^{2+} fluxes. *Neuropharmacology* 34: 1423-1442.

[33] Palecek J, Lips MB and Keller BU (1999). Calcium dynamics and buffering in motoneurones of the mouse spinal cord. *J. Physiol.* 520: 485–502.

[34] Von Lewinski F and Keller BU (2005). Ca^{2+}, mitochondria and selective motoneuron vulnerability: implications for ALS. *Trends Neurosci. 28*: 494-500.

[35] Ladewig T and Keller BU (2000). Simultaneous patch-clamp recording and calcium imaging in a rhythmically active neuronal network in the brainstem slice preparation from mouse. *Pflugers Arch.* 440: 322–332.

[36] Rothstein JD, Van Kammen M, Levey AI, Martin LJ and Kuncl RW (1995). Selective loss of glial glutamate transporter GLT-1 in amyotrophic lateral sclerosis. Ann. Neurol. 38(1): 73-84.

[37] Carriedo SG, Yin HZ, Sensi SL and Weiss JH (1998). Rapid Ca^{2+} entry through Ca^{2+} - permeable AMPA/Kainate channels triggers marked intracellular Ca2+ rises and consequent oxygen radical production. *J. Neurosci.* 18:7727-38.

[38] Shaw PJ and Ince PG (1997). Glutamate, excitotoxicity and amyotrophic lateral sclerosis. J. Neurol. 244 (Suppl 2): S3-14.

[39] Cleveland DW (1999). From charcot to SOD1: Mechanisms of selective motor neuron death in ALS. *Neuron* 24:515–520.

[40] Nägerl UV and Mody I (1998). Calcium-dependent inactivation of high-threshold calcium currents in human dentate gyrus granule cells. *J. Physiol.* 509:39–45.

[41] Simpson EP, Yen AA and Appel SH (2003). Oxidative Stress: a common denominator in the pathogenesis of amyotrophic lateral sclerosis. *Curr. Opin. Rheumatol.* 15(6): 730-736.

[42] Goodall EF and Morrison KE (2006).Amyotrophic lateral sclerosis (motor neuron disease): proposed mechanisms and pathways to treatment. *Expert Rev. Mol. Med* .Vol. 8, Issue 11, 24 May, DOI: 10.1017/S1462399406010854.

[43] Von Lewinski F and Keller BU (2005). Ca^{2+}, mitochondria and selective motoneuron vulnerability: implications for ALS. *Trends Neurosci. 28*: 494-500.

[44] Elliott JL and Snider WD (1995). Parvalbumin is a marker of ALS-resistant motor neurons. *Neuroreport* 6(3): 449-52.

[45] Zhou Z and Neher E (1993). Mobile and immobile calcium buffers in bovine adrenal chromaffin cells. *J. Physiol.* 469: 245-273.

[46] Klingauf J and Neher E (1997). Modeling buffered Ca^{2+} diffusion near the membrane: implications for secretion in neuroendocrine cells. *Biophys J.* 72: 674-690.

[47] Lips MB and Keller BU (1999). Activity-related calcium dynamics in motoneurons of the nucleus hypoglossus from mouse. *J. Neurophysiol.* 82: 2936–2946.

[48] Beers DR, Ho, BK, Siklos L, Alexianu ME, Mosier DR, Habib Mohamed A, Otsuka Y, Kozovska ME, Smith RE, McAlhany RG and Appel SH (2001). Parvalbumin overexpression alters immune-mediated increases in intracellular calcium, and delays disease onset in a transgenic model of familial amyotrophic lateral sclerosis. *J. Neurochem.* 79: 499-509.

[49] Roy J, Minotti S, Dong L, Figlewicz DA and Durham HD (1998). Glutamate potentiates the toxicity of mutant Cu/Zn-superoxide dismutase in motor neurons by postsynaptic calcium-dependent mechanisms. *J. Neurosci.* 18: 9673-9684.

[50] Maragakis NJ and Rothstein JD (2001). Glutamate transporters in neurologic disease. *Arch. neurol.* 58(3): 365-70.

[51] Appel SH, Smith RG, Alexianu M, Siklos L, Engelhardt J, Colom LV and Stefani E (1995). Increased intracellular calcium triggered by immune mechanisms in amyotrophic lateral sclerosis. *Clin. Neurosci.* (6): 368-74.

[52] Tateno M, Sadakata H, Tanaka M, Itohara S, Shin RM, Miura M, Masuda M, Aosaki T, Urushitani M, Misawa H and Takahashi R (2004). Calcium-permeable AMPA receptors promote misfolding of mutant SOD1 protein and development of amyotrophic lateral sclerosis in a transgenic mouse model. *Hum. Mol. Genet* 13: 2183-2196.

[53] Stout AK, Raphael HM, Kanterewicz BI, Klann E and Reynolds IJ (1998). Glutamate-induced neuron death requires mitochondrial calcium uptake. Nat. Neurosci. 1(5): 366-73.

[54] Beal MF (2002). Oxidatively modified proteins in aging and disease. *In Free Radic. Biol. Med.* pp. 797-803.

[55] Strong MJ (2003). The basic aspects of therapeutics in amyotrophic lateral sclerosis. *Pharmacol. Ther 98*: 379-414.

[56] Beal MF (2000). Mitochondria and the pathogenesis of ALS. *Brain* 123: 1291-1292.

[57] Bowling AC, Schulz JB, Brown RH Jr and Beal MF (1993). Superoxide dismutase activity, oxidative damage, and mitochondrial energy metabolism in familial and sporadic amyotrophic lateral sclerosis. *J. Neurochem.* 61(6): 2322-5.

[58] Browne SE, Bowling AC, Baik MJ, Gurney M, Brown RH and Beal MF (1998). Metabolic dysfunction in familial, but not sporadic, amyotrophic lateral sclerosis. *J. Neurochem.* 71: 281-287.

[59] Jaarsma D, Rognoni F, Duijn WV, Verspaget HW, Haasdijk ED and Holstege JC (2001). Cu- Zn superoxide dismutase (SOD1) accumulates in vacuolated mitochondria in transgenic mice expressing amyotrophic lateral sclerosis-linked SOD1 mutations. *Acta Neuropath.* 102: 293-305.

[60] Hirano A, Nakano I, Kurland LT, Mulder DW, Holley PW and Saccomanno G (1984). Fine structural study of neurofibrillary changes in a family with amyotrophic lateral sclerosis. *J. Neuropathol. Exp. Neurol.* 43: 471–80.

[61] Hirano A (1991). Cytopathology of amyotrophic lateral sclerosis. *Adv. Neurol.* 56: 91-101.

[62] Siklos L, Engelhardt J, Harati Y, Smith RG, Joo F and Appel SH (1996). Ultrastructural evidence for altered calcium in motor nerve terminals in amyotrophic lateral sclerosis. *Ann. Neurol.* 39: 203-16.

[63] Jaiswal MK, Zech W, Goos M, Leutbecher C, Ferri A, Zippelius A, Carrì MT, Nau R and Keller BU (2009). Impairment of mitochondrial calcium handling in a mtSOD1 cell culture model of motoneuron disease. *BMC Neurosci* 2009, 10:64.

[64] Wiedemann FR, Winkler K, Kuznetsov AV, Bartels C, Vielhaber S, Feistner H and Kunz WS (1998). Impairment of mitochondrial function in skeletal muscle of patients with amyotrophic lateral sclerosis. *J. Neurol. Sci.* 156(1): 65-72.

[65] Vielhaber S, Kunz D, Winkler K, Wiedemann FR, Kirches E, Feistner H, Heinze HJ, Elger CE, Schubert W and Kunz WS (2000). Mitochondrial DNA abnormalities in

skeletal muscle of patients with sporadic amyotrophic lateral sclerosis. *Brain* 123 (Pt 7): 1339-48.

[66]   Swerdlow RH, Parks JK, Cassarino DS, Trimmer PA, Miller SW, Maguire DJ, Sheehan JP, Maguire RS, Pattee G and Juel VC (1998). Mitochondria in sporadic amyotrophic lateral sclerosis. *Exp Neurol* 153: 135-142.

[67]   Kruman II, Pedersen WA, Springer JE, and Mattson MP (1999). ALS-linked Cu/Zn-SOD mutation increases vulnerability of motor neurons to excitotoxicity by a mechanism involving increased oxidative stress and perturbed calcium homeostasis. *Exp. Neurol.* 160: 28-39.

[68]   Bergmann F and Keller BU (2004). Impact of mitochondrial inhibition on excitability and cytosolic Ca^{2+} levels in brainstem motoneurons from mouse. *J. Physiol.* 555: 45–59.

[69]   Kirkinezos IG, Bacman SR, Hernandez D, Oca-Cossio J, Arias LJ, Perez-Pinzon MA, Bradley WG and Moraes CT (2005). Cytochrome c association with the inner mitochondrial membrane is impaired in the CNS of G93A-SOD1 mice. *J. Neurosci.* 5(25): 164-72.

[70]   Dal Canto MC and Gurney ME (1995). Neuropathological changes in two lines of mice carrying a transgene for mutant human Cu,Zn SOD, and in mice overexpressing wild type human SOD: a model of familial amyotrophic lateral sclerosis (fALS). *Brain Res.* 676: 25-40.

[71]   Bendotti C, Calvaresi N, Chiveri L, Prelle A, Moggio M, Braga M, Silani V and De Biasi S (2001). Early vacuolization and mitochondrial damage in motor neurons of FALS mice are not associated with apoptosis or with changes in cytochrome oxidase histochemical reactivity. *J. Neurol. Sci.* 191: 25-33.

[72]   Higgins CMJ, Jung C and Xu Z (2003). ALS-associated mutant SOD1[G93A] causes mitochondrial vacuolation by expansion of the intermembrane space and by involvement of SOD1 aggregation and peroxisomes. *BMC Neurosci* 4:16.

[73]   Xu Z, Jung C, Higgins C, Levine J and Kong J (2004). Mitochondrial degeneration in amyotrophic lateral sclerosis. *J. Bioenerg Biomembr.* 36: 395-399.

[74]   Liu J, Lillo C, Jonsson PA, Velde CV, Ward CM, Miller TM, Subramaniam JR, Rothstein JD, Marklund S, Andersen PM, Brannstrom T, Gredal O, Wong PC, Williams DS and Cleveland DW (2004). Toxicity of familial ALS-linked SOD1 mutants from selective recruitment to spinal mitochondria. *Neuron* 43: 5–17.

[75]   Kaal EC, Vlug AS, Versleijen MW, Kuilman M, Joosten EA and Bar PR (2000). Chronic mitochondrial inhibition induces selective motoneuron death in vitro: a new model for amyotrophic lateral sclerosis. *J. Neurochem.* 74: 1158-65.

[76]   Oosthuyse B, Moons L, Storkebaum E, Beck H, Nuyens D, Brusselmans K, Van Dorpe J, Hellings P, Gorselink M and Heymans S (2001). Deletion of the hypoxia-response element in the vascular endothelial growth factor promoter causes motor neuron degeneration. *Nat Genet* 28: 131-138.

[77]   Lambrechts D, Storkebaum E, Morimoto M, Del-Favero J, Desmet F, Marklund SL, Wyns S, Thijs V, Andersson J and Van Marion I (2003). VEGF is a modifier of amyotrophic lateral sclerosis in mice and humans and protects motoneurons against ischemic death. *Nat. Genet.* 34: 383-394.

[78]   Zheng C, Nennesmo I, Fadeel B and Henter JI (2004). Vascular endothelial growth factor prolongs survival in a transgenic mouse model of ALS. *Ann. Neurol.* 56: 564-567.

[79]   Azzouz M, Ralph GS, Storkebaum E, Walmsley LE, Mitrophanous KA, Kingsman SM, Carmellet P and Mazarakis ND (2004). VEGF delivery with retrogradely transported lentivector prolongs survival in a mouse ALS model. *Nature* 429: 413-417.

[80]   Wang Y, Ou Mao X, Xie L, Banwait S, Marti HH, Greenberg DA and Jin K (2007). Vascular Endothelial Growth Factor Overexpression Delays Neurodegeneration and Prolongs Survival in Amyotrophic Lateral Sclerosis Mice. *J. Neurosci.* 27: 304-307.

[81]   Choi D, Koh J and Peters S (1988). Pharmacology of glutamate neurotoxicity in cortical cell culture: attenuation by NMDA antagonists. *J. Neurosci.* 8: 185-196.

[82]   Shaw PJ, Forest V, Ince PG, Richardson JP and Wastell HJ (1995). CSF and plasma amino acid levels in motor neuron disease: elevation of CSF glutamate in a subset of patients. *Neurodegeneration* 4(2): 209-216.

[83]   Carriedo SG, Yin H Z and Weiss JH (1996). Motor Neurons Are Selectively Vulnerable to AMPA/Kainate Receptor-Mediated Injury In Vitro. *J. Neurosci.* 16: 4069-4079.

[84]   Jia Z, Agopyan N, Miu P, Xiong Z, Henderson J, Gerlai R, Taverna FA, Velumian A, MacDonald J and Carlen P (1996). Enhanced LTP in mice deficient in the AMPA receptor GluR2. *Neuron* 17: 945-956.

[85]   Rothstein JD, Dykes-Hoberg M, Pardo CA, Bristol LA, Jin L, Kuncl RW, Kanai Y, Hediger MA, Wang Y, Schielke JP and Welty DF (1996). Knockout of glutamate transporters reveals a major role for astroglial transport in excitotoxicity and clearance of glutamate. *Neuron* 16: 675-686.

[86]   Gurney ME, Cutting FB, Zhai P, Doble A, Taylor CP, Andrus PK and Hall ED (1996). Benefit of vitamin E, riluzole, and gabapentin in a transgenic model of familial amyotrophic lateral sclerosis. Ann. Neurol. 39(2): 147-57.

[87]   Higuchi M, Maas S, Single FN, Hartner J, Rozov A, Burnashev N, Feldmeyer D, Sprengel R and Seeburg PH (2000). Point mutation in an AMPA receptor gene rescues lethality in mice deficient in the RNA-editing enzyme ADAR2. *Nature* 406: 78-81.

[88]   Kuner R, Groom AJ, Bresink I, Kornau HC, Stefovska V, Muller G, Hartmann B, Tschauner K, Waibel S and Ludolph AC (2005). Late-onset motoneuron disease caused by a functionally modified AMPA receptor subunit. *Proc. Natl. Acad. Sci. USA* 102: 5826-5831.

[89]   Strong MJ, Sashi K and Pant HC (2005). The Pathobiology of Amyotrophic Lateral Sclerosis: A Proteinopathy. *J. Neuropath Exp. Neurol.* 64(8): 649-664.

[90]   Wetzel R (1994). Mutations and off-pathway aggregation of proteins. *Trends Biotech.* 12: 193-198.

[91]   Soto C (2003). Unfolding the role of protein misfolding in neurodegenerative diseases. *Nat Rev Neurosci* 4: 49-60.

[92]   Sherman MY and Goldberg AL (2001). Cellular defenses against unfolded proteins: a cell biologist thinks about neurodegenerative diseases. *Neuron* 29: 15-32.

[93]   Valentine JS and Hart PJ (2003). Bioinorganic chemistry special feature: misfolded Cu,Zn, SOD and amyotrophic lateral sclerosis. *Proc. Natl. Acad. Sci. USA* 100: 3617-3622.

[94] Hoffman EK, Wilcox HM, Scott RW and Siman R (1996). Proteasome inhibition enhances the stability of mouse Cu/Zn superoxide dismutase with mutations linked to familial amyotrophic lateral sclerosis. J. Neurol. Sci. 139(1): 15-20.

[95] Bruijn LI, Miller TM and Cleveland DW (2004). Unraveling the mechanisms involved in motor neuron degeneration in ALS. *Ann. Rev. Neurosci.* 27: 723-749.

[96] Ince PG, Tomkins J, Slade JY, Thatcher NM and Shaw PJ (1998). Amyotrophic lateral sclerosis associated with genetic abnormalities in the gene encoding Cu/Zn superoxide dismutase: molecular pathology of five new cases, and comparison with previous reports and 73 sporadic cases of ALS. *J. Neuropathol. Exp. Neurol.* 57(10): 895-904.

[97] Julien JP and Beaulieu JM (2000). Cytoskeletal abnormalities in amyotrophic lateral sclerosis: beneficial or detrimental effects? *J. Neurol. Sci.* 180: 7-14.

[98] Xu Z, Cork LC, Griffin JW and Cleveland DW (1993). Increased expression of neurofilament subunit NF-L produces morphological alterations that resemble the pathology of human motor neuron disease. *Cell* 73: 23-33.

[99] Williamson TL, Bruijn LI, Zhu Q, Anderson KL, Anderson SD, Julien JP and Cleveland DW (1998). Absence of neurofilaments reduces the selective vulnerability of motor neurons and slows disease caused by a familial amyotrophic lateral sclerosis-linked superoxide dismutase 1 mutant. *Proc. Natl. Acad. Sci. USA* 95: 9631-9636.

[100] Ching GY, Chien CL, Flores R and Liem RKH (1999). Overexpression of alpha-internexin causes abnormal neurofilamentous accumulations and motor coordination deficits in transgenic mice. *J. Neurosci.* 19: 2974-2986.

[101] Robertson J, Doroudchi MM, Nguyen MD, Durham HD, Strong MJ, Shaw G, Julien JP and Mushynski WE (2003). A neurotoxic peripherin splice variant in a mouse model of ALS. *J. Cell Biol.* 160: 939-949.

[102] Sasaki S, Warita H, Abe K and Iwata M (2005). Impairment of axonal transport in the axon hillock and the initial segment of anterior horn neurons in transgenic mice with a G93A mutant SOD1 gene. *Acta Neuropathol.* (Berl) 110: 48-56.

[103] Kieran D, Hafezparast M, Bohnert S, Dick JRT, Martin J, Schiavo G, Fisher EMC and Greensmith L (2005). A mutation in dynein rescues axonal transport defects and extends the life span of ALS mice. *J. Cell Biol.* 169: 561-567.

[104] Puls I, Jonnakuty C, LaMonte BH, Holzbaur ELF, Tokito M, Mann E, Floeter MK, Bidus K, Drayna D, Oh SJ, Brown RH, Ludlow CL and Fischbeck KH (2003). Mutant dynactin in motor neuron disease. *Nat. Genet* 33: 455-456.

[105] Hafezparast M, Klocke R, Ruhrberg C, Marquardt A, Ahmad-Annuar A, Bowen S, Lalli G, Witherden AS, Hummerich H, Nicholson S, *et al.* (2003). Mutations in dynein link motor neuron degeneration to defects in retrograde transport. *Science* 300: 808-812.

[106] LaMonte BH, Wallace KE, Holloway BA, Shelly SS, Ascano J, Tokito M, Van Winkle T, Howland DS and Holzbaur ELF (2002). Disruption of dynein/dynactin inhibits axonal transport in motor neurons causing late-onset progressive degeneration. *Neuron* 34: 715-727.

[107] Holzbaur ELF (2004). Motor neurons rely on motor proteins. *Trends Cell Biol.* 14: 233-240.

[108] Caviston JP and Holzbaur ELF (2006). Microtubule motors at the intersection of trafficking and transport. *Trends Cell Biol.* 16: 530-537.

[109] Herrington J, Park YB, Babcock DF and Hille B (1996). Dominant role of mitochondria in clearance of large Ca^{2+} loads from rat adrenal chromaffin cells. *Neuron* 16: 219-228.

[110] Schinder AF, Olson EC, Spitzer NC and Montal M (1996). Mitochondrial dysfunction is a primary event in glutamate neurotoxicity. *J. Neurosci.* 16: 6125-33.

[111] Arnaudeau S, Kelley WL, Walsh JV Jr. and Demaurex N (2001). Mitochondria recycle Ca^{2+} to the endoplasmic reticulum and prevent the depletion of neighboring endoplasmic reticulum regions. *J. Biol. Chem.* 276: 29430-29439.

[112] Szabadkai G, Simoni AM and Rizzuto R (2003). Mitochondrial Ca^{2+} uptake requires sustained Ca^{2+} release from the endoplasmic reticulum. *J. Biol. Chem.* 278: 15153-15161.

[113] Rothstein JD, Martin LJ and Kuncl RW (1992). Decreased glutamate transport by the brain and spinal cord in amyotrophic lateral sclerosis. *N. Engl. J. Med.* 326(22): 1464-8.

[114] Seifert G, Schilling K and Steinhauser C (2006). Astrocyte dysfunction in neurological disorders: a molecular perspective. *Nat. Rev. Neurosci.* 7(3):194-206.

[115] Clement AM, Nguyen MD, Roberts EA, Garcia ML, Boillee S, Rule M, McMahon AP, Doucette W, Siwek D, Ferrante RJ, Brown RH Jr, Julien JP, Goldstein LS and Cleveland DW(2003). Wild-type nonneuronal cells extend survival of SOD1 mutant motor neurons in ALS mice. *Science* 302(5642):113-7.

[116] Urushitani M, Sik A, Sakurai T, Nukina N, Takahashi R and Julien JP (2006). Chromogranin-mediated secretion of mutant superoxide dismutase proteins linked to amyotrophic lateral sclerosis. *Nat. Neurosci.* 9: 108-118.

[117] Marin-Teva JL, Dusart I, Colin C, Gervais A, van Rooijen N and Mallat M (2004). Microglia Promote the Death of Developing Purkinje Cells. *Neuron* 41: 535-547.

[118] Henkel JS, Engelhardt JI, Siklós L, Simpson EP, Kim SH, Pan T, Goodman JC, Siddique T, Beers DR and Appel SH (2004). Presence of dendritic cells, MCP-1, and activated microglia/macrophages in amyotrophic lateral sclerosis spinal cord tissue. *Annals Neurol.* 55: 221-235.

[119] Turner MR, Cagnin A, Turkheimer FE, Miller CCJ, Shaw CE, Brooks DJ, Leigh PN and Banati RB (2004). Evidence of widespread cerebral microglial activation in amyotrophic lateral sclerosis: an [11C](R)-PK11195 positron emission tomography study. *Neurobiol. Dis.* 15: 601-609.

[120] Hall ED, Jo AO and Gurney ME (1998). Relationship of microglial and astrocytic activation to disease onset and progression in a transgenic model of familial ALS. *Glia* 23: 249-256.

[121] Kriz J, Nguyen MD and Julien JP (2002). Minocycline slows disease progression in a mouse model of amyotrophic lateral sclerosis. *Neurobiol. Dis.* 10: 268-278.

[122] Zhu S, Stavrovskaya IG, Drozda M, Kim BYS, Ona V, Li M, Sarang S, Liu AS, Hartley DM, Wu DC, *et al.* (2002). Minocycline inhibits cytochrome c release and delays progression of amyotrophic lateral sclerosis in mice. *Nature* 417: 74-78.

[123] Baron KT, Wang GJ, Padua RA, Campbell C and Thayer SA (2003). NMDA-evoked consumption and recovery of mitochondrially targeted aequorin suggests increased Ca^{2+} uptake by a subset of mitochondria in hippocampal neurons. *Brain Res.* 993: 124-32.

[124] Malli R, Frieden M, Osibow K, Zoratti C, Mayer M, Demaurex N and Graier WF (2003). Sustained Ca^{2+} transfer across mitochondria is essential for mitochondrial Ca^{2+} buffering, store-operated Ca^{2+} entry, and Ca^{2+} store refilling. *J. Biol. Chem.* 45: 44769-79.

[125] Rizzuto R, Bernardi P and Pozzan T (2000). Mitochondria as all-round players of the calcium game. *J. Physiol.* 529: 37-47.

[126] Rizzuto R, Duchen MR and Pozzan T (2004). Flirting in little space: the ER/mitochondria Ca^{2+} liaison. *Sci STKE* 13; 2004(215):re1.

[127] De Leon M, Covenas R, Narvaez JA, Aguirre JA and Gonzalez-Baron S (1993). Distribution of parvalbumin immunoreactivity in the cat brain stem. *Brain Res. Bull* 32: 639-46.

[128] Vanselow BK and Keller BU (2000). Calcium dynamics and buffering in oculomotor neurones from mouse those are particularly resistant during amyotrophic lateral sclerosis (ALS)-related motoneuron disease. *J. Physiol.* 525: 433-445.

[129] Rizzuto R, Brini M and Pozzan T (1993). Intracellular targeting of the photoprotein aequorin: a new approach for measuring, in living cells, Ca^{2+} concentrations in defined cellular compartments. *Cytotechnology* 11: 44-6.

[130] Gunter TE, Yule DI, Gunter KK, Eliseev RA and Salter JD (2004). Calcium and mitochondria. *FEBS Lett* 567: 6-102.

[131] Rizzuto R, Bastianutto C, Brini M, Murgia M and Pozzan T (1994). Mitochondrial Ca^{2+} homeostasis in intact cells. *J. Cell Biol.* 126: 1183-94.

[132] Rizzuto R (2003). Calcium mobilization from mitochondria in synaptic transmitter release. *J. Cell Biol.* 163: 441-443.

[133] Rutter GA, Burnett P, Rizzuto R, Brini M, Murgia M, Pozzan T, Tavare JM and Denton RM (1996). Subcellular imaging of intramitochondrial Ca^{2+} with recombinant targeted aequorin: Significance for the regulation of pyruvate dehydrogenase activity. *Proc. Natl. Acad. Sci. USA* 93: 5489-5494.

[134] Ladewig T, Kloppenburg P, Lalley PM, Zipfel WR, Webb WW and Keller BU (2003). Spatial profiles of store-dependent calcium release in motoneurones of the nucleus hypoglossus from newborn mouse. *J. Physiol.* 547: 775–787.

[135] Sen I, Nalini A, Joshi NB and Joshi PG (2005). Cerebrospinal fluid from amyotrophic lateral sclerosis patients preferentially elevates intracellular calcium and toxicity in motor neurons via AMPA/kainate receptor. J. Neurol. Sci. 235: 45-54.

[136] Duchen MR (2000). Mitochondria and Ca^{2+} in cell physiology and pathophysiology. *Cell Calcium* 28: 339-348.

[137] Pivovarova NB, Nguyen HV, Winters CA, Brantner CA, Smith CL and Andrews SB (2004). Excitotoxic calcium overload in a subpopulation of mitochondria triggers delayed death in hippocampal neurons. *J. Neurosci.* 24: 5611-22.

[138] Rosenstock TR, Carvalho AC, Jurkiewicz A, Frussa-Filho R and Smaili SS (2004). Mitochondrial calcium, oxidative stress and apoptosis in a neurodegenerative disease model induced by 3-nitropropionic acid. J. Neurochem. 88(5): 1220-8.

[139] Shaw PJ (2005). Molecular and cellular pathways of neurodegeneration in motor neurone disease. *J. Neurol. Neurosurg. Psychiatry* 76: 1046-1057.

[140] Kaspar BK, Llado J, Sherkat N, Rothstein JD and Gage FH (2003). Retrograde viral delivery of IGF-1 prolongs survival in a mouse ALS model. *Science* 301: 839-842.

[141] Zhang W, Narayanan M and Friedlander RM (2003). Additive neuroprotective effects of minocycline with creatine in a mouse model of ALS. *Ann. Neurol.* 53: 267-270.

[142] Garbuzova-Davis S, Willing A E, Zigova T, Saporta S, Justen EB, Lane JC, Hudson JE, Chen N, Davis CD and Sanberg PR (2003). Intravenous administration of human umbilical cord blood cells in a mouse model of amyotrophic lateral sclerosis:

distribution, migration, and differentiation. *J. Hematotherapy Stem Cell Res.* 12: 255-270.

[143] Lepore AC and Maragakis NJ (2007). Targeted stem cell transplantation strategies in ALS. *Neurochem. Internat* 50: 966-975.

In: Motor Neuron Diseases
Editors: Bradley J. Turner and Julie B. Atkin

ISBN 978-1-61470-101-9
© 2012 Nova Science Publishers, Inc.

Chapter IV

TREATMENT OF ALS UTILIZING A STEM CELL STRATEGY

Xiufang Guo[1] and James J. Hickman[1,2]

[1]Hybrid Systems Laboratory, NanoScience Technology Center,
University of Central Florida, Orlando, FL, U. S.
[2]College of Medicine, University of Central Florida, Orlando, FL, U. S.

ABSTRACT

Amyotrophic lateral sclerosis is a devastating neurodegenerative disorder that results in motoneuron loss, paralysis and ultimately death due to respiratory failure within 3-5 years after disease onset. Currently, there is no effective treatment that exists despite the substantial numbers of approaches that are under investigation.

The development of the stem cell field brings promise due to the fact that these cells are self-replenishable and either pluripotent or multipotent and give rise to various cell types. This review will focus on the *in vivo* applications of these stem cells for ALS treatment. The progress, as well as the advantages and limitations of utilizing each variety of stem cell or their derivatives for ALS treatment, is reviewed in this book chapter. Transplantation of these cells may benefit the diseased tissue by cell replacement therapy or by non-cell replacement functions such as delivery of trophic support. The generation of MNs from stem cells *in vitro* could enable a significant contribution to cell replacement therapy. However, the need to protect grafted cells highlights the importance of developing an effective trophic therapy.

The recent development of induced pluripotent stem cells and the mobilization of endogenous stem cells shed light on the possibility of autologous treatment. However, several challenges need to be overcome to achieve an effective treatment including timing of transplantation, immune system attack, systematic delivery of the cells and their integration, and especially the hostile environment that would exist in a individual with ALS disease.

GENERAL INTRODUCTION OF ALS

Amyotrophic Lateral Sclerosis (ALS, also known as Lou Gehrig's Disease) is a relentlessly progressive, adult-onset fatal neurodegenerative disease characterized by motoneuron (MN) loss in the cerebral cortex, brain stem and spinal cord, which leads to muscle wasting and eventually death within 5 years of clinical onset [1]. ALS symptoms usually begin between 50 to 60 years of age as a weakness in the extremities and progress to complete paralysis [1-3]. ALS affects 2-3 per 100,000 individuals, which ranks it as the most frequent adult-onset motoneuron disease, and the most serious neurodegenerative disease after Alzheimer's and Parkinson's disease. ALS is both a sporadic and familial disease and the origin of most incidences of ALS is unknown. Familial ALS (fALS) accounts for approximately 5-10% of all individuals with the disease, and about 20% of fALS is the result of mutations in the SOD1 gene (the cytosolic Cu, Zn superoxide dismutase gene). Currently there is no cure for ALS. The only licensed therapy available for ALS treatment is the anti-glutamatergic agent Riluzole, and it has limited therapeutic effects.

Collective evidence concerning ALS etiology indicates that the disease process is clearly non-cell autonomous [4], and there is evidence that pathological events occurring outside the MNs, especially in muscle and glia cells, can cause MN death and neuromuscular junction (NMJ) destruction [5, 6]. Muscle cells, as the direct targets of MNs, retrogradely provide a pleiotropic group of growth factors to modulate MN development and function [7]. Although it is still controversial whether muscle pathology in ALS is the initiator [5, 8-10] or victim [11, 12] of MN loss, muscle clearly can be considered a therapeutic target [13]. Glia cells are the other possible targets in understanding ALS etiology, and under normal conditions, there are essential interactions between glia and neurons [14]. Astrocytes affect MN survival by releasing growth/trophic factors and removing glutamate from the synaptic cleft. They also determine certain functional characteristics of MNs, such as the composition of α-amino-3-hydroxy-5-methyl-4-isoxazolepropionic acid (AMPA) receptors on MNs, and hence their vulnerability to excitotoxicity. Reciprocally, MNs affect the functional characteristics of astrocytes including glutamate uptake capability and the spectrum of factors they secrete [15]. Activation of astrocytes in ALS leads to a disturbance of this crosstalk, which may contribute to MN death [16, 17]. Microglia activation, an indicator of neuroinflammation, can initially slow ALS disease progression, but later may contribute to the acceleration of the disease, probably due to the production and release of reactive oxygen species (ROS) and augment the inflammatory cytokine cascade [18].

Currently, the more accepted hypothesis regarding ALS etiology [19], based on ALS animal studies, is that the pathology in MNs initiates the disease [20], either in MN death or MN distress that leads to NMJ deterioration. The selective degeneration of the MNs is believed to be at least partly due to their vulnerability, i.e. high metabolic activity, low levels of reduced glutathione and high levels of unsaturated lipids on the large membrane surfaces along their axons, which increase their susceptibility to oxidative damage. The pathologically activated astrocytes and microglia accelerate ALS progression by releasing neurotoxins, inflammatory factors, reactive oxygen species and nitrogen species (ROS/RNS), as well as increasing the level of glutamate, all of which produce an environment toxic to MNs [12, 20, 21]. This hostile environment can accelerate the process of MN degeneration, leading to neurodegeneration and eventually death.

STEM CELLS AND THEIR APPLICATION IN ALS TREATMENT

Stem cells are defined as cells that have the ability to renew themselves and possess pluripotent or multipotent ability to differentiate into various cell types [22]. Pluripotent stem cells (PSCs), such as embryonic stem cells (ESCs), can give rise to all tissue types and cells of the three germ layers (endoderm, mesoderm and ectoderm) [23, 24]. Multipotent stem cells are from a more advanced developmental stage, with a more restricted differentiation potential. They can be isolated from various tissues such as bone marrow, umbilical cord blood, adipose, muscle and the nervous system. The self-renew and multi-potent properties of stem cells have generated a tremendous amount of enthusiasm for the treatment of many diseases and injuries. Clinical trials are already under way for stem cell treatment of MS with ESCs and the treatment of ALS with fetal stem cells (Neuralstem). *In vitro*, human stem cells and/or their derivatives become important tools in developing functional models for drug screening and etiological studies [25-27] to avoid trans-species problems, which will not be covered in this review. *In vivo* applications in regenerative medicine are being considered by implanting *in vitro*-expanded cells so that they can replace lost cells, or provide trophic support to either delay the degeneration or enhance the regeneration process (Figure 1).

The use of stem cells overcomes the need for synchronization between donation and transplant, the problem of limited donor-cell numbers, and reveals the possibility of using autologous non-neuronal sources. The application of multiple types of stem cells to the treatment of ALS has been explored extensively and numerous studies have contributed to the fast progress of this field. This review will cite only some of these studies as a representative group.

Pluripotent stem cells: PSCs can be isolated from either the inner cell mass of a blastocyst (ESCs) or from the primordial germ cells of the gonadal ridge from post-implantation embryos (embryonic germ cells, EGCs) [23]. A considerable advantage of ESCs over adult stem cells are that ESC-derived neural progenitor cells (NPCs) have a higher plasticity and efficiency to be differentiated into regional specific neurons, while the directed differentiation from adult SCs-derived NPCs has not been shown to be effective [28]. However, a major concern for the clinical application of PSCs is its high risk of forming cancerous structures after transplantation [29]. For this reason, a number of studies [30-33] have focused on the development of the methods for pre-differentiation of human hESCs into neural or neuronal precursors. Currently, most *in vivo* studies involving PSCs in the animal models of diseases and injuries have used the derivatives from ESCs [34-36] or EGCs [37] rather than the undifferentiated cells alone. Other concerns include ethical issues associated with the use of embryonic tissue, and the unavoidable immunological rejection problems due to the lack of autologous ESCs or EGCs from an adult patient.

Mesenchymal stem cells (MSCs): MSCs can be isolated from many types of tissues including bone marrow and umbilical cord blood. They have been investigated for ALS treatment due to their feasible availability that lacks any ethical issues and the possibility for autologous transplantation, which may avoid problems due to immune rejection. MSCs can differentiate into various types of mesenchymal cells, such as cardiomyocytes [38-40]. Certain studies have suggested that they could also trans-differentiate into neural cells [41, 42], while others suggested this was not possible [43, 44].

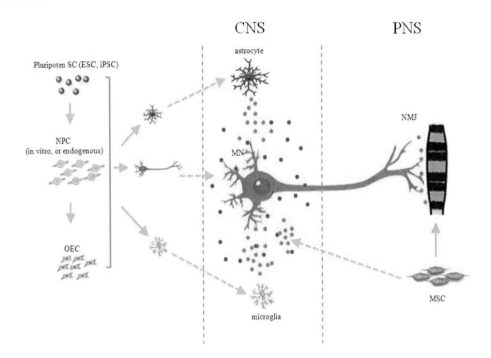

Figure 1. Depiction of the general strategies of stem cell therapy for ALS. In the CNS of ALS patients, MNs are damaged by the toxic environment generated by a plethora of factors including the activated astrocyte and microglia. ESC, iPSC, NPC (in vitro or endogenous) and OEC all have the potential to give rise to cells in the CNS. The derived MNs can replace the damaged MNs after transplantation (replacement therapy), while the derived astrocytes or microglia can alleviate the toxicity of host environment by releasing trophic factors or removing stress factors such as glutamate (trophic support therapy). MSCs can give rise to cells in the peripheral including muscle to preserve the endangered NMJ, or can provide trophic support to the CNS by releasing trophic factors or regulating cell activity in the CNS.

The transplantation of human umbilical blood cells (via retro-ocular injection) have been shown to extend the life of SOD1 mice by ~20 days [45]. A 4-year clinical trial with autologous bone marrow MSCs in 9 ALS patients (via intraspinal injection) indicated the safety of this stem cell treatment as well as their efficacy in decreasing the linear decline of the forced vital capacity and of the ALS-FRS (functional rating scale) score [46]. A subsequent Phase I clinical trial with similar procedures and cells in 10 ALS patients confirmed the safety of MSC transplantation into the spinal cord of ALS patients. However, the lack of post mortem material prevents any definitive conclusion concerning the vitality of the transplanted MSCs [47]. Despite these encouraging results, there are some limitations, such as the difficulty of targeting the central nervous system (CNS) [48, 49] and concern about how well these stem cells can differentiate into neural cells. One study utilizing GFP/YFP-labeled bone marrow cells intraperitonially transplanted in mice revealed very few donor-derived cells in the CNS, except microglia and a few labeled cells from cell fusion [50]. However, transplanted cells were found to participate in the regeneration of skeletal and cardiac muscles, and the disease onset was delayed and the life span was increased in the animals receiving transplantation [50]. This suggests the beneficial effects could be from a non-neuronal environment (i.e. NMJ preservation) rather than the neuronal replenishment. Conversely, positive effects have been observed by employing MSCs as a vehicle for the delivery of trophic factors [49], especially into muscle for preserving NMJ connections [51, 52]. In general, currently, the mechanism for the therapeutic effects of MSCs is not considered to be through cell replacement, but rather through neuronal protection by either providing trophic support [53-55] or modulating the inflammation process [56, 57].

Olfactory ensheathing cells (OECs): OECs are glial cells that reside in the olfactory bulb and olfactory nasal mucosa. They ensheath olfactory axons and assist axonal extension of the olfactory sensory neurons from the peripheral nervous system (PNS) to the CNS [58]. Advantages of OECs are that they are easily accessible, present the possibility for autologous treatment, have a neural lineage (unlike MSCs), and are capable of enhancing axonal regeneration [59]. It has been shown that OECs can promote regeneration and remyelination of injured spinal pathways and enhance motor recovery in experimental animal models with spinal cord injury [60-64]. Indeed, OECs from patients with spinal cord lesions were grafted autologously in a clinical trial in Australia [65]. However, the intrathecal implantation of OECs into the spinal cord did not show any beneficial effect in ALS mice [66]. In comparison, another study used MNs that were differentiated from NPCs from the mouse olfactory bulb demonstrated improved motor function and enlongated the life span of ALS mice [67]. Although, histological analysis later indicated that the functional improvement was not attributed to MN replacement but to the trophic support from the OEC-derived cells, this suggests that pre-treatment of OECs with NPCs or even MNs may improve the therapeutic effect.

Neural Progenitor Cells (NPCs) or Neural Stem Cells (NSCs): NPCs are multipotent cells with the potential to differentiate into neurons, oligodendrocytes, and astrocytes and can be efficiently propagate *in vitro* [68, 69]. NPCs can be isolated from late-term embryos or adult tissues. In the adult CNS, the tissue adjacent to ventricles and the ependymal cells directly lining the lateral ventricles are known to be rich sources of multipotent NPCs [70]. In the spinal cord, these cells are located in the ependymal zone surrounding the central canal [71]. *In vitro*, the NSCs can maintain their capacity for self-renewal after several passages and are capable of secreting neurotrophic factors [72, 73]. NSCs account for the enhanced neurogenesis that occurs at earlier stages of ALS based on a study with SOD1 transgenic mice [74]. An endoscopic neurosurgical approach has been developed for isolating NPCs from the ventricular wall of the human brain [75]. Focal transplantation of human NSCs into the lumber spinal cord of rats resulted in successful survival, differentiation and integration of these cells with the host neural circuits [76]. However, very few MNs were differentiated from the grafted cells, suggesting the host environment does not facilitate MN differentiation. Despite this, grafted cells in the spinal cord of SOD1 rats caused a delayed onset and progression of the disease, probably through the secretion of Glial cell-derived neurotrophic factor (GDNF) and Brain-derived neurotrophic factor (BDNF), factors that are known to protect MNs [77, 78]. A part of the scientific community believes that NSCs are more preferable than hESCs for clinical applications because they are considered safer for cell therapy, as NSCs have less potential to form teratomas compared to ESCs [73]. One disadvantage of *in vitro*-derived NSCs for clinical therapies is their decreased potential of differentiation after several passages [79].

MNs or glia cells differentiated from stem cells: Cell replacement therapy proposes to replenish the lost MNs with stem cells or their derivatives, hoping that the transplanted cells can survive, integrate with the host neuronal circuitry, send out axons to the periphery and form NMJs a with target muscle group and this strategy has attracted major interest. Previous transplantation studies with PSCs or NPCs all indicated that MN differentiation did not occur in the adult spinal cord [76, 80, 81]. Thus, *in vitro* MN differentiation before implantation could be an option to achieve successful implantation. Critical progress in recent years has demonstrated the successful differentiation of MNs from ESCs [33, 82, 83]. Our group has successfully differentiated MNs from human fetal spinal cord stem cells (NSI-566RSC) [84] (Figure 2). Transplantation of this cell line has been proven effective in the treatment of spinal cord injury and ALS in rat models [77, 85], and is currently the first human stem cell line approved by the FDA for clinical trials in ALS patients.

Multiple studies have evaluated the integration of grafted cells with the host system as well. ESC–derived MNs transplanted into embryonic chick spinal cord extended axons into the periphery and formed NMJs [82]. Human neural stem cell-derived MNs can innervate muscle in MN-deficient rats [86]. A series of studies by Kerr and his colleagues indicated that mouse ESC-derived MNs could survive direct parenchymal transplantation into the ventral gray matter of adult rats and could extend axons into the ventral roots of animals treated with a cAMP analog or Rho kinase inhibitor to overcome myelin-mediated inhibition [87].

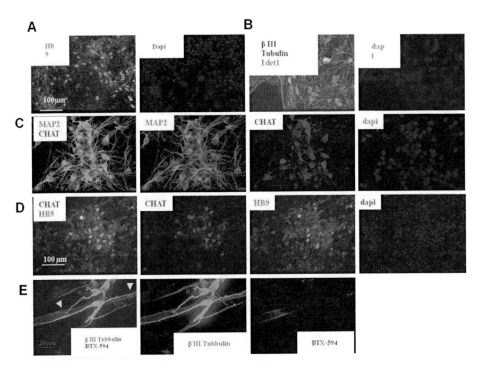

Figure 2. MN differentiation from human fetal NPCs. MNs were successfully differentiated from the human fetal NPC (NSI-566RSC) in vitro in a defined system as demonstrated by the immunostaining of MN marker HB9 (A), Islet1 co-stained with neuronal marker β III Tubulin (B), CHAT (Choline Acetyl Transferase) co-stained with neuronal marker MAP2 (C) and the co-staining of HB9 and CHAT (D). The corresponding Dapi staining was provided to show the total number of cells in each image. E. Differentiated MNs can form NMJs with rat embryonic skeletal myotubes in vitro in a defined system as displayed by the co-staining of Bungarotoxin-Alexa 488 (bind to Acetyl choline receptor on the myotube) and the` antibody against β III Tubulin which stains axonal terminal. (Guo X. et al., Tissue Engineering and Regenerative Medicine 2010; 4:181-193, and Guo X. et al., Tissue Engineering Part C 2010; 16(6):1347-1355).

It was further demonstrated that the axons of these grafted MNs could exit the spinal cord, extend along the sciatic nerve toward the hind limb musculature and form functional NMJs [88]. This was achieved by blocking the myelin-mediated axon repulsion and providing an attractive cue, GDNF, in peripheral nerves (Figure 3).

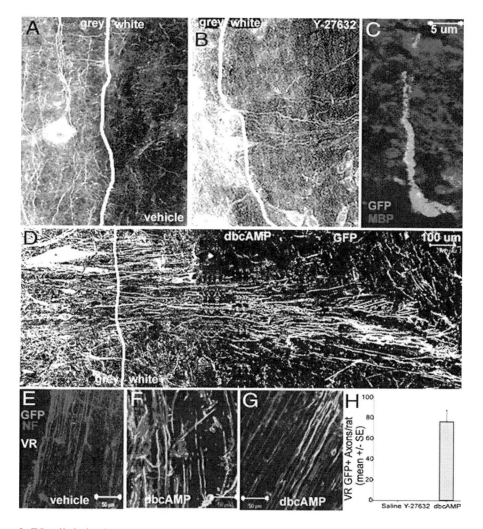

Figure 3. ES cell-derived MNs extend axons into white matter and ventral roots in the presence of dbcAMP or Y27632 (a Rho kinase inhibitor). MN-committed ES cells were transplanted into the spinal cord of NSV (Neuroadapted Sindbis virus)-paralyzed rats. (A) In vehicle-infused rats, GFP+ axons extend rostrally and caudally but only rarely extend into the surrounding white matter (sagittal section). (B) In Y27632-infused rats, GFP+ axons traverse surrounding white matter. (C) Dual-color confocal microscopy confirms that GFP+ axons extend into surrounding white matter, defined by immunoreactivity to myelin basic protein (red). (D) In dbcAMP-infused rats, axonal processes extend 1.3 mm to the surface of the spinal cord. (E–H) Ventral roots from the lumbar spinal cord were examined for the presence of GFP+ axons at 1 month after transplantation. No GFP+ axons are detected in vehicle-infused rats (E), whereas GFP+ axons are detected within ventral roots of dbcAMP-infused rats (F and G). (H) Quantification of GFP+ axons within ventral roots of transplanted animals. No GFP+ axons within ventral roots were observed in paralyzed rats infused with either saline or with Y-27632, but a mean of 76 ± 10.69 GFP+ axons were observed per transplanted rat infused with dbcAMP. (Harper JM et al. PNAS 2004; 101:7123-7128). In compliance with the PNAS copyright notice.

However, the poor survival of the transplanted MNs in the spinal cord of the ALS models emerged to be a critical hurdle [19]. One study using MNs differentiated from NPCs from the mouse olfactory bulb demonstrated that the grafted MNs could integrate into the neural circuits and even send out axons to the peripheral nervous system after transplantation into the lumber spinal cord of pre-symptomatic mice, but demonstrated distal axonopathy and failed to form any NMJs [67]. Another study with MNs derived from mouse ESCs demonstrated a transient recovery in a rat model of fALS after cell transplantation. Immunohistochemistry analysis revealed no survival of the transplanted cells in the spinal cords of the end-stage animals, suggesting the transgenic hSOD1 (G93A) environment was detrimental to grafted MNs for long term applications [34]. Therefore, the toxic host environment would need to be modified for a successful MN transplantation.

Considering the non-cell autologous feature of ALS, transplantation of healthy glia cells could be beneficial [89, 90]. Glial-restricted precursors (GRPs) from fetal rat spinal cord promoted MN survival in a slice culture model of chronic glutamate excitotoxicity [91]. Focal transplantation of lineage-restricted astrocyte precursors into the respiratory MN pools at the cervical spinal cord was able to protect the MNs, probably by increasing glutamate uptake, and correspondingly delayed the disease progression and extended the animal life span [92]. Transplantation of wild-type microglia slowed MN loss and extended survival in mice with fALS [93].

Induced Pluripotent stem cells (iPSC): The recent development of iPSC technology provides the possibility to reprogram somatic cells into PSCs and offers additional avenues for autologous transplantation [94-96]. Characterization to date indicates that iPSCs are similar to ESCs in karyotype integrity, transcriptome patterns, epigenome modification and development potential [97]. They have the potential to differentiate into all cell types, including neurons, glia, NPCs, and MNs [98, 99]. The successful generation of iPSCs from the fibroblasts of an ALS patient has been reported and these patient-derived iPSCs were shown to have the capacity to be differentiated into MNs [98] (Figure 4). These advances have the potential to generate patient-specific PSCs from adult somatic cells, which could then be differentiated into a desired cell type for transplantation. Particularly, a national ALS patient-derived iPSCs bank for MNs and astroglia is in development and expected to be available in the near future [100]. In general, this technology could potentially overcome two important hurdles associated with human stem cells: immune rejection after transplantation due to the autologous nature of the cell source and ethical concerns regarding the use of human embryos.

However, clinical applications of iPSCs still face certain obstacles. One that is similar to ESCs is teratoma formation, as even a small number of undifferentiated cells may result in their formation after transplantation. The other two obstacles are unique to iPSCs: 1) The method of nuclear reprogramming was originally carried out by virus-mediated gene transduction [101], but there are serious safety concerns with this methodology such as gene activation induced by multiple viral gene integration, or possible transgene reactivation. New approaches are being developed for reprogramming to overcome these difficulties including utilizing of non-integrating viruses [102], plasmids [103], chemicals or small molecules [104], and proteins [105]. 2) Regardless of the methodology of re-programming, current technology still cannot efficiently identify and exclude aberrant reprogramming, which can induce the cells refractory to differentiation and cause tumors after transplantation [106].

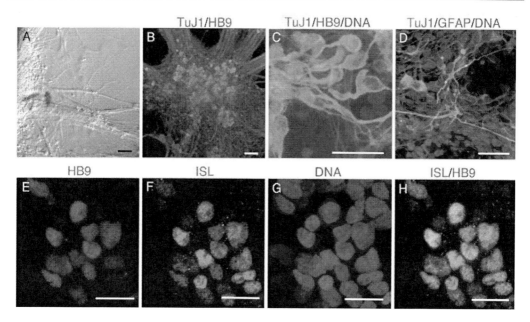

Figure 4. iPS cells generated from ALS patients can be differentiated into motoneurons. A29b iPS cell EBs were patterned with RA and SHH, then plated on laminin, either whole (A and B) or after dissociation (C to H), and allowed to mature for 7 to 15 days. (A) Neuron-like outgrowths are visible from whole A29b patient-specific iPS cell EBs. (B) Extensive TuJ1-positive neuronal processes grow out from plated whole iPS EBs, which contain a high proportion of HB9-stained nuclei. (C) Neuronal identity of HB9-expressing cells is confirmed by high-magnification image of HB9 and TuJ1 coexpression in dissociated patient-specific motoneuron cultures. (D) GFAP-expressing glial cells can be found in addition to TuJ1-expressing neurons in differentiated patient-specific iPS cell cultures. [(E) to (H)] The motoneuron identity of HB9- and TuJ1-positive cells is confirmed by the coexpression of HB9 and ISL. HB9 (E) and ISL (F) localization is nuclear (G) and highly coincident (H). Scale bars, 100 μm [(A) to (D)], 75 μm [(E) to (H)]. (Dimos JT et al. Science 2008;321:1218-1221).

Therefore, it may be necessary to differentiate the iPSCs into the required cell type and eliminate undifferentiated cells before transplantation. In addition, if utilizing cells derived from autologous iPSCs, any genetic defects associated with ALS etiology should be corrected before transplantation.

Endogenous stem cells: In comparison to strategies of delivering extrinsic stem cells for therapeutic applications, there are also efforts aiming to mobilize endogenous stem cells. This strategy is attractive due to its non-invasive nature and lack of an immunological reaction. In humans, the existence of NSCs with multipotent differentiation capability has been reported in the embryonic and adult human brain [107-110]. However, the endogenous environment of the CNS does not appear to be favorable under certain circumstances to efficiently recruit these innate stem cells. This is evidenced by the failure of the natural repair mechanisms in multiple neurodegenerative diseases as well as with injuries. To date, almost all the findings on the mobilization of endogenous NPCs for ALS treatment are from animal models. The endogenous NPCs (most likely from the subventricular zone) in adult rats can generate mature pyramidal neurons in cortical layer V following targeted apoptotic degeneration of the host corticospinal MNs. A subset of these neurons can extend axons to the spinal cord and survive beyond a year [111]. An increase in NPC (from the ependymal zone surrounding the central canal) proliferation, migration, and neurogenesis in lumber spinal cord in SOD1 mice has also been reported during disease onset and progression. These cells initially migrate toward the dorsal horn and later move to the ventral horn region, suggesting an attempt to induce repair mechanisms [112] (Figure 5).

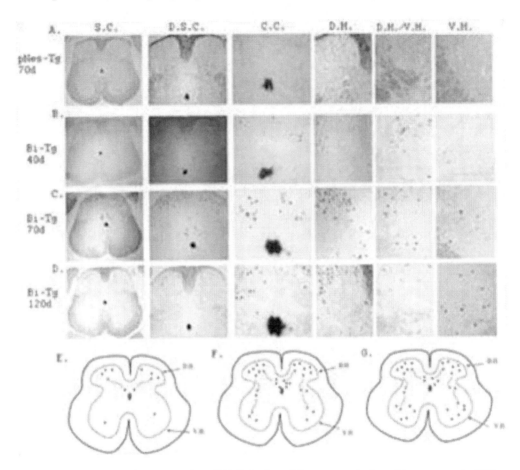

Figure 5. Migration and migratory paths of NPCs in the adult mouse spinal cord in response to MN degeneration in an ALS mouse model which containing human mutant SOD1 transgene (G93A) and Nestin promoter-driven LacZ reporter transgene. The migration of NPCs was characterized by LacZ staining from the ependymal zone surrounding central canal region to the dorsal direction and subsequently to ventral direction in control pNes-Tg mice (A) (70 days of age) and in ALS-like BiTg mice during disease-free (B) (40 days of age), disease-onset (C) (70 days of age), and disease-progression (D) (120 days of age) stages. The migratory paths of NPCs at normal and clinical disease-free (E), disease-onset (F), and disease-progression (G) stages are shown. Abbreviations: BiTg, amyotrophic lateral sclerosis-like; NPC, neural progenitor cell; pNes-Tg, age-matched littermate control. S.C., spinal cord; D.S.C., dorsal spinal cord; C.C. central canal; D.H., dorsal horn; V.H., ventral horn. (Chi L, et al. Stem Cells 2006. 24(1):34-43).

In addition, the activation of NPCs, as well as the neuronal differentiation of NPCs in SOD1 mice, was greatly enhanced by intrathecal treatment with EGF and FGF2 [113]. Characterization of extracellular matrix (ECM) proteins in the spinal anterior horn of an ALS mouse model suggested that although the spinal anterior horn in ALS loses MNs, it initially possesses the capability to self-regenerate, but displays a gradual loss of the ability to regenerate new effective synapses [114]. It has been suggested that reactive gliosis accompanied by the up-regulation of inhibitory molecules in the ECM, such as Chondroitin Sulfate Proteoglycans (CSPGs), creates a non-permissive environment for regeneration [115] [116]. Moreover, due to the nature of this neurodegenerative disease, regenerated neurons and glia have the potential to face the same pathological fate if the microenvironment is not improved. Therefore, the major challenges are not only how to reactivate the proliferation of endogenous stem cells, guide their migration, induce MN differentiation, re-establish neuro-circuitry, but also how to protect them from noxious environments created by disease or injury.

CELL REPLACEMENT STRATEGY VS. TROPHIC SUPPORT STRATEGY

There are two major strategies in utilizing stem cells for applications in the treatment of ALS [89]. One is to replace lost MNs, another is to protect the MNs from degeneration and death. For replacement therapy, MN supply is no longer a problem and immunological rejection can also be bypassed with the development of iPSC technology. Residual challenges are the systematic distribution of the replenished cells, their circuit integration, and MN survival within a hostile spinal environment. Grafted or recruited cells will not be able to survive if the hostile spinal, and even muscular, environment is not modified to increase the chances for survival and integration. Therefore, how to protect implanted MNs would be a more short-term and urgent goal for ALS treatment. It is also more feasible considering the multiple challenges that cell replacement therapy still faces [117].

The primary approach to modify the host environment would be by supplying various biological or chemical factors with a spectrum of functions. Neurotrophic factors and related proteins, which have an ability to protect MNs, have been reviewed by Ekestern [118]. Stem cells and their derivatives are either the natural source of these molecules [67] or can act as a vehicle for their delivery after genetic modification [119].

Various targets have been investigated for the modification of the host environment. Treatments targeting glial cells, both astrocytes [90, 120, 121] and microglia [18, 122], has been proven effective in ALS animal models. Suppressing microglial activation by utilizing small molecules or chemicals is neuro-protective as it delays disease onset and prolongs the lifespan in transgenic ALS models [123, 124]. Modifying aberrant glial cell activity with virus-mediated factors (IGF-1) can also extend survival in ALS mice [125]. NPCs [77, 126] and non-neural stem cells such as MSCs [54-57], can also benefit the local environment by either delivering trophic support or regulating the immune response.

Treatments targeting the muscle provide another avenue by preserving NMJs and MNs [13]. Muscle expression of a local IGF-1 isoform protected MNs in an ALS mouse model [127], and intramuscular grafts of myoblasts genetically modified to secrete GDNF prevented MN loss and disease progression in a mouse model of fALS [128]. Another effective approach explored was to enhance axonal regeneration by removing the cause of myelin-mediated repulsion [129, 130] or by providing attractive cues in the PNS or muscle [87, 88, 131]. Manipulating the expression of cell adhesion molecules in ECM is also an emerging approach to the modification of the local environment so as to enhance regeneration [132]. Generally, the parameters that need to be optimized for trophic support therapy are the optimal cell source, the most effective gene(s)/factor(s) to be delivered, the optimal vector and method of gene delivery into the cells as well as the most efficient route for the delivery of the cells/factors into the patient [119].

CHALLENGES FOR STEM CELL THERAPY

Timing of transplantation: Transplantation in most animal studies is normally applied before the onset of ALS as a preventative therapy. However, in human ALS, no treatment is incurred before the onset of the disease and pre-onset treatment would not be possible if there is no availability of pre-onset diagnosis. Pre-onset diagnosis is extremely hard for sporadic cases of ALS since no genetic correlation can be traced to generate a prediction of disease pathology. Thus, the outcome of post-onset treatment should be given more weight when evaluating the effectiveness of a therapy.

Route of delivery: As MNs distribute throughout the entire CNS, replenishment of stem cells by focal injection would not be ideal for the treatment of ALS. Various cell delivery methods have been investigated and have provided valuable insights [133]. However, these methods are still in the preliminary stage of establishing a reliable method to deliver each type of cell systematically as well as to facilitate the integration of the implanted cells.

Immunological barriers: Long-term immune suppression is never a desirable variable for any treatment. Fortunately, the possibility of autologous transplantation provided by novel stem cell technologies, especially utilizing iPSC technology, could enable the avoidance of immune rejection and the administration of immunosuppresent drugs.

A hostile environment: An inescapable obstacle for any cell therapy of ALS is the environment in the area for cellular delivery [19, 34]. Extensive studies, both *in vivo* and *in vitro*, have focused on this issue and studies are ongoing. Breakthrough approaches to combat the aberrant activation of astrocytes and microglia should rely heavily on understanding the etiology of ALS. Essential questions include the mechanisms for glial activation, and the interactions between glia cells and MNs etc. *In vitro* ALS models developed with stem cells, especially patient-derived stem cells, combined with *in vivo* experiments, are expected to make substantial contributions to this task [19, 134].

CONCLUSION

In summary, the development of the stem cell field has brought great promise for the treatment of ALS. Each type of stem cell or their derivatives has its own advantages and limitations, and could be employed to work through different mechanisms. ESCs and NPCs are good sources for the derivation of MNs and glia cells. MSCs and OECs can benefit by providing trophic support. The development of iPSCs technology offers the potential for autologous therapy with the cell source derived from the adult with the disease. The therapy of recruiting endogenous stem cells is attractive although still at a preliminary stage. While replacement therapy is a distinct possibility now due to successful *in vitro* derivation of MNs from stem cells, it is still a distant goal with multiple challenges. The major immediate hurdle is how to correct the hostile local environment in the individuals with ALS so that the transplanted cells can survive. Trophic support therapy holds the promise for resolving this problem, and is a short-term goal with more urgency, but feasible avenues of investigation. Stem cell therapy can participate in this mission through multiple applications. Ultimately, the combination of these two strategies should be able to effectively combat the MN loss in ALS and finally treat the disease.

REFERENCES

[1]   Zeitlhofer J. [Clinical aspects of amyotrophic lateral sclerosis]. Wien Med Wochenschr 1996; 146(9-10): 182-5.

[2]   Engel AG, Lambert EH, Mulder DM, Torres CF, Sahashi K, Bertorini TE, et al. A newly recognized congenital myasthenic syndrome attributed to a prolonged open time of the acetylcholine-induced ion channel. *Ann. Neurol.* 1982; 11(6): 553-69.

[3]   Rowland LP and Shneider NA. Medical progress: Amyotrophic lateral sclerosis. *New England Journal of Medicine* 2001; 344(22): 1688-1700.

[4]   Boillée S, Vande Velde C and Cleveland Don W. ALS: A Disease of Motor Neurons and Their Nonneuronal Neighbors. *Neuron* 2006; 52(1): 39-59.

[5]   Dupuis L and Loeffler J-P. Neuromuscular junction destruction during amyotrophic lateral sclerosis: insights from transgenic models. *Current Opinion in Pharmacology* 2009; 9(3): 341-346.

[6]   Di Giorgio FP, Carrasco MA, Siao MC, Maniatis T and Eggan K. Non-cell autonomous effect of glia on motor neurons in an embryonic stem cell-based ALS model. *Nat. Neurosci.* 2007; 10(5): 608-614.

[7]   Gould TW and Enomoto H. Neurotrophic Modulation of Motor Neuron Development. *The Neuroscientist* 2009; 15(1): 105-116.

[8]   Jokic N, Gonzalez de Aguilar JL, Dimou L, Lin S, Fergani A, Ruegg MA, et al. The neurite outgrowth inhibitor Nogo-A promotes denervation in an amyotrophic lateral sclerosis model. *EMBO Rep* 2006; 7(11): 1162-7.

[9]   Jokic N, Gonzalez de Aguilar JL, Pradat PF, Dupuis L, Echaniz-Laguna A, Muller A, et al. Nogo expression in muscle correlates with amyotrophic lateral sclerosis severity. *Ann. Neurol.* 2005; 57(4): 553-6.

[10]   Wong M and Martin LJ. Skeletal muscle-restricted expression of human SOD1 causes motor neuron degeneration in transgenic mice. *Hum. Mol. Genet.*; 19(11): 2284-2302.

[11]   Miller TM, Kim SH, Yamanaka K, Hester M, Umapathi P, Arnson H, et al. Gene transfer demonstrates that muscle is not a primary target for non-cell-autonomous toxicity in familial amyotrophic lateral sclerosis. *Proceedings of the National Academy of Sciences* 2006; 103(51): 19546-19551.

[12]   Ilieva H, Polymenidou M and Cleveland DW. Non–cell autonomous toxicity in neurodegenerative disorders: ALS and beyond. *The Journal of Cell Biology* 2009; 187(6): 761-772.

[13]   Dupuis L and Echaniz-Laguna A. Skeletal muscle in motor neuron diseases: therapeutic target and delivery route for potential treatments. *Curr. Drug Targets*; 11(10): 1250-61.

[14]   Allen NJ and Barres BA. Signaling between glia and neurons: focus on synaptic plasticity. *Current Opinion in Neurobiology* 2005; 15(5): 542-548.

[15] Van Den Bosch L and Robberecht W. Crosstalk between astrocytes and motor neurons: what is the message? *Exp. Neurol.* 2008; 211(1): 1-6.

[16] Marchetto MC, Muotri AR, Mu Y, Smith AM, Cezar GG and Gage FH. Non-cell-autonomous effect of human SOD1 G37R astrocytes on motor neurons derived from human embryonic stem cells. *Cell Stem Cell* 2008; 3(6): 649-57.

[17] Nagai M, Re DB, Nagata T, Chalazonitis A, Jessell TM, Wichterle H, et al. Astrocytes expressing ALS-linked mutated SOD1 release factors selectively toxic to motor neurons. *Nat. Neurosci.* 2007; 10(5): 615-622.

[18] Henkel JS, Beers DR, Zhao W and Appel SH. Microglia in ALS: the good, the bad, and the resting. *J. Neuroimmune Pharmacol.* 2009; 4(4): 389-98.

[19] Thonhoff JR, Ojeda L and Wu P. Stem cell-derived motor neurons: applications and challenges in amyotrophic lateral sclerosis. *Curr. Stem Cell Res. Ther.* 2009; 4(3): 178-99.

[20] Boillée Sv, Yamanaka K, Lobsiger CS, Copeland NG, Jenkins NA, Kassiotis G, et al. Onset and Progression in Inherited ALS Determined by Motor Neurons and Microglia. *Science* 2006; 312(5778): 1389-1392.

[21] Yamanaka K, Chun SJ, Boillee S, Fujimori-Tonou N, Yamashita H, Gutmann DH, et al. Astrocytes as determinants of disease progression in inherited amyotrophic lateral sclerosis. *Nat. Neurosci.* 2008; 11(3): 251-253.

[22] Kim SU and de Vellis J. Stem cell-based cell therapy in neurological diseases: a review. *J. Neurosci. Res.* 2009; 87(10): 2183-200.

[23] Thomson JA, Itskovitz-Eldor J, Shapiro SS, Waknitz MA, Swiergiel JJ, Marshall VS, et al. Embryonic stem cell lines derived from human blastocysts. *Science* 1998; 282(5391): 1145-1147.

[24] Donovan PJ and Gearhart J. The end of the beginning for pluripotent stem cells. Nature 2001; 414(6859): 92-97.

[25] Schnabel J. Neuroscience: Standard model. *Nature* 2008; 454(7205): 682-5.

[26] Rubin LL. Stem Cells and Drug Discovery: The Beginning of a New Era? *Cell* 2008; 132(4): 549-552.

[27] Janne J, Johan H and Petter B. Human embryonic stem cell technologies and drug discovery. *Journal of Cellular Physiology* 2009; 219(3): 513-519.

[28] Mohammad R, Slaven E, Victoria M-M and Miodrag S. Challenges of Stem Cell Therapy for Spinal Cord Injury: Human Embryonic Stem Cells, Endogenous Neural Stem Cells, or Induced Pluripotent Stem Cells? *Stem Cells*; 28(1): 93-99.

[29] Li J-Y, Christophersen NS, Hall V, Soulet D and Brundin P. Critical issues of clinical human embryonic stem cell therapy for brain repair. *Trends in Neurosciences* 2008; 31(3): 146-153.

[30] Chambers SM, Fasano CA, Papapetrou EP, Tomishima M, Sadelain M and Studer L. Highly efficient neural conversion of human ES and iPS cells by dual inhibition of SMAD signaling. *Nat. Biotech* 2009; 27(3): 275-280.

[31] Zhao Y, Xiao Z, Gao Y, Chen B, Zhao Y, Zhang J, et al. Insulin rescues ES cell-derived neural progenitor cells from apoptosis by differential regulation of Akt and ERK pathways. *Neuroscience Letters* 2007; 429(1): 49-54.

[32] Erceg S, LaÑez S, Ronaghi M, Stojkovic P, Pérez-Aragó MA, Moreno-Manzano V, et al. Differentiation of Human Embryonic Stem Cells to Regional Specific Neural Precursors in Chemically Defined Medium Conditions. *PLoS ONE* 2008; 3(5): e2122.

[33] Li XJ, Hu BY, Jones SA, Zhang YS, LaVaute T, Du ZW, et al. Directed Differentiation of Ventral Spinal Progenitors and Motor Neurons from Human Embryonic Stem Cells by Small Molecules. *Stem Cells* 2008: 2007-0620.

[34] Lopez-Gonzalez R, Kunckles P and Velasco I. Transient recovery in a rat model of familial amyotrophic lateral sclerosis after transplantation of motor neurons derived from mouse embryonic stem cells. *Cell Transplant* 2009; 18(10): 1171-81.

[35] Aharonowiz M, Einstein O, Fainstein N, Lassmann H, Reubinoff B and Ben-Hur T. Neuroprotective Effect of Transplanted Human Embryonic Stem Cell-Derived Neural Precursors in an Animal Model of Multiple Sclerosis. *PLoS ONE* 2008; 3(9): e3145.

[36] Keirstead HS, Nistor G, Bernal G, Totoiu M, Cloutier F, Sharp K, et al. Human Embryonic Stem Cell-Derived Oligodendrocyte Progenitor Cell Transplants Remyelinate and Restore Locomotion after Spinal Cord Injury. *J. Neurosci.* 2005; 25(19): 4694-4705.

[37] Kerr DA, Llado J, Shamblott MJ, Maragakis NJ, Irani DN, Crawford TO, et al. Human Embryonic Germ Cell Derivatives Facilitate Motor Recovery of Rats with Diffuse Motor Neuron Injury. *J. Neurosci.* 2003; 23(12): 5131-5140.

[38] Choi YH, Kurtz A and Stamm C. Mesenchymal stem cells for cardiac cell therapy. *Hum. Gene Ther*; 22(1): 3-17.

[39] Chamberlain G, Fox J, Ashton B and Middleton J. Concise Review: Mesenchymal Stem Cells: Their Phenotype, Differentiation Capacity, Immunological Features, and Potential for Homing. *Stem Cells* 2007; 25(11): 2739-2749.

[40] Makino S, Fukuda K, Miyoshi S, Konishi F, Kodama H, Pan J, et al. Cardiomyocytes can be generated from marrow stromal cells in vitro. *The Journal of Clinical Investigation* 1999; 103(5): 697-705.

[41] Woodbury D, Schwarz EJ, Prockop DJ and Black IB. Adult rat and human bone marrow stromal cells differentiate into neurons. *J. Neurosci. Res.* 2000; 61(4): 364-70.

[42] Boucherie C and Hermans E. Adult stem cell therapies for neurological disorders: Benefits beyond neuronal replacement? *Journal of Neuroscience Research* 2009; 87(7): 1509-1521.

[43] Neuhuber B, Gallo G, Howard L, Kostura L, Mackay A and Fischer I. Reevaluation of in vitro differentiation protocols for bone marrow stromal cells: Disruption of actin cytoskeleton induces rapid morphological changes and mimics neuronal phenotype. *Journal of Neuroscience Research* 2004; 77(2): 192-204.

[44] Lu P, Blesch A and Tuszynski MH. Induction of bone marrow stromal cells to neurons: Differentiation, transdifferentiation, or artifact? *Journal of Neuroscience Research* 2004; 77(2): 174-191.

[45] Ende N, Weinstein F, Chen R and Ende M. Human umbilical cord blood effect on sod mice (amyotrophic lateral sclerosis). *Life Sciences* 2000; 67(1): 53-59.

[46] Mazzini L, Mareschi K, Ferrero I, Vassallo E, Oliveri G, Nasuelli N, et al. Stem cell treatment in Amyotrophic Lateral Sclerosis. *Journal of the Neurological Sciences* 2008; 265(1-2): 78-83.

[47] Mazzini L, Ferrero I, Luparello V, Rustichelli D, Gunetti M, Mareschi K, et al. Mesenchymal stem cell transplantation in amyotrophic lateral sclerosis: A Phase I clinical trial. *Experimental Neurology*; 223(1): 229-237.

[48] Habisch HJ, Janowski M, Binder D, Kuzma-Kozakiewicz M, Widmann A, Habich A, et al. Intrathecal application of neuroectodermally converted stem cells into a mouse

model of ALS: limited intraparenchymal migration and survival narrows therapeutic effects. *J. Neural. Transm.* 2007; 114(11): 1395-406.

[49]   Azari MF, Mathias L, Ozturk E, Cram DS, Boyd RL and Petratos S. Mesenchymal Stem Cells for Treatment of CNS Injury. *Current Neuropharmacology*; 8(4): 316-323.

[50]   Corti S, Locatelli F, Donadoni C, Guglieri M, Papadimitriou D, Strazzer S, et al. Wild-type bone marrow cells ameliorate the phenotype of SOD1-G93A ALS mice and contribute to CNS, heart and skeletal muscle tissues. *Brain* 2004; 127(11): 2518-2532.

[51]   Suzuki M, McHugh J, Tork C, Shelley B, Hayes A, Bellantuono I, et al. Direct Muscle Delivery of GDNF With Human Mesenchymal Stem Cells Improves Motor Neuron Survival and Function in a Rat Model of Familial ALS. *Mol. Ther.* 2008; 16(12): 2002-2010.

[52]   Kaspar BK. Mesenchymal Stem Cells as Trojan Horses for GDNF Delivery in ALS. *Mol. Ther.* 2008; 16(12): 1905-1906.

[53]   Joyce N, Annett G, Wirthlin L, Olson S, Bauer G and Nolta JA. Mesenchymal stem cells for the treatment of neurodegenerative disease. *Regen Med*; 5(6): 933-46.

[54]   Crigler L, Robey RC, Asawachaicharn A, Gaupp D and Phinney DG. Human mesenchymal stem cell subpopulations express a variety of neuro-regulatory molecules and promote neuronal cell survival and neuritogenesis. *Experimental Neurology* 2006; 198(1): 54-64.

[55]   Lanza C, Morando S, Voci A, Canesi L, Principato MC, Serpero LD, et al. Neuroprotective mesenchymal stem cells are endowed with a potent antioxidant effect in vivo. *Journal of Neurochemistry* 2009; 110(5): 1674-1684.

[56]   Ren G, Zhang L, Zhao X, Xu G, Zhang Y, Roberts AI, et al. Mesenchymal Stem Cell-Mediated Immunosuppression Occurs via Concerted Action of Chemokines and Nitric Oxide. *Cell Stem Cell* 2008; 2(2): 141-150.

[57]   Zhang J, Li Y, Chen JL, Cui YS, Lu M, Elias SB, et al. Human bone marrow stromal cell treatment improves neurological functional recovery in EAE mice. *Experimental Neurology* 2005; 195(1): 16-26.

[58]   Doucette R. Olfactory ensheathing cells: potential for glial cell transplantation into areas of CNS injury. *Histol. Histopathol.* 1995; 10(2): 503-7.

[59]   Ramon-Cueto A and Avila J. Olfactory ensheathing glia: properties and function. *Brain Res. Bull.* 1998; 46(3): 175-87.

[60]   Lopes A. Olfactory ensheathing cells for human spinal cord injury. *Neurorehabil Neural Repair;* 24(8): 772-3; author reply 772-3.

[61]   Bretzner F, Plemel JR, Liu J, Richter M, Roskams AJ and Tetzlaff W. Combination of olfactory ensheathing cells with local versus systemic cAMP treatment after a cervical rubrospinal tract injury. *J. Neurosci. Res.*; 88(13): 2833-46.

[62]   Ramon-Cueto A and Nieto-Sampedro M. Regeneration into the spinal cord of transected dorsal root axons is promoted by ensheathing glia transplants. *Exp. Neurol.* 1994; 127(2): 232-44.

[63]   Ramon-Cueto A, Plant GW, Avila J and Bunge MB. Long-distance axonal regeneration in the transected adult rat spinal cord is promoted by olfactory ensheathing glia transplants. *J. Neurosci.* 1998; 18(10): 3803-15.

[64]   Li Y, Field PM and Raisman G. Repair of Adult Rat Corticospinal Tract by Transplants of Olfactory Ensheathing Cells. *Science* 1997; 277(5334): 2000-2002.

[65]   Feron F, Perry C, Cochrane J, Licina P, Nowitzke A, Urquhart S, et al. Autologous olfactory ensheathing cell transplantation in human spinal cord injury. *Brain* 2005; 128(Pt 12): 2951-60.

[66]   Morita E, Watanabe Y, Ishimoto M, Nakano T, Kitayama M, Yasui K, et al. A novel cell transplantation protocol and its application to an ALS mouse model. *Experimental Neurology* 2008; 213(2): 431-438.

[67]   Martin LJ and Liu Z. Adult olfactory bulb neural precursor cell grafts provide temporary protection from motor neuron degeneration, improve motor function, and extend survival in amyotrophic lateral sclerosis mice. *J. Neuropathol. Exp. Neurol.* 2007; 66(11): 1002-18.

[68]   Cattaneo E and McKay R. Proliferation and differentiation of neuronal stem cells regulated by nerve growth factor. *Nature* 1990; 347(6295): 762-765.

[69]   Neural Stem Cells, Neural Progenitors, and Neurotrophic Factors. *Cell Transplantation* 2007; 16: 133-150.

[70]   Johansson CB, Momma S, Clarke DL, Risling M, Lendahl U and Frisén J. Identification of a Neural Stem Cell in the Adult Mammalian Central Nervous System. *Cell* 1999; 96(1): 25-34.

[71]   Thuret S, Moon LDF and Gage FH. Therapeutic interventions after spinal cord injury. *Nat. Rev. Neurosci.* 2006; 7(8): 628-643.

[72]   Lladó J, Haenggeli C, Maragakis NJ, Snyder EY and Rothstein JD. Neural stem cells protect against glutamate-induced excitotoxicity and promote survival of injured motor neurons through the secretion of neurotrophic factors. *Molecular and Cellular Neuroscience* 2004; 27(3): 322-331.

[73]   Coutts M and Keirstead HS. Stem cells for the treatment of spinal cord injury. *Experimental Neurology* 2008; 209(2): 368-377.

[74]   Lee JC, Jin Y, Jin J, Kang BG, Nam DH, Joo KM, et al. Functional neural stem cell isolation from brains of adult mutant SOD1 (SOD1(G93A)) transgenic amyotrophic lateral sclerosis (ALS) mice. *Neurological Research*; 33(1): 33-37.

[75]   Westerlund U, Moe MC, Varghese M, Berg-Johnsen J, Ohlsson M, Langmoen IA, et al. Stem cells from the adult human brain develop into functional neurons in culture. *Experimental Cell Research* 2003; 289(2): 378-383.

[76]   Yan J, Leyan X, Welsh AM, Hatfield G, Hazel T, Johe K, et al. Extensive Neuronal Differentiation of Human Neural Stem Cell Grafts in Adult Rat Spinal Cord. *PLoS Medicine* 2007; 4(2): 318-332.

[77]   Xu L, Yan J, Chen D, Welsh AM, Hazel T, Johe K, et al. Human Neural Stem Cell Grafts Ameliorate Motor Neuron Disease in SOD-1 Transgenic Rats. *Transplantation* 2006; 82(7): 865-875 10.1097/01.tp.0000235532.00920.7a.

[78]   Leyan X, David KR, Tan P, Karl J and Vassilis EK. Human neural stem cell grafts in the spinal cord of SOD1 transgenic rats: Differentiation and structural integration into the segmental motor circuitry. *The Journal of Comparative Neurology* 2009; 514(4): 297-309.

[79]   Wright LS, Prowse KR, Wallace K, Linskens MHK and Svendsen CN. Human progenitor cells isolated from the developing cortex undergo decreased neurogenesis and eventual senescence following expansion in vitro. *Experimental Cell Research* 2006; 312(11): 2107-2120.

[80] Kerr DA, Llado J, Shamblott MJ, Maragakis NJ, Irani DN, Crawford TO, et al. Human
      embryonic germ cell derivatives facilitate motor recovery of rats with diffuse motor
      neuron injury. *Journal of Neuroscience* 2003; 23(12): 5131-5140.

[81] Marques SA, Almeida FM, Fernandes AM, dos Santos Souza C, Cadilhe DV, Rehen
      SK, et al. Predifferentiated embryonic stem cells promote functional recovery after
      spinal cord compressive injury. *Brain Research*; 1349: 115-128.

[82] Wichterle H, Lieberam I, Porter JA and Jessell TM. Directed Differentiation of
      Embryonic Stem Cells into Motor Neurons. *Cell* 2002; 110(3): 385-397.

[83] Li X-J, Du Z-W, Zarnowska ED and czzz. Specification of motoneurons from human
      embryonic stem cells. *Nat. Biotech.* 2005; 23(2): 215-221.

[84] Guo X, Johe K, Molnar P, Davis H and Hickman J. Characterization of a human fetal
      spinal cord stem cell line, NSI-566RSC, and its induction to functional motoneurons. *J.
      Tissue Eng. Regen. Med.*; 4(3): 181-93.

[85] Cizkova D, Kakinohana O, Kucharova K, Marsala S, Johe K, Hazel T, et al. Functional
      recovery in rats with ischemic paraplegia after spinal grafting of human spinal stem
      cells. *Neuroscience* 2007; 147(2): 546-560.

[86] Gao J, Coggeshall RE, Tarasenko YI and Wu P. Human neural stem cell-derived
      cholinergic neurons innervate muscle in motoneuron deficient adult rats. *Neuroscience*
      2005; 131(2): 257-262.

[87] Harper JM, Krishnan C, Darman JS, Deshpande DM, Peck S, Shats I, et al. Axonal
      growth of embryonic stem cell-derived motoneurons in vitro and in motoneuron-injured
      adult rats. *PNAS* 2004; 101(18): 7123-7128.

[88] Deepa M. Deshpande Y-SKTMJCSDISLLRJDCKAHNMJSJDR. Recovery from
      paralysis in adult rats using embryonic stem cells. *Annals of Neurology* 2006; 60(1): 32-
      44.

[89] Silani V, Calzarossa C, Cova L and Ticozzi N. Stem cells in amyotrophic lateral
      sclerosis: motor neuron protection or replacement? *CNS Neurol. Disord. Drug Targets*;
      9(3): 314-24.

[90] Blackburn D, Sargsyan S, Monk PN and Shaw PJ. Astrocyte function and role in motor
      neuron disease: a future therapeutic target? *Glia* 2009; 57(12): 1251-64.

[91] Maragakis NJ, Rao MS, Llado J, Wong V, Xue H, Pardo A, et al. Glial restricted
      precursors protect against chronic glutamate neurotoxicity of motor neurons in vitro.
      Glia 2005; 50(2): 145-159.

[92] Lepore AC, Rauck B, Dejea C, Pardo AC, Rao MS, Rothstein JD, et al. Focal
      transplantation-based astrocyte replacement is neuroprotective in a model of motor
      neuron disease. *Nat. Neurosci.* 2008; 11(11): 1294-301.

[93] Beers DR, Henkel JS, Xiao Q, Zhao W, Wang J, Yen AA, et al. Wild-type microglia
      extend survival in PU.1 knockout mice with familial amyotrophic lateral sclerosis.
      Proceedings of the National Academy of Sciences 2006; 103(43): 16021-16026.

[94] Takahashi K, Tanabe K, Ohnuki M, Narita M, Ichisaka T, Tomoda K, et al. Induction
      of Pluripotent Stem Cells from Adult Human Fibroblasts by Defined Factors. *Cell*
      2007; 131(5): 861-872.

[95] Li C, Zhou J, Shi G, Ma Y, Yang Y, Gu J, et al. Pluripotency can be rapidly and
      efficiently induced in human amniotic fluid-derived cells. *Hum. Mol. Genet.* 2009;
      18(22): 4340-4349.

[96] Goldman S and Sim F, *Stem Cells: Nuclear Programming and Therapeutic Applications*. Novartis Foundation Symposium 265. 2005.

[97] Amabile G and Meissner A. Induced pluripotent stem cells: current progress and potential for regenerative medicine. *Trends in Molecular Medicine* 2009; 15(2): 59-68.

[98] Dimos JT, Rodolfa KT, Niakan KK, Weisenthal LM, Mitsumoto H, Chung W, et al. Induced Pluripotent Stem Cells Generated from Patients with ALS Can Be Differentiated into Motor Neurons. *Science* 2008; 321(5893): 1218-1221.

[99] Wernig M, Zhao J-P, Pruszak J, Hedlund E, Fu D, Soldner F, et al. Neurons derived from reprogrammed fibroblasts functionally integrate into the fetal brain and improve symptoms of rats with Parkinson's disease. *Proceedings of the National Academy of Sciences* 2008; 105(15): 5856-5861.

[100] Theme 4 Human Cell Biology and Pathology. *Amyotrophic Lateral Sclerosis*; 11(S1): 96-109.

[101] Takahashi K and Yamanaka S. Induction of Pluripotent Stem Cells from Mouse Embryonic and Adult Fibroblast Cultures by Defined Factors. *Cell* 2006; 126(4): 663-676.

[102] Stadtfeld M, Nagaya M, Utikal J, Weir G and Hochedlinger K. Induced Pluripotent Stem Cells Generated Without Viral Integration. *Science* 2008; 322(5903): 945-949.

[103] Okita K, Nakagawa M, Hyenjong H, Ichisaka T and Yamanaka S. Generation of Mouse Induced Pluripotent Stem Cells Without Viral Vectors. Science 2008; 322(5903): 949-953.

[104] Huangfu D, Osafune K, Maehr R, Guo W, Eijkelenboom A, Chen S, et al. Induction of pluripotent stem cells from primary human fibroblasts with only Oct4 and Sox2. *Nat. Biotech.* 2008; 26(11): 1269-1275.

[105] Zhou H, Wu S, Joo JY, Zhu S, Han DW, Lin T, et al. Generation of Induced Pluripotent Stem Cells Using Recombinant Proteins. *Cell Stem Cell* 2009; 4(5): 381-384.

[106] Yamanaka S. A Fresh Look at iPS Cells. *Cell* 2009; 137(1): 13-17.

[107] Sah DWY, Ray J and Gage FH. Bipotent progenitor cell lines from the human CNS. *Nature Biotechnology* 1997; 15(6): 574-580.

[108] Kim SU. Human neural stem cells genetically modified for brain repair in neurological disorders. *Neuropathology* 2004; 24(3): 159-171.

[109] Flax JD, Aurora S, Yang CH, Simonin C, Wills AM, Billinghurst LL, et al. Engraftable human neural stem cells respond to developmental cues, replace neurons, and express foreign genes. *Nature Biotechnology* 1998; 16(11): 1033-1039.

[110] Eriksson PS, Perfilieva E, Bjork-Eriksson T, Alborn AM, Nordborg C, Peterson DA, et al. Neurogenesis in the adult human hippocampus. *Nature Medicine* 1998; 4(11): 1313-1317.

[111] Chen J, Magavi SSP and Macklis JD. Neurogenesis of corticospinal motor neurons extending spinal projections in adult mice. *Proceedings of the National Academy of Sciences of the United States of America 2004*; 101(46): 16357-16362.

[112] Chi L, Ke Y, Luo C, Li B, Gozal D, Kalyanaraman B, et al. Motor Neuron Degeneration Promotes Neural Progenitor Cell Proliferation, Migration, and Neurogenesis in the Spinal Cords of Amyotrophic Lateral Sclerosis Mice. *Stem Cells* 2006; 24(1): 34-43.

[113] Ohta Y, Nagai M, Nagata T, Murakami T, Nagano I, Narai H, et al. Intrathecal injection of epidermal growth factor and fibroblast growth factor 2 promotes proliferation of

neural precursor cells in the spinal cords of mice with mutant human SOD1 gene. *Journal of Neuroscience Research* 2006; 84(5): 980-992.

[114] Miyazaki K, Nagai M, Morimoto N, Kurata T, Takehisa Y, Ikeda Y, et al. Spinal anterior horn has the capacity to self-regenerate in amyotrophic lateral sclerosis model mice. *Journal of Neuroscience Research* 2009; 87(16): 3639-3648.

[115] Mizuno H, Warita H, Aoki M and Itoyama Y. Accumulation of chondroitin sulfate proteoglycans in the microenvironment of spinal motor neurons in amyotrophic lateral sclerosis transgenic rats. *Journal of Neuroscience Research* 2008; 86(11): 2512-2523.

[116] Guan Y-j, Wang X, Wang H-y, Kawagishi K, Ryu H, Huo C-f, et al. Increased stem cell proliferation in the spinal cord of adult amyotrophic lateral sclerosis transgenic mice. *Journal of Neurochemistry* 2007; 102(4): 1125-1138.

[117] Lindvall O and Kokaia Z. Stem cells for the treatment of neurological disorders. *Nature* 2006; 441(7097): 1094-1096.

[118] Ekestern E. Neurotrophic Factors and Amyotrophic Lateral Sclerosis. *Neurodegenerative Diseases* 2004; 1(2-3): 88-100.

[119] Taha MF. Cell based-gene delivery approaches for the treatment of spinal cord injury and neurodegenerative disorders. *Curr Stem Cell Res Ther*; 5(1): 23-36.

[120] Vargas MR, Johnson DA, Sirkis DW, Messing A and Johnson JA. Nrf2 activation in astrocytes protects against neurodegeneration in mouse models of familial amyotrophic lateral sclerosis. *J. Neurosci.* 2008; 28(50): 13574-81.

[121] Suzuki M, McHugh J, Tork C, Shelley B, Klein SM, Aebischer P, et al. GDNF Secreting Human Neural Progenitor Cells Protect Dying Motor Neurons, but Not Their Projection to Muscle, in a Rat Model of Familial ALS. *PLoS ONE* 2007; 2(8): e689.

[122] Napoli I and Neumann H. Protective effects of microglia in multiple sclerosis. *Exp. Neurol*; 225(1): 24-8.

[123] West M, Mhatre M, Ceballos A, Floyd RA, Grammas P, Gabbita SP, et al. The arachidonic acid 5-lipoxygenase inhibitor nordihydroguaiaretic acid inhibits tumor necrosis factor α activation of microglia and extends survival of G93A-SOD1 transgenic mice. *Journal of Neurochemistry* 2004; 91(1): 133-143.

[124] Kim H-S and Suh Y-H. Minocycline and neurodegenerative diseases. *Behavioural Brain Research* 2009; 196(2): 168-179.

[125] Dodge JC, Haidet AM, Yang W, Passini MA, Hester M, Clarke J, et al. Delivery of AAV-IGF-1 to the CNS extends survival in ALS mice through modification of aberrant glial cell activity. *Mol. Ther.* 2008; 16(6): 1056-64.

[126] Klein SM, Behrstock S, McHugh J, Hoffmann K, Wallace K, Suzuki M, et al. GDNF Delivery Using Human Neural Progenitor Cells in a Rat Model of ALS. *Human Gene Therapy* 2005; 16(4): 509-521.

[127] Dobrowolny G, Giacinti C, Pelosi L, Nicoletti C, Winn N, Barberi L, et al. Muscle expression of a local Igf-1 isoform protects motor neurons in an ALS mouse model. *The Journal of Cell Biology* 2005; 168(2): 193-199.

[128] Mohajeri MH, Figlewicz DA and Bohn MC. Intramuscular grafts of myoblasts genetically modified to secrete glial cell line-derived neurotrophic factor prevent motoneuron loss and disease progression in a mouse model of familial amyotrophic lateral sclerosis. *Hum. Gene Ther.* 1999; 10(11): 1853-66.

[129] Spencer T, Domeniconi M, Cao ZX and Filbin MT. New roles for old proteins in adult CNS axonal regeneration. *Current Opinion in Neurobiology* 2003; 13(1): 133-139.

[130] Schwab ME. Functions of Nogo proteins and their receptors in the nervous system. *Nature Reviews Neuroscience*; 11(12): 799-811.

[131] Hou ST, Jiang SX and Smith RA, *Permissive and repulsive cues and signalling pathways of axonal outgrowth and regeneration*, in *International Review of Cell and Molecular Biology, Vol 267*. 2008, Elsevier Academic Press Inc: San Diego. p. 125-181.

[132] Lavdas AA, Papastefanaki F, Thomaidou D and Matsas R. Cell Adhesion Molecules in Gene and Cell Therapy Approaches for Nervous System Repair. *Curr Gene Ther*.

[133] Lepore AC and Maragakis NJ. Targeted stem cell transplantation strategies in ALS. *Neurochem Int* 2007; 50(7-8): 966-75.

[134] Marchetto MCN, Winner B and Gage FH. Pluripotent stem cells in neurodegenerative and neurodevelopmental diseases. *Human Molecular Genetics*.

In: Motor Neuron Diseases
Editors: Bradley J. Turner and Julie B. Atkin

ISBN 978-1-61470-101-9
© 2012 Nova Science Publishers, Inc.

Chapter V

TDP-43-Immunoreactive Pathology in Frontotemporal Lobar Degeneration with TDP Proteinopathy (FTLD-TDP) with and without Associated Motor Neuron Disease (MND)

R. A. Armstrong[*]
Vision Sciences, Aston University,
Birmingham B4 7ET, UK

Abstract

A proportion of patients with motor neuron disease (MND) exhibit frontotemporal dementia (FTD) and some patients with FTD develop the clinical features of MND. Frontotemporal lobar degeneration (FTLD) is the pathological substrate of FTD and some forms of this disease (referred to as FTLD-U) share with MND the common feature of ubiquitin-immunoreactive, tau-negative cellular inclusions in the cerebral cortex and hippocampus. Recently, the transactive response (TAR) DNA-binding protein of 43 kDa (TDP-43) has been found to be a major protein of the inclusions of FTLD-U with or without MND and these cases are referred to as FTLD with TDP-43 proteinopathy (FTLD-TDP). To clarify the relationship between MND and FTLD-TDP, TDP-43 pathology was studied in nine cases of FTLD-MND and compared with cases of familial and sporadic FTLD–TDP without associated MND. A principal components analysis (PCA) of the nine FTLD-MND cases suggested that variations in the density of surviving neurons in the frontal cortex and neuronal cytoplasmic inclusions (NCI) in the dentate gyrus (DG) were the major histological differences between cases. The density of surviving neurons in FTLD-MND was significantly less than in FTLD-TDP cases

[*] Corresponding Author: Dr. R.A. Armstrong, Vision Sciences, Aston University, Birmingham B4 7ET, UK. Tel: 0121-359-3611; Fax 0121-333-4220; EMail R.A.Armstrong@aston.ac.uk.

without MND, and there were greater densities of NCI but fewer neuronal intranuclear inclusions (NII) in some brain regions in FTLD-MND. A PCA of all FTLD-TDP cases, based on TDP-43 pathology alone, suggested that neuropathological heterogeneity was essentially continuously distributed. The FTLD-MND cases exhibited consistently high loadings on PC2 and overlapped with subtypes 2 and 3 of FTLD-TDP. The data suggest: (1) FTLD-MND cases have a consistent pathology, variations in the density of NCI in the DG being the major TDP-43-immunoreactive difference between cases, (2) there are considerable similarities in the neuropathology of FTLD-TDP with and without MND, but with greater neuronal loss in FTLD-MND, and (3) FTLD-MND cases are part of the FTLD-TDP 'continuum' overlapping with FTLD-TDP disease subtypes 2 and 3.

Keywords: Motor neuron disease (MND), TAR DNA-binding protein of 43 kDa (TDP-43), Frontotemporal lobar degeneration (FTLD) with TDP-43 proteinopathy (FTLD-TDP), Principal components analysis (PCA), Disease overlap.

INTRODUCTION

Motor neuron disease (MND) describes a group of neurological disorders in which there is a selective loss of upper and lower motor neurons, the cells responsible for controlling voluntary muscle activity. The classic symptoms of MND include progressive weakness, muscle wasting, muscle fasciculations, stiffness in the arms and legs, and overactive tendon reflexes. Cognitive changes, however, occur in a proportion of patients with MND, including MND dementia (MND-D) while some patients develop the signs and symptoms of frontotemporal dementia (FTD) (Forman et al., 2004). Furthermore, some patients with FTD develop the clinical features of MND (FTD-MND) (Garraux et al., 1999, Miller et al., 1999) with some studies suggesting that approximately 38% of neuropathologically confirmed FTD may have MND (Lipton et al., 2004). Hence, there is considerable overlap between MND and FTD and therefore, whether FTD-MND represents the chance association of relatively common diseases or a single multifaceted disease remains to be determined (Talbot et al., 1995; Talbot, 1996; Gentileschi et al., 1999; Bigio et al., 2004).

Motor Neuron Disease (MND)

In MND loss of upper and lower motor neurons results in problems with speaking, walking, breathing, swallowing, and in general movement of the body. Hence, MND is closely related to other 'motor neuron' disorders such as spinobulbar muscular atrophy, spinal muscular atrophy, and Charcot-Marie-Tooth disease. It was J-M Charcot in 1869 who first suggested grouping together the various diseases affecting the lateral horn of the spinal cord. Approximately 90% of cases of MND are sporadic and both genetic risk factors and environmental factors are likely to be involved in their aetiology. About 10% of cases are familial and a variety of different genes have been implicated including Cu/Zn superoxide dismutase (*SOD1*), *ALS2*, senataxin (*SETX*), and vesicle associated protein B (*VAPB*), *SOD1* being the most common cause of familial MND. The neuropathology of MND is characterized by the degeneration of the ventral horns of the spinal cord accompanied by atrophy of the ventral roots while in the cerebral cortex, there is degeneration of the frontal and temporal lobes. Histological features include vacuolation, astrocytosis, and skein-like cellular inclusions called 'Bunina bodies'.

Frontotemporal Lobar Degeneration (FTLD)

Frontotemporal lobar degeneration (FTLD) is the neuropathological substrate of FTD and is the second commonest form of cortical dementia of early-onset after Alzheimer's disease (AD) (Tolnay and Probst, 2002; Josephs, 2006). The disorder is associated with a heterogeneous group of clinical syndromes including in addition, to FTD, FTD-MND, progressive non-fluent aphasia (PNFA), semantic dementia (SD), and progressive apraxia (PAX) (Snowden et al., 2007). The presence of ubiquitin-immunoreactive, tau-negative cellular inclusions in the cortex, hippocampus and motor cortex is a feature of a proportion of cases of FTLD (referred to as FTLD-U) and MND (Bergmann et al., 1996). In addition, neuropsychiatric studies and single photon emission computed-tomography (SPECT) show a common pattern of cerebral involvement in MND, FTD and FTD-MND suggesting that these diseases represent the clinical range of a pathological continuum (Talbot et al., 1995). Recently, transactive response (TAR) DNA-binding protein of 43kDa (TDP-43) has been found to be a major protein of the inclusions of FTLD-U with or without associated MND (Davidson et al., 2007; Grossman et al., 2007; Neumann et al., 2007; Kwong et al., 2007). FTLD with TDP-43-immunoreactive inclusions (FTLD-TDP) is characterized by variable neocortical and allocortical atrophy principally affecting the frontal and temporal lobes. In addition, there is neuronal loss, microvacuolation of the superficial cortical laminae, and a reactive astrocytosis (Cairns et al., 2007a). A variety of TDP-43-immunoreactive inclusions are present in FTLD-TDP including neuronal cytoplasmic inclusions (NCI), neuronal intranuclear inclusions (NII), oligodendroglial inclusions (GI), and dystrophic neurites (DN) (Armstrong et al., 2010).

Pathological Heterogeneity within FTLD-TDP

FTLD-TDP is a heterogeneous molecular disorder (Armstrong et al., 2010). First, there are sporadic (sFTLD-TDP) and familial (fFTLD-TDP) forms of the disease, the majority of the latter being caused by mutations in the *progranulin* (*GRN*) gene (Baker et al., 2006; Cruts et al., 2006; Mukherjee et al., 2006; Mackenzie et al., 2006a, Behrens et al., 2007; Rademakers and Hutton, 2007; Van der Zee et al., 2007; Van Deerlin et al., 2007). In addition, cases with valosin-containing protein *(VCP)* gene mutation (Forman et al., 2006), variants in the ubiquitin-associated binding protein 1 *(UBAP1)* gene (Luty et al., 2008; Rollinson et al., 2009), and common variants at the 7p21 locus have also been shown to be associated with FTLD-TDP (Van Deerlin et al., 2010).

Second, four or five pathological subtypes of FTLD-TDP have been proposed based on the predominant type of inclusion present originally detected with anti-ubiquitin immunohistochemistry (IHC), and the distribution and density of the pathological changes in the cortex (Mackenzie et al., 2006b; Sampathu et al., 2006; Cairns et al., 2007b; Josephs, 2008; Mackenzie et al., 2009). Patterns of histology based solely on cortical pathology include the systems of Sampathu et al. (2006) and Neumann et al. (2007) whereas Mackenzie et al. (2006b) proposed a system that includes both cortical and dentate gyrus (DG) inclusions. The same descriptors are often used to define subtypes, but the numbering of each subtype varies between schemes. Using a composite system proposed by Cairns et al. (2007b): type 1 cases (Mackenzie-type 2) are characterized by long DN in superficial cortical laminae with few or no NCI or NII, type 2 (Mackenzie-type 3) by numerous NCI in superficial and deep cortical laminae with infrequent DN and sparse or no NII, type 3 (Mackenzie-type 1) by pathology predominantly affecting the superficial cortical laminae with numerous NCI, DN, and varying numbers of NII, and type 4 by numerous NII, and infrequent NCI and DN especially in neocortical areas. More recently, Josephs (2008) has proposed five subtypes of FTLD and Mackenzie et al. (2009) four subtypes plus a group containing unclassifiable cases.

Third, FTLD-TDP can occur in combination with MND (FTLD-MND) and such cases may be associated with a more localized pattern of frontal lobe atrophy (Whitwell et al., 2006). Fourth, a proportion of FTLD-TDP cases have coexisting hippocampal sclerosis (HS) in which there is neuronal loss in the subiculum and sector CA1 of the hippocampus (Josephs et al., 2006; Amandir-Ortiz et al., 2007). A significant degree of Alzheimer's disease (AD) pathology, viz., senile plaques (SP) and neurofibrillary tangles (NFT) may also be present in some cases (Armstrong et al., 2010).

Objectives

The major objective of the present study is to clarify the relationship between FTLD-TDP and MND. Hence, the following quantitative studies were carried out: (1) the density and distribution of the TDP-43 immunoreactive inclusions together with abnormally enlarged neurons (EN), surviving neurons, and vacuolation were studied in the frontal and temporal lobes of nine cases of FTLD-MND, (2) a principal components analysis (PCA) was performed to study neuropathological variations within the nine FTLD-MND cases, (3) the densities of the TDP-43-immunoreactive inclusions, EN, surviving neurons, and vacuolation were compared in FTLD-MND, and in fFTLD-TDP and sFTLD-TDP without associated MND, and (4) a PCA was peformed on all FTLD-TDP cases based on TDP-43-immunoreactive pathology to examine the relationship between the FTLD-MND cases and FTLD-TDP.

MATERIALS AND METHODS

Cases

Ninety-four cases of FTLD-TDP were obtained from dementia centers in the USA and Canada: Washington University School of Medicine, St. Louis, MO (32 cases), University of California, Davis, CA (15 cases), University of Pittsburgh, Pittsburgh, PA (15 cases), Vancouver General Hospital, Vancouver, Canada (11 cases), Harvard Brain Tissue Resource Center, Belmont, MA (9 cases), Emory University, Atlanta, GA (6 cases), University of

Washington, Seattle, WA (2 cases), Columbia University, New York, NY (2 cases), University of California, Irvine, CA (1 case), and University of Michigan, Ann Arbor, MI (1 case). All cases exhibited FTLD with neuronal loss, microvacuolation in the superficial cortical laminae, and reactive astrocytosis consistent with the proposed criteria for FTLD (Mackenzie et al., 2006b; Cairns et al., 2007b). A variety of TDP-43-immunoreactive lesions was present in these cases including NCI, NII, DN, and GI consistent with a diagnosis of FTLD-TDP (Cairns et al., 2007b). Of the 94 cases, 37 were identified as fFTLD-TDP (at least one or more first degree relatives affected) and 57 were sFTLD-TDP. Of the fFTLD-TDP cases, 14 cases had *GRN* mutations (Baker et al., 2006; Cruts et al., 2006; Beck et al., 2008), one had a *VCP* gene mutation (Forman et al., 2006), and one case was associated with *UBAP1* (Rollinson et al., 2009), a presumptive gene on chromosome 9 (9p21). The genetic defects in the remaining familial cases have not been identified to date. Nine of the sFTLD-TDP cases had coexisting motor neuron disease (FTLD-MND) (Josephs et al 2005, Kersaitis et al., 2006) (see Table 1). Cases were assigned to the four subtypes of FTLD-U/FTLD-TDP based on the composite scheme of Cairns et al. (2007b). Staging of cases was based on the Braak score of neurofibrillary pathology (Braak et al., 2006).

Table 1. Demographic features and gross brain weight of the nine cases of frontotemporal lobar dementia with TDP-43 proteinopathy (FTLD-TDP) with associated motor neuron disease (MND). Braak score is based on density and distribution of neurofibrillary tangles. (M = male, F = female)

Case	Gender	Age (yrs)	Onset (yrs)	Duration (yrs)	Brain weight (gm)	Braak score
A	M	66	71	5	1230	2
B	M	69	72	3	570	0
C	M	70	71	1	1140	4
D	F	67	68	1	1180	2
E	M	80	-	-	1200	1
F	M	47	48	1	1370	0
G	M	56	59	3	1160	0
H	F	60	61	1	1344	0
J	M	88	89	1	1278	2

Histological Methods

After death, the consent of the next-of-kin was obtained for brain removal, following local Ethical Committee procedures and the 1995 Declaration of Helsinki (as modified in Edinburgh, 2000). Tissue blocks were taken from the frontal lobe at the level of the genu of the corpus callosum to study the middle frontal gyrus (MFG) and the temporal lobe at the level of the lateral geniculate body to study the inferior temporal gyrus (ITG), parahippocampal gyrus (PHG), CA1/2 sectors of the hippocampus, and DG. Tissue was fixed in 10% phosphate buffered formal-saline and embedded in paraffin wax. IHC was performed on 4 to 10μm sections with a rabbit polyclonal antibody that recognizes TDP-43 epitopes (dilution 1:1000; ProteinTech Inc., Chicago, IL). Sections were counterstained with haematoxylin.

Morphometric Methods

In the MFG, ITG, and PHG of each case, histological features were counted along strips of tissue (1600 to 3200μm in length) located parallel to the pia mater, using 250 x 50μm sample fields arranged contiguously. The sample fields were located both in the upper and lower cortex, the short edge of the sample field being orientated parallel with the pia mater and aligned with guidelines marked on the slide. Between 32 and 64 sample fields were necessary to sample each region. In the hippocampus, the features were counted in the cornu ammonis (CA) in a region extending from the prosubiculum/CA boundary to the maximum point of curvature of the pyramidal layer before it extends to join the dentate fascia via CA3 and CA4. Hence, the region sampled encompassed approximately sectors CA1 and CA2, the short dimension of the contiguous sample field being aligned with the alveus. Very little pathology was observed to extend into sectors CA3/4 in the cases studied and these areas were not sampled. NCI have been commonly observed in the DG in FTLD-TDP (Mackenzie et al., 2006b; Woulfe et al., 2001; Kovari et al., 2004) and the sample field was aligned with the upper edge of the granule cell layer.

The NCI (Figure 1) were rounded, spicular, or skein-like in shape (Yaguchi et al., 2004; Davidson et al., 2007), while the GI morphologically resembled the 'coiled bodies' reported in various tauopathies such as corticobasal degeneration (CBD), progressive supranuclear palsy (PSP), and argyrophilic grain disease (AGD).

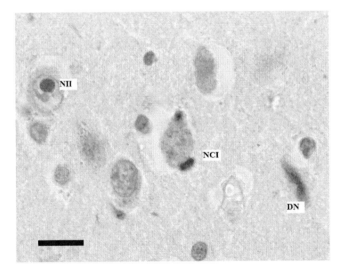

Figure 1. Frontotemporal lobar degeneration with TDP-43 proteinopathy (FTLD-TDP): TDP-43 immunoreactive lesions in the frontal cortex including neuronal cytoplasmic inclusion (NCI), neuronal intranuclear inclusions (NII), and a dystrophic neurite (DN) (TDP-43 immunohistochemistry, bar = 50μm).

The NII (Figure 1) were lenticular or spindle-shaped (Pirici et al., 2006) and the DN (Figure 1) were characteristically long and contorted (Hatanpaa et al., 2008). Surviving neurons were identified as cells containing at least some stained cytoplasm in combination with larger shape and non-spherical outline (Armstrong, 1996).

Small spherical or asymmetrical nuclei without cytoplasm but with the presence of a thicker nuclear membrane and more heterogeneous chromatin were regarded as glial cells. EN had enlarged perikarya, lacked NCI, had a shrunken nucleus displaced to the periphery of the cell, and the maximum cell diameter was at least three times the diameter of the nucleus (Armstrong, 1996). The number of discrete vacuoles greater than 5μm in diameter was also recorded in each sample field. It can be difficult to differentiate microvacuolation of the neuropil from vacuolation around neurons and blood vessels attributable to artifacts of processing. Hence, vacuoles clearly associated with such structures were not counted.

Data Analysis

All data analyses were carried out using STATISTICA Software (Statsoft Inc., Tulsa, OK, USA). Data analysis was carried out using analysis of variance (ANOVA) with subsequent comparisons between brain regions using Fisher's 'protected least significant difference' (PLSD) as a *post-hoc* procedure. First, in the nine FTLD-MND cases alone, the densities of each histological feature in the upper cortical laminae of neocortical regions were compared with those in sectors CA1/2 and the DG using a one-way ANOVA. A similar analysis was then carried out but substituting densities in the lower cortical laminae. Second, densities of each pathological feature in each brain region were compared between three groups of cases, viz. FTLD-MND, sFTLD-TDP, and fFTLD-TDP using one-way ANOVA and Fisher's PLSD as a *post-hoc* procedure.

Neuropathological differences between cases were also studied using PCA. PCA enables the similarity and dissimilarity between the cases to be studied based on their quantitative neuropathological characteristics (Armstrong et al., 2000, Armstrong 2003). Two separate analyses were carried out using the FTLD-TDP cases as variables: (1) PCA-1 was carried out on the nine FTLD-MND cases using all neuropathological features as defining characteristics and (2) PCA-2 was carried out on all 94 cases of FTLD-TDP based on the densities of TDP-43-immunoreactive inclusions alone.

Preliminary analysis of the data suggested a significant degree of skew and kurtosis was present suggesting non-normality. Hence, each PCA was carried out on the raw data and on data transformed to logarithms. Initially, all PC were extracted which had eigenvalues (λ) > 1 but usually in a PCA, only the first two or three PC account for significant proportions of the original variance (Armstrong et al., 2000). The result of each PCA is a scatter plot of the FTLD-TDP cases in relation to the extracted PC in which the distance between cases reflects their similarity or dissimilarity, based on the defining histological features. Such a plot can reveal whether neuropathological variation is continuously distributed or whether discrete clusters of cases are present. Correlations (Pearson's 'r') were calculated between the 'loadings' (the coordinates of the case in relation to the PCs) of each FTLD-TDP case on the PC and demographic and neuropathological variables to determine which features could account best for the distribution of the cases.

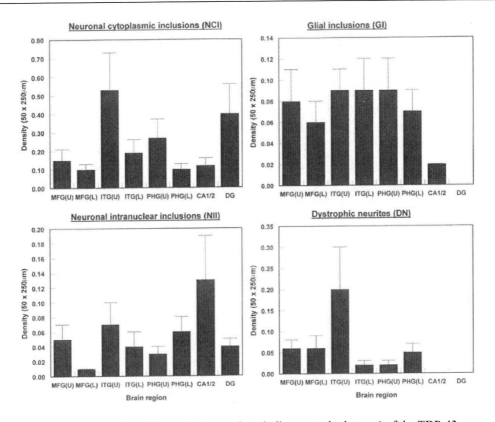

Figure 2. Mean densities (50 x 250μm field, error bars indicate standard errors) of the TDP-43 immunoreactive pathological features in the frontal and temporal lobe (MFG = Middle frontal gyrus, ITG = Inferior temporal gyrus, PHG = Parahippocampal gyrus, CA1/2 = Sectors CA/2 of the hippocampus, DG = Dentate gyrus), U = Upper cortex, L = Lower cortex) of nine cases of frontotemporal lobar dementia with TDP proteinopathy (FTLD-TDP) with associated motor neuron disease (FTLD-MND). Analysis of variance (ANOVA) (1-way) Significant differences only: (1) Comparing upper cortex, NCI: ITG > MFG, NII: HC > PHG. (2) Comparing lower cortex, NCI: DG > MFG, PHG, CA1/2; NII: CA1/2 > MFG.

DENSITIES OF PATHOLOGICAL FEATURES IN FTLD-MND

The densities of the TDP-43-immunoreactive inclusions in each brain region, averaged over the nine FTLD-MND cases, are shown in Figure 2. Moderate densities of NCI were present but densities of GI, NII, and DN were significantly lower.

In the upper cortex, densities of NCI were greater in the ITG compared with the MFG and in the lower cortex, densities of the NCI were greater in the DG than in the MFG, PHG and CA1/2. Apart from the DG, in which no GI were recorded, there were no significant differences in GI density between regions when either the upper cortex or lower cortex data were analyzed. In both the upper and lower cortex, densities of the NII were greater in sectors CA1/2 than in the PHG and MFG respectively. Excluding the DG, there were no significant differences in DN density between brain regions when either the upper cortex data or lower cortex data were included in the analysis.

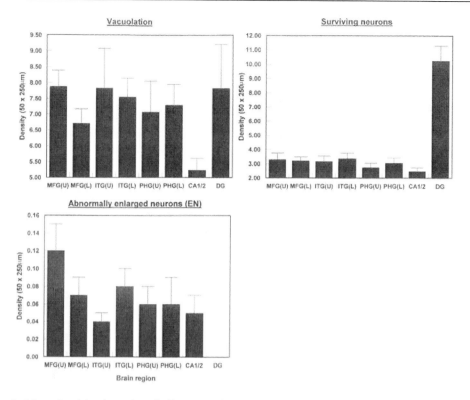

Figure 3. Mean densities (error bars indicate standard errors) of the vacuolation, surviving neurons, and enlarged neurons (EN) in the frontal and temporal lobe (MFG = Middle frontal gyrus, ITG = Inferior temporal gyrus, PHG = Parahippocampal gyrus, CA1/2 = Sectors CA/2 of the hippocampus, DG = Dentate gyrus), U = Upper cortex, L = lower cortex) of nine cases of frontotemporal lobar dementia with TDP proteinopathy (FTLD-TDP) with associated motor neuron disease (FTLD-MND). Analysis of variance (ANOVA) (1-way) Significant differences only: (1) Comparing upper cortex, RN: MFG> ITG,CA1/2, DG; Vacuolation: MFG > ITG,PHG,CA1/2; ITG < CA1/2, DG, DG > CA1/2; (2) Comparing lower cortex, EN: DG < MFG, ITG; Vacuolation: ITG > CA1/2, DG > CA1/2.

The densities of the EN, surviving neurons, and vacuoles in each brain region, averaged over the nine FTLD-MND cases, are shown in Figure 3. When the upper cortex data were analysed, there were significantly lower densities of vacuoles in CA1/2 compared with all other brain regions and when lower cortex data were analyzed, there were significantly lower densities of vacuoles in CA1/2 compared with the ITG and DG. There were significantly greater densities of EN in the MFG compared with the ITG, CA1/2, and DG and in the lower cortex, in the MFG and ITG compared with the DG. Excluding CA1/2 and the DG, there were no significant differences in the densities of surviving neurons between cortical gyri.

The data suggest that the neuropathology of the nine FTLD-MND cases can be characterized by the following features: (1) the presence of moderate numbers of NCI especially in the upper laminae of the ITG and in the DG, (2) generally low densities of GI and NII, although NII may be observed more consistently in sectors CA1/2 of the hippocampus, (3) low densities of DN with the possible exception of the upper laminae of the ITG, (4) extensive vacuolation throughout the superficial laminae of frontal and temporal cortex (Mimura et al., 1998) although with less vacuolation in sectors CA1/2 of the hippocampus, and (5) low densities of EN in all brain regions.

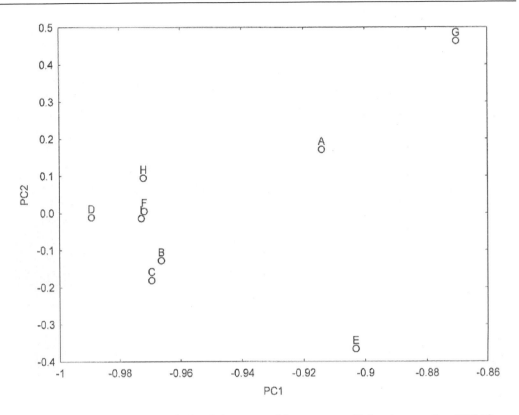

Figure 4. Principal components analysis of nine cases of frontotemporal lobar degeneration (FTLD) with associated motor neuron disease (FTLD-MND) based on all histological features (PCA-1). Correlations between neuropathological variables and PC1: Middle frontal gyrus-upper laminae (MFG-U) r = 0.82 (P < 0.01) surviving neurons r = 0.82 (P < 0.01), Dentate gyrus (DG) r = 0.68 (P < 0.05). There were no significant correlations with PC2.

Previous studies suggest that FTLD-TDP cases lacking MND are associated with a more widespread pattern of atrophy affecting the frontal and temporal lobes while FTLD-MND has more localized frontal lobe atrophy (Josephs et al., 2005). In addition, NCI are frequently present in the DG in FTLD-MND with 66% of cases having NCI in this region compared with 58% in the temporal lobe and 32% in the frontal lobe (Kovari et al., 2004), results consistent with the present data. Relatively few NII have been observed in sFTLD-TDP with associated MND (Woulfe et al., 2001; Bigio et al., 2004) consistent with the present data, but more significant numbers of NII may be observed in fFTLD-TDP with associated MND (Mackenzie and Feldman, 2003). In addition, ubiquitin-immunoreactive neurites have been observed in superficial laminae of the frontal cortex in FTLD-MND and were present in dendritic branches, dendritic spines, and in smooth slender neurites (Tolnay and Probst, 1995). Nevertheless, very few TDP-43-immunoreactive DN were observed in the present cases and hence, this type of neuritic pathology may not be revealed by TDP-43 IHC.

PCA OF THE FTLD-MND CASES BASED ON ALL HISTOLOGICAL FEATURES (PCA-1)

Similar PCA results were obtained using untransformed and transformed data and only the results of the untransformed data are reported. The first two PCs accounted for 93.8% of the total variance (PC1 = 89%, PC2 = 4.8%). Hence, most of the variance was associated with PC1 suggesting the presence of a single 'dominant' defining axis. A plot of the FTLD-MND cases in relation to PC1 and PC2 is shown in Figure 4. Six of the cases cluster towards the left of the plot with the remaining three cases scattered at varying distances from the main cluster. There were no significant correlations between disease onset, duration, age at death, Braak tangle score, or disease subtype with PC1. The density of surviving neurons in the upper cortex of the MFG and the NCI in the DG, however, was positively correlated with PC1. Hence, the data suggest that the nine FTLD-MND cases have a consistent neuropathology, differences in the density of NCI in the DG being the most significant source of variation in TDP-43-immunoreactive pathology between cases.

COMPARISON OF FTLD-MND WITH FAMILIAL AND SPORADIC CASES OF FTLD-TDP

The densities of the various histological features in FTLD-MND compared with familial and sporadic FTLD-TDP without associated MND are shown in Table 2. The density of surviving neurons in the MFG, ITG and DG were significantly lower in FTLD-MND compared with both fFTLD-TDP and sFTLD-TDP (MFG-upper laminae, DG) or compared with fFTLD-TDP only (MFG-lower laminae, ITG-lower laminae).

In addition, there were greater densities of NCI in the upper laminae of the ITG of FTLD-MND compared with fFTLD-TDP and sFTLD-TDP and fewer NII in the lower laminae of the MFG and upper laminae of the PHG in FTLD-MND compared with fFTLD-TDP. The densities of the GI, DN, EN and vacuoles were similar in all regions studied in the FLTD-MND cases compared with FTLD-TDP without associated MND.

Hence, there are considerable quantitative similarities in the neuropathological features of FTLD-TDP cases with and without associated MND, the most noticeable difference being lower densities of surviving neurons and therefore presumably, greater neuronal loss in FTLD-MND. In addition, there is evidence for quantitative variation in TDP-43-immunoreactive pathology in FTLD-TDP with and without MND, but none of these differences were consistent enough to be regarded as characteristic of FTLD-MND. Shi et al. (2005) studied 70 consecutive clinical cases of FTD and found that the pathology was neither highly linked nor pathologically diagnostic of any part of the clinical range of the disease including FTD-MND emphasizing the close relationship between MND and FTLD. The greater neuronal losses in the FTLD-MND cases may reflect the cumulative effect of neuronal losses from both disorders viz., FTLD and MND, and therefore, provide support for the hypothesis that FTLD-MND represents the chance association of both disorders.

Table 2. Mean densities (50 x 250μm field, error bars indicate standard errors) of the histological features (NCI = Neuronal cytoplasmic inclusions, GI = Glial inclusions, NII = Neuronal intranuclear inclusions, DN = Dystrophic neurites, V = vacuolation, SN = surviving neurons, EN = enlarged neurons) in the frontal and temporal lobe (MFG = Middle frontal gyrus, ITG = Inferior temporal gyrus, PHG = Parahippocampal gyrus, CA1/2 = Sectors CA/2 of the hippocampus, DG = Dentate gyrus), U = Upper cortex, L = Lower cortex) of cases of familial and sporadic frontotemporal lobar dementia (fFTLD-TDP and sFTLD-TDP) and cases of FTLD-TDP associated with motor neuron disease (MND)

Region	Group	Histological features						
		NCI	GI	NII	DN	EN	SN	V
MFG-U	fFTLD-TDP	0.21	0.06	0.12	0.35	0.10	4.96	9.92
	sFLTD	0.11	0.05	0.10	0.22	0.06	4.14	9.78
	FTLD-MND	0.15	0.08	0.05	0.06	0.12	3.30	7.88
MFG-L	fFTLD-TDP	0.13	0.05	0.17	0.22	0.07	4.56	7.03
	sFLTD	0.11	0.05	0.12	0.15	0.06	4.23	9.78
	FTLD-MND	0.10	0.06	0.01	0.06	0.07	3.21	6.71
ITG-U	fFTLD-TDP	0.16	0.06	0.10	0.41	0.05	4.99	8.27
	sFLTD	0.18	0.06	0.08	0.28	0.03	4.27	10.12
	FTLD-MND	0.53	0.09	0.07	0.20	0.04	3.17	7.83
ITG-L	fFTLD-TDP	0.11	0.05	0.10	0.14	0.12	4.55	6.99
	sFLTD	0.11	0.06	0.15	0.12	0.09	4.33	8.24
	FTLD-MND	0.19	0.09	0.04	0.02	0.08	3.38	7.55
PHG-U	fFTLD-TDP	0.15	0.06	0.12	0.34	0.07	3.96	8.71
	sFLTD	0.17	0.06	0.07	0.22	0.07	3.96	10.12
	FTLD-MND	0.27	0.09	0.03	0.02	0.06	2.75	7.07
PHG-L	fFTLD-TDP	0.10	0.06	0.15	0.08	0.11	3.87	6.47
	sFLTD	0.12	0.05	0.15	0.12	0.10	3.78	8.45
	FTLD-MND	0.10	0.07	0.06	0.05	0.06	3.06	7.30
CA1/2	fFTLD-TDP	0.08	0.07	0.15	0.11	0.11	2.53	5.71
	sFLTD	0.07	0.04	0.21	0.05	0.12	2.22	6.11
	FTLD-MND	0.12	0.02	0.13	0	0.05	2.48	5.24
DG	fFTLD-TDP	0.23	0	0.06	0.01	0	13.65	7.01
	sFLTD	0.41	0	0.04	0	0	11.56	6.60
	FTLD-MND	0.40	0	0.04	0	0	10.24	7.83

Analysis of variance (ANOVA) (1-way): Significant effects only. MFG-U, SN F = 4.28 ($P < 0.05$), MFG-L, NII F = 3.84 ($P < 0.05$); SN F = 2.70 ($P < 0.05$); ITG-U MNI F = 6.51 ($P < 0.01$), SN F = 4.02 ($P < 0.05$); ITG-L SN F = 2.99 ($P < 0.05$); PHG-U NII F = 2.54 ($P < 0.05$); DG SN F = 6.32 ($P < 001$).

Nevertheless, although FTLD-TDP cases with coexisting MND have the shortest survival times (Kersaitis et al., 2006) the severity of the pathology is the same in FTLD-TDP with or without MND, which is not consistent with this hypothesis.

PCA OF ALL FTLD-TDP CASES BASED ON TDP-43-IMMUNOREACTIVE INCLUSIONS (PCA-2)

The first three PC accounted for 30.35% of the total variance (PC1 =16.98%, PC2 =13.37%, PC3 = 10.51%). A PCA of all FTLD-TDP cases studied in relation to PC1 and PC2 is shown in Figure 5. Cases were scattered uniformly in relation to the extracted PC suggesting that neuropathological variation within this group of cases was continuously distributed. fFTLD-TDP cases were scattered throughout the plot and therefore as a whole did not have a neuropathology distinctly different from that of sFTLD-TDP. By contrast, the FTLD-MND cases cluster towards the upper region of the plot suggesting that they overlap with a specific subgroup of FTLD-TDP cases. Examination of the data suggests that the FTLD-MND cases overlap with FTLD-TDP subtypes 2 and 3. The correlations between neuropathological features and PC1 and PC2 are shown in Table 3. First, the density of NCI in the upper and lower laminae of the ITG and in the DG was negatively correlated with PC1 while the density of NII in the lower laminae of the MFG and the upper laminae of the PHG was positively correlated with PC1. Second, the density of DN in the upper and lower laminae of the MFG, ITG, and PHG was negatively correlated with PC2. In addition, disease duration and disease subtype were negatively correlated with PC2.

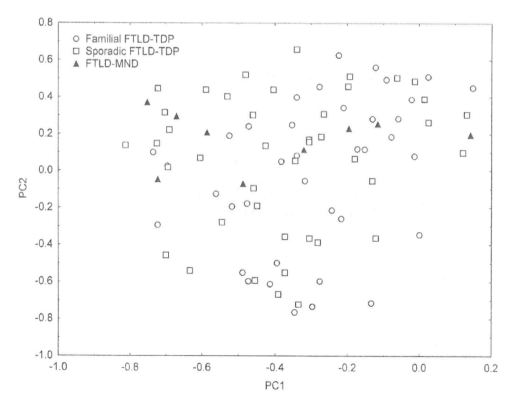

Figure 5. Principal components analysis of all 94 cases of frontotemporal lobar degeneration with TDP-43 proteinopathy (FTLD-TDP) based on TDP-43 pathology only (PCA-2) showing the relationship between cases with associated motor neuron disease (FTLD-MND) and FTLD-TDP as a whole.

Table 3. Correlations (Pearson's 'r') between the pathological features (NCI = neuronal cytoplasmic inclusions, GI = oligodendroglial inclusions, NII = neuronal intranuclear inclusions (NII), DN = dystrophic neurites, EN = abnormally enlarged neurons, N = surviving neurons, V = vacuolation), demographic variables, familial status, and Braak score based on the distribution of neurofibrillary tangles (NFT) and the first three principal components (PC) in various brain regions (MFG = superior frontal cortex, ITG = inferior temporal gyrus, PHG = parahippocampal gyrus, CA1/2 = sectors CA1 and 2 of the hippocampus, DG = dentate gyrus, II/III = laminae II/III, V/VI = laminae V/VI) in cases of frontotemporal lobar degeneration with TDP-43 proteinopathy (FTLD-TDP) (All significant correlations are indicated in bold)

Region	PC	Correlations with PC						
		NCI	GI	NII	DN	EN	SN	V
MFG-U	PC1	-0.16	-0.01	**0.21**	-0.06	-0.02	-0.16	-0.08
	PC2	0.02	-0.12	0.07	**-0.62**	0.02	-0.14	-0.12
MFG-L	PC1	-0.18	-0.11	**0.30**	0.03	-0.08	-0.08	-0.16
	PC2	0.08	-0.12	**0.24**	**-0.41**	0.14	-0.05	-0.17
ITG-U	PC1	**-0.47**	**-0.25**	0.17	**-0.27**	0.11	-0.08	-0.12
	PC2	0.06	0	**0.28**	**-0.68**	-0.02	-0.10	**-0.34**
ITG-L	PC1	**-0.26**	-0.14	0.16	-0.10	0.01	-0.05	0
	PC2	-0.10	**-0.22**	0.16	**-0.64**	0.14	-0.10	**-0.29**
PHG-U	PC1	**-0.51**	-0.18	**0.28**	0.05	0.07	-0.02	0
	PC2	0.19	-0.17	0.18	**-0.44**	0.07	-0.07	**-0.31**
PHG-L	PC1	**-0.27**	**-0.28**	0.12	0.03	0.01	-0.02	0.06
	PC2	-0.05	-0.27	**0.32**	**-0.40**	-0.03	0.07	-0.10
CA1/2	PC1	-0.08	-0.05	0.09	0.13	-0.07	0.03	0.14
	PC2	0.04	-0.19	**0.38**	**-0.29**	-0.15	0.15	-0.02
DG	PC1	**-0.65**	-	0.12	-0.16	0.10	-0.02	-0.16
	PC2	0	-	0.14	-0.05	-0.12	0.01	**-0.29**

Correlations with demographic features: PC2 disease duration r = -0.35 (P < 0.05).

These results suggest that the FLTD-MND cases belong to the spectrum of FTLD-TDP but have a more restricted pathology compared with the FTLD-TDP cases as a whole. FTLD-MND cases appear to segregate within a part of the continuum occupied by FTLD-TDP subtypes 2 and 3, i.e. those cases characterized by numerous NCI in superficial and deep cortical laminae with infrequent DN and sparse or no NII (Type 2), or by pathology predominantly affecting the superficial cortical laminae with numerous NCI, DN, and varying numbers of NII (Type 3). Hence, neuropathologists should be especially vigilant in the diagnosis of potential FTLD-TDP cases that fall within the range of subtypes 2 and 3 as they may overlap extensively with MND.

CONCLUSION

There are considerable similarities in quantitative neuropathology between FTLD-MND and FTLD-TDP cases without associated MND. Nevertheless, there appears to be greater neuronal loss in FTLD-MND compared with FTLD-TDP alone. In addition, there may be greater densities of NCI and lower densities of NII in some brain regions in FTLD-MND. The nine FTLD-MND cases studied have a consistent neuropathology, variations in the densities of surviving neurons in the MFG and NCI in the DG being the major source of variation between cases. In addition, PCA suggests that FTLD-TDP cases as a whole form a 'continuum' and although FTLD-MND forms a part of this continuum, these cases have a more restrictive pathology, cases of FTLD-MND overlapping with those of FTLD-TDP subtypes 2 and 3.

ACKNOWLEDGMENTS

I thank clinical, genetic, pathology, and technical staff of Washington University School of Medicine, St. Louis, MO, University of California, Davis, CA, University of Pittsburgh, Pittsburgh, PA, Vancouver General Hospital, Vancouver, Canada, Harvard Brain Tissue Resource Center, Belmont, MA, Emory University, Atlanta, GA), University of Washington, Seattle, WA, Columbia University, New York, NY, University of California, Irvine, CA, and University of Michigan, Ann Arbor, MI. for making information and tissue samples available for this study and we thank the families of patients whose generosity made this research possible.

REFERENCES

Amandor-Ortiz C, Lin WL, Ahmed Z, Personett D, Davies P, Duara R, Graff-Radford NR, Hutton ML, Dickson DW. TDP-43 immunoreactivity in hippocampal sclerosis and Alzheimer's disease. *Annals of Neurology*, 2007, 61, 435-445.

Armstrong RA. Correlations between the morphology of diffuse and primitive β-amyloid (Aβ) deposits and the frequency of associated cells in Down's syndrome. *Neuropathology and Applied Neurobiology*, 1996, 22, 527-530.

Armstrong RA. Quantifying the pathology of neurodegenerative disorders: quantitative measurements, sampling strategies and data analysis. *Histopathology* 2003, 42, 521-529.

Armstrong RA, Nochlin D, Bird TD. Neuropathological heterogeneity in Alzheimer's disease: A study of 80 cases using principal components analysis. *Neuropathology*, 2000, 20: 31-37.

Armstrong RA, Ellis W, Hamilton RL, Mackenzie IRA, Hedreen J, Gearing M, Montine T, Vonsattel J-P, Head E, Lieberman AP, Cairns NJ. Neuropathological heterogeneity in frontotemporal lobar degeneration with TDP-43 proteinopathy: a quantitative study of 94 cases using principal components analysis. *Journal of Neural Transmission*, 2010, 117: 227-239.

Baker M, Mackenzie IR, Pickering-Brown SM, Gass J, Rademakers R, Lindholm C, Snowden J, Adamson J, Sadovnick AD, Rollinson S, Cannon A, Dwosh E, Neary D, Melquist S, Richardson A, Dickson D, Berger Z, Eriksen J, Robinson T, Zehr C, Dickey CA, Crook R, McGowan E, Mann D, Boeve B, Feldman H, Hutton M. Mutations in progranulin cause tau-negative frontotemporal dementia linked to chromosome 17. *Nature*, 2006, 442, 916-919.

Beck J, Rohrer JD, Campbell T, Isaacs A, Morrison KE, Goodall EF, Warrington EK, Stevens J, Revesz T, Hoton J, Al-Sarraj S, King A, Scabill R, Warren JD, Rossor MN, Collinge J, Mead S. A distinct clinical, neuropsychological and radiological phenotype is associated with progranulin gene mutation in a large UK series. *Brain* 2008, 131, 706-720.

Behrens MI, Mukherjee O, Tu PH, Liscic RM, Grinberg LT, Carter D, Paulsmeyer K, Taylor-Reinwald L, Gitcho M, Norton JB, Chakraverty S, Goate AM, Morris JC, Cairns NJ. Neuropathologic heterogeneity in HDDD1: a familial frontotemporal lobar degeneration with ubiquitin-positive inclusions and progranulin mutation. *Alzheimer's Disease and Associated Disorders,* 2007, 21, 1-7.

Bergmann M, Kuchelmiester K, Schmid KW, Kretzschmar HA, Schroder R. Dtfferent variants of frontotemproal dementia: a neuropathological and immunohistochemical study. *Acta Neuropathologica* 1996, 92, 170-179.

Bigio EH, Lipton AM, White CL, Dickson DW, Hirano A. Frontotemporal dementia and motor neurone degeneration with neurofilament inclusion bodies: additional evidence for overlap between FTD and ALS. *Neuropathology and Applied Neurobiology* 2003, 29, 239-253.

Bigio EH, Johnsan NA, Rademaker AW, Fung BB, Mesulam MM, Siddique N, Dallafave L, Caliendo J, Freeman S, Siddique T. Neuronal ubiquinated intranuclear inclusions in familial and non-familial frontotemporal dementia of the monitor neuron disease type associated with amylotrophic lateral sclerosis. *Journal of Neuropathology and Experimental Neurology* 2004, 63, 801-811.

Braak H, Alafuzoff I, Arzberger T, Kretzschmar H, Del Tredici K. Staging of Alzheimer disease-associated neurofibrillary pathology using paraffin sections and immunocytochemistry. *Acta Neuropathologica*, 2006, 112, 389-404.

Cairns NJ, Neumann M, Bigio EH, Holm IE, Troost D, Hatanpaa KJ, Foong C, White CL III, Schneider JA, Kretzschmar HA, Carter D, Taylor-Reinwald L, Paulsmeyer K, Strider J, Gitcho M, Goate AM, Morris JC, Mishra M, Kwong LK, Steiber A, Xu Y, Forman MS, Trojanowski JQ, Lee VMY, Mackenzie IRA. TDP-43 familial and sporadic frontotemporal lobar degeneration with ubiquitin inclusions. *American Journal of Pathology* 2007a, 171, 227-240.

Cairns NJ, Bigio EH, Mackenzie IRA, Neumann M, Lee VMY, Hatanpaa KJ, White CL, Schneider JA, Grinberg LT, Halliday G, Duyckaerts C, Lowe JS, Holm IE, Tolnay M, Okamoto K, Yokoo H, Murayama S, Woulfe J, Munoz DG, Dickson DW, Ince PG, Trojanowski JQ, Mann DMA. Neuropathologic diagnostic and nosological criteria for frontotemporal lobar degeneration: consensus of the Consortium for Frontotemporal Lobar Degeneration. *Acta Neuropathologica*, 2007b, 114, 5-22.

Cruts M, Gijselink I, van der ZJ, Engelborgs S, Wils H, Pirici D, Radamakers R, Vandenberghe R, Dermaut B, Martin JJ, van Duijn C, Peeters K, Sciot R, Santens P, De pooter T, Mattheijssens M, van den BM, Cuijt I, Vennekens K, De Deyn PP, Kumar-Singh S, Van Broeckhoven C. Null mutations in progranulin cause ubiquitin-positive frontotemporal dementia linked to chromosome 17q21. *Nature* 2006, 442, 920-924.

Davidson Y, Kelley T, Mackenzie IRA, Pickering Brown S, Du Plessis D, Neary D, Snowden JS, Mann DMA. Ubiquinated pathological lesions in frontotemporal lobar degeneration contain TAR DNA-binding protein, TDP-43. *Acta Neuropathologica*, 2007, 113, 521-533.

Forman MS, Trojanowski JQ, Lee VM-Y. Neurodegenerative diseases: a decade of discoveries paves the way for therapeutic breakthroughs. *Nature Med* 2004; **10**: 1055-1063.

Forman MS, Mackenzie IR, Cairns NJ, Swanson E, Boyer PJ, Drachman DA, Jhaveri BS, Karlawish JH, Pestrvik A, Smith TN, Tu PH, Watts GDJ, Markesbery WR, Smith CD, Kimonis VE. Novel ubiquitin neuropathology in frontotemporal dementia with valosin-containing protein gene mutations. *Journal of Neuropathology and Experimental Neurology*, 2006, 65, 571-581.

Garraux G, Salmon E, Degueldre C, Lemaire C, Frank G. medial temporal lobe metabolic impairment in dementia associated with motor neuron disease. *Journal of Neurological Science* 1999, 168, 145-150.

Gentileschi V, Muggia S, Poloni W, Spinner H. Fronto-temporal dementia and motor neuron disease: a neuropsychological study. *Archives of Neurology of Scandanavia* 1999, 100, 341-349.

Grossman M, Wood EM, Moore P, Neumann M, Kwong L, Forman MS, Clark CM, McCluskey LF, Miller BL, Lee VMY, Trojanowski JQ. TDP-43 pathologic lesions and clinical phenotype in frontotemporal lobar degeneration with ubiquitin positive inclusions. *Archives of Neurology,* 2007, 64, 1449-1454.

Hatanpaa KJ, Bigio EH, Cairns NJ, Womack KB, Weintraub S, Morris JC, Foong C, Xiao GH, Hladik C, Mantanona TY, White CL. TAR DNA-binding protein 43 immunohistochemistry reveals extensive neuritic pathology in FTLD-U: A Midwest-Southwest Consortium for FTLD-U study. *Journal of Neuropathology and Experimental Neurology*, 2008, 67, 271-279.

Josephs KA. Frontotemporal dementia and related disorders: Deciphering the enigma. *Annals of Neurology,* 2008, 64, 4-14.

Josephs KA, Knopman DS, Whitwell JL, Boeve BF, Parisi JE, Petersen RC, Dickson DW. Survival in the two variants of tau negative FTLD: FTLD-U versus FTLD-MND. *Neurology*, 2005, 65, 645-647.

Josephs KA, Whitwell JL, Jack CR, Parisi JE, Dickson DW. Frontotemporal lobar degeneration without lobar atrophy. *Archives of Neurology,* 2006, 63, 1632-1638.

Kersaitis C, Holliday GM, Xuereb JH, Pamphlett R, Bak TH, Hodges JR, Kril JJ. Ubiquitin-posiitve inclusions and progression of pathology in FTD and MND identifies a group with mainly early pathology. *Neuropathology and Applied Neurobiology*, 2006, 32, 83-91.

Kovari E, Gold G, Giannakopoulos P, Bouras C. Cortical ubiquitin positive inclusions in frontotemporal dementia without motor neuron disease: a quantitative immunocytochemical study. *Acta Neuropathologica*, 2004, 108, 207-212.

Kwong LK, Neumann M, Sampathu DM, Lee VMY, Trojanowski JQ. TDP-43 proetinopathy: the neuropathology underlying major forms of sporadic and familial frontotemporal lobar degeneration and motor neuron disease. *Acta Neuropathologica* 2007, 114, 63-70.

Lipton AM, White CL, Bigio EH. Frontotemporal lobar degeneration with motor neuron disease-type inclusions predominates in 76 cases of frontotemporal dementia. *Acta Neuropathologica* 2004, 108, 379-385.

Luty AA, Kwok JBJ, Thompson EM, Blumsbergs P, Brooks WS, Loy CT, Dobson-Stone C, Panegyres PK, Hecker J, Nicholson GA, Halliday GM, Schofield PR. Pedigree with frontotemporal lobar degeneration-motor neuron disease and Tar DNA binding protein-43 positive neuropathology: genetic linkage to chromosome 9. *BMC Neurology*, 2008, 8, 32.

Mackenzie IRA, Feldman H. Neuronal intranuclear inclusions distinguish familial FTD-MND type from sporadic cases. *Acta Neuropathologica* 2003, 105, 543-548.

Mackenzie IRA, Baker M, Pickering-Brown S, Hsinng GYR, Lindholm C, Dwosh E, cannon A, Rademakers R, Hutton M, Feldman HH. The neuropathology of frontotemporal lobar degeneration caused by mutations in the progranulin gene. *Brain* 2006a, 129, 3081-3090.

Mackenzie IRA, Baborie A, Pickering-Brown S, Du Plessis D, Jaros E, Perry RH, Neary D, Snowden JS, Mann DMA. Heterogeneity of ubiquitin pathology in frontotemporal lobar degeneration: classification and relation to clinical phenotype. *Acta Neuropathologica*, 2006b, 112, 539-549.

Mackenzie IRA, Neumann M, Bigio EH, Cairns NJ, Alafuzoff I, Kril J, Kovacs GG, Ghetti B, Halliday G, holm IE, Ince PG, Kamphorst W, Revesz T, Rozemuller AJM, Kumar-Singh S, Akiyama H, Baborie A, Spina S, Dickson D, Trojanowski JQ, Mann DMA. Nomenclature for neuropathologic subtypes of frontotemporal degeneration: consensus recommendations. *Acta Neuropathologica*, 2009, 117, 15-18.

Miller BL, Boone K, Geschwind D, Wilheimsen K. Pick's disease and frontotemporal dementias: emerging clinical and molecular concepts. *Neurology* 1999, 5, 205-212.

Mimura M, Tominaga I, Kashima H. Honda M, Kosaka K, Kata Y. Presenile non-Alzheimer dementia with motor neuron disease and laminar spongiform degeneration. *Neuropathology* 1998, 18, 19-26.

Mukherjee O, Pastor P, Cairns NJ, Chakraaverty S, Kauwe JSK, Shears S, Behrens MI, Budde J, Hinrichs AL, Norton J, Levitch D, Taylor-Reinwald L, Gitcho M, Tu PH, Grinberg LT, Liscic RM, Armendariz J, Morris JC, Goate AM. HDDD2 is a familial frontotemporal lobar degeneration with ubiquitin-positive tau-negative inclusions caused by a missense mutation in the signal peptide of progranulin. *Annals of Neurology*, 2006, 60, 314-322.

Neumann M, Igaz LM, Kwong LK, Nakashima-Yasuda H, Kolb SJ, Dreyfuss G, Kretzschmar HA, Trojanowski JQ, Lee VMY. Absence of heterogeneous nuclear riboproteins and survival neuron protein (TDP-43) positive inclusions in frontotemporal lobar degeneration. *Acta Neuropathologica*, 2007, 113, 543-548.

Pirici D, Vandenberghe R, Rademakers R, Dermant B, Cruts M, Vennekens K, Cuijt I, Lubke U, Centerick C, Martin JJ, Van Broeckhoven C, Kumar-Singh S. Characterization of ubiquinated intraneuronal inclusions in a novel Belgian frontotemporal lobar degeneration family. *Journal of Neuropathology and Experimental Neurology* 2006, 65, 289-301.

Rademakers R, Hutton M. The genetics of frontotemporal lobar degeneration. *Current Neurology and Neuroscience Reports,* 2007, 7, 434-442.

Rollinson S, Rizzu P, Sikkink S, Baker M, Halliwell N, Snowden J, Traynor BJ, Ruano D, cairns N, Rohrer JD, Mead S, Collinge J, Rossor M, Akay E, Gueireiro R, Rademakers R, Morrison KE, Pastor P, Alonso E, Martinez-Lage P, Graff-Radford N, Neary D, Henlink P, Mann DMA, Van Swieten J, Pickering-Brown SM. Ubiquitin associated protein 1 is a risk factor for frontotemporal lobar degeneration. *Neurobiology of Aging,* 2009, 30, 656-665.

Sampathu DM, Neumann M, Kwong LK, Chou TT, Micsenyi M, Truax A, Bruce J, Grossman M, Trojanowski JQ, Lee VM. Pathological heterogeneity of frontotemporal lobar degeneration with ubiquitin-positive inclusions delineated by ubiquitin immonohistochemistry and novel monoclonal antibodies. *American Journal of Pathology,* 2006, 189, 1343-1352.

Shi J, Shaw CL Du Plessis, Richardson AMT, Bailey KL, Julien C, Stoppard C, Thompson J, Varma A, Cranford D, Tian JZ, Pickering-Brown S, Neary D, Snowden JS, Mann DMA. Histopathological changes underlying frontotemporal lobar degeneration with clinicopathological correlation. *Acta Neuropathologica* 2005, 110, 501-512.

Snowden J, Neary D, Mann D. Frontotemporal lobar degeneration: clinical and pathological relationships. *Acta Neuropathologica,* 2007, 114, 31-38.

Talbot PR. Frontal lobe dementia and motor neuron disease. *Journal of Neural Transmission (supple.)* 1996, 47, 125-132.

Talbot PR, Goulding PJ, Lloyd JJ, Snowden JS, Neary D, Testa HJ. Interrelation between classic motor neuron disease and fronto-temporal dementia: Neuropsychological and single-photon emission computed-tomography study. *Journal of Neurology, Neurosurgery and Psychiatry.* 1995, 58, 541-547.

Tolnay M, Probst A. Frontal lobe degeneration: Novel ubiquitin-immunoreactive neurites within frontotemporal cortex. *Neuropathology and Applied Neurobiology* 1995, 21, 492-497.

Tolnay M, Probst A. Frontotemporal lobar degeneration- tau as a pied piper? *Neurogenetics,* 2002, 4, 63-75.

Van Deerlin VM, Wood EM, Moore P, Yuan W, Forman MS, Clark CM, Neumann M, Kwong LK, Trojanowski JQ, Lee VMY, Grossman M. Clinical, genetic and pathologic characteristics of patients with frontotemporal dementia and progranulin mutation. *Archives of Neurology* 2007; 64: 1148-1153.

Van Deerlin VM, Sleiman PMA, Martinez-Lage M, Chen-Plotkin A, Wang LS, Graff-Radford NR, Dickson DW, Rademakers R, Boeve BF, Grossman M, Arnold SE, Mann DMA, Pickering-Brown SM, Seelaar H, Heutink P, van Swieten JC, Murrell JR, Ghetti B, Spina S, Grafman J, Hodges J, Spillantini MG, Gilman S, Lieberman AP, Kaye JA, Woltjer RL, Bigio EH, Mesulam M, al-Sarraj S, Troakes C, Rosenberg RN, White CL, Ferrer I, Lado A, Neumann M, Kretzschmar HA, Hulette CM, Welsh-Bohmer KA, Miller BL, Alzualde A, de Munain AL, McKee AC, Gearing M, Levey AI, Lah JJ, Hardy J, Rohrer JD, Lashley T, Mackenzie IRA, Feldman HH, Hamilton RL, Dekosky ST, van der Zee J, Kumar-Singh S, Van Broeckhoven C, Mayeux R, Vonsattel JPG, Troncoso JC,

Kril JJ, Kwok JBJ, Halliday GM, Bird TD, Ince PG, Shaw PJ, Cairns NJ, Morris JC, McLean CA, DeCarli C, Ellis WG, Freeman SH, Frosch MP, Growdon JH, Perl DP, Sano M, Bennett DA, Schneider JA, Beach TG, REiman EM, Woodruff BK, Cummings J, Vinters HV, Miller CA, Chui HC, Alafuzoff I, Hartilainen P, Seilhean D, Galasko D, Masliah E, Cotman CW, Tunon MT, Martinez MCC, Munoz DG, Carroll SL, Marson D, Riederer PF, Bogdanovic N, Schellenberg GD, Hakonarson H, Trajanowski JQ, Lee VMY. Common variants of 7p21 are associated with frontotemporal lobar degeneration with TDP-43 inclusions. *Nature Genetics* 2010; 42: 234-U34.

Van der Zee J, Gyselinck I, Pirici D, Kumar-Singh S, Cruts M, van Broeckhoven C. Frontotemporal lobar degeneration with ubiquitin-positive inclusions: A molecular genetic update. *Neurodegenerative diseases,* 2007, 4, 227-235.

Whitwell JL, Jack CR, Serijeni ML, Josephs KA. Patterns of atrophy in pathologically confirmed FTLD with or without motor neuron degeneration. *Neurology*, 2006, 66, 102-104.

Woulfe J, Kertesz A, Munoz DG. Frontotemporal dementia with ubiquinated cytoplasmic and intranuclear inclusions. *Acta Neuropathologica,* 2001, 102, 94-102.

Yaguchi M, Fujita Y, Amari M, Takatama M, Al-Sarraj S, Leigh PN, Okamoto K. Morphological differences of intraneural ubiquitin positive inclusions in the dentate gyrus and parahippocampal gyrus of motor neuron disease with dementia. *Neuropathology,* 2004, 24, 296-301.

In: Motor Neuron Diseases
Editors: Bradley J. Turner and Julie B. Atkin

ISBN 978-1-61470-101-9
© 2012 Nova Science Publishers, Inc.

Chapter VI

EXCITOTOXICITY AND SELECTIVE MOTOR NEURON DEGENERATION

K. A. Staats[1,2] and L. Van Den Bosch[1,2]
[1]Department of Neurobiology, K.U. Leuven, Belgium
[2]Vesalius Research Center, VIB, Belgium

ABSTRACT

Being a well-establishedand important player in neuronal death, excitotoxicity is a solid basis for understanding selective motor neuron degeneration during amyotrophic lateral sclerosis (ALS). The only available drug for ALS, riluzole, offers patients a moderate increase in survival by targeting this process of excitotoxicity. The overstimulation of glutamate receptors induces calcium influx that leads to detrimental levels of cytosolic calcium, which cause motor neuron loss. Glutamate binds to a number of receptors including the calcium permeable AMPA receptors which facilitate excessive amounts of extracellular calcium to enter the neuron. Glutamate transporters expressed by astrocytes remove this neurotransmitter to limit the effect of glutamate in the synaptic cleft. Interestingly, these processes are impaired or dysregulated in ALS, influencing excitotoxic motor neuron loss. A large number of factors influence excitotoxicity including the inherent characteristics of motor neurons (low intracellular calcium buffering) and their receptors (AMPA receptor subunit combinations), but also their neighbouring cell types, such as astrocytes, play a crucial role. This chapter aims to provide a clear overview of the known players and their interactions and their role in the selective motor neuron loss detected in ALS.

INTRODUCTION

Amyotrophic Lateral Sclerosis (ALS) is a devastating progressive neurodegenerative disease, due to the loss of motor neurons and denervation of muscle fibres, resulting in increasing muscle weakness and paralysis. The disease has an incidence of 2.7 cases per

100,000 people in Europe [1]. It is diagnosed from teen years on, but is more prevalent in the later years of life. In lack of a medical cure, average life expectancy post diagnosis is between 2 and 5 years, but 10% of all patients live longer than 10 years. Patients mainly succumb to the disease by respiratory insufficiency or may opt for euthanasia where legislature permits. Although ALS is characterised by degeneration of central nervous system tissue, mental functions remain largely unaffected resulting in a locked-in state; the patient is mentally conscious while motor function further declines [2]. Regretfully, there is only one medicine on the market today to treat the disease, riluzole, which merely slows disease progression by an estimated 12% [3].

Mutations in the ubiquitously expressed Cu/Zn superoxide dismutase 1 (SOD1) gene are a well known cause of ALS. SOD1 detoxifies potentially cell damaging free radicals and its mutations account for 20% of the ALS patients suffering from the familial variant of the disease (fALS). The remaining 90% of ALS patients suffer from the disease by unknown sporadic origins (sALS), though due to indistinguishable clinical phenotypes a common disease mechanism is hypothesised. Overexpression of mutant forms of human SOD1 causes an ALS phenotype in transgenic mice or rats and this disease model has made a large contribution to ALS research [4]. Many hallmarks of the disease are shared by patients and mice, including specific motor neuron loss, aggregate formation, astrogliosis, microgliosis and progressive paralysis. The progression of the disease in ALS model rodents is divided into three stages, namely a pre-symptomatic stage, a symptomatic stage and end stage. As the genetic ablation of SOD1 does not produce an ALS-like phenotype in mice [5, 6] the mechanism, in which SOD1 causes the disease, is described as a toxic gain of function. This gain of function exerts itself by mechanisms including protein misfolding, aggregation, impaired proteasome functioning, impaired retrograde transport, excitotoxic cell death and many more (reviewed in [7]). Mutations in a number of other genes also cause familial ALS, including mutations in vesicle-associated membrane protein-associated protein B (VAPB), TAR DNA binding protein (TDP-43), fused in sarcoma/translocated in liposarcoma (FUS/TLS), optineurin and valsolin containing protein (VCP) have been identified as causes of familial ALS [8-14], although the frequency of these mutations is unknown. Unfortunately, the discovery of these mutant genes has not yet progressed into useful ALS model organisms, allowing most work described below to have been conducted on mutant SOD1 cells, rodents or on patients (both familial and sporadic).

ALS is a non cell-autonomous disease [15], which means that not only one single cell type is involved in the disease process. By addition or deletion of mutant SOD1 in specific cell types, it is known that a number of cell types can influence the disease, including astrocytes [16], microglia [17], Schwann cells [18] and motor neurons [19]. Although ALS is a non-cell autonomous disease, the cell type that directly leads to the loss of movement are the motor neurons and it is shown that mutant SOD1 expressed solely in this cell type is sufficient to initiate the disease, although disease progression is slow compared to ubiquitous expression of mutant SOD1 [19]. In patients, motor neurons in the motor cortex, brain stem and spinal cord undergo cell death selectively. There are a number of hypotheses that explain this cell type selectivity, including the exceptional long axons of these cells, the large cell soma and the poor intracellular calcium buffering capacity. It is the latter hypothesis that shall be elaborated on in this chapter and motor neuronal vulnerability to excitotoxicity, the only mechanism proved to play a role in patients.

Although neurons are characterised by their ability to stimulate and to be stimulated, overstimulation of neurons can cause neurodegeneration and this mechanism is called excitotoxicity. Neurons communicate with each other by releasing neurotransmitters into the synaptic cleft that bind to receptors on the post synaptic neuron initiating a cascade of reactions allowing the post-synaptic neuron to propagate the signal. In the case of motor neurons, the neurotransmitter is glutamate that binds to the N-methyl D-aspartate (NMDA) or α-amino-3-hydroxy-5-methyl-4-isoxazole proprionic acid (AMPA) receptors, that allows extracellular sodium and/or extracellular calcium to flow into the motor neuron. It is the increased levels of calcium in the cytosol that can eventually cause cell death.

The importance of excitotoxicity in ALS has been deduced from the beneficial effects obtained by treating patients with riluzole. Although the precise working mechanism of this drug is yet unknown, it is reported that this drug inhibits glutamate release by blocking voltage-gated sodium channels [20], blocks AMPA and NMDA receptors and enhances the re-uptake of glutamate from the synaptic cleft, thus preventing the overstimulation of the motor neurons [21]. Administration of riluzole to patients increases their predicted lifespan with a significant 12% [3, 22], but unfortunately does not stop the disease.

A description of the most important players in excitotoxicity, which are glutamate and other excitotoxins, AMPA receptor mediated calcum influx, glutamate re-uptake from the synaptic cleft and their role in selective motor neuron degeneration will be discussed in more detail in the next part of this chapter.

THE INITIAL CULPRIT:
GLUTAMATE AND OTHER EXCITOTOXINS

Glutamate is the neurotransmitter used to excite motor neurons that is the initiator of excitotoxicity in ALS. This neurotransmitter is the most abundant excitatory neurotransmitter in the brain and binds to ionotropic (NMDA, AMPA, kainate) and metabotropic glutamate receptors (mGluR). Packaged into vesicles in the pre-synaptic neuron, glutamate is released into the synaptic cleft by the fusion of vesicles to the membrane of the neuron to excite the post-synaptic neuron.

The amount of glutamate present in the spinal cord of patients, controls and ALS model organisms has been investigated. Increased levels of this neurotransmitter have been detected in familial and sporadic patients compared to controls [23, 24]. This has also been confirmed in spinal cords of ALS model mice and rats, implying its potential role in the disease process.

The detrimental role of glumate in the disease is demonstrated by the pronounced cell death that occurs to primary cultured neurons in vitro when exposed to low levels of glutamate, even as low as physiologically detected in cerebrospinal fluid (CSF) [25]. A further illustration of the negative role of glutamate in ALS is that administration of compounds that block the formation of glutamate in the pre-synaptic neuron increase cell survival, both in vivo and in vitro [25]. Decreasing vesicular glutamate transporter 2 (VGLUT2) extends survival of motor neurons in ALS mice, but did not extend lifespan in vivo of ALS mice [26]. Unfortunately, it is unclear whether the decrease in VGLUT2 in these mice indeed decreased the amount of glutamate in the synaptic cleft.

Although not glutamate itself, a small number of substances have similarly been linked to being excitotoxic and are known to cause motor neuropathies and/or neurodegeneration. To begin, domoic acid has been reported to cause a motor neuropathy in some patients that suffered from food poisoning after consumption of mussels containing high levels of such compound [27]. Domoic acid has also been associated with epileptic seizures in, among other species, humans [28], sea lions [29], rats [30] and lowers the threshold for seizure in adult rats when exposed to it at neonatal stages [31]. Another substance causing excitotoxicity is β-N-oxalyl-amino-L-alanine (BOAA) also known as β-oxalyl-L-α,β-diaminopropionic acid (ODAP). BOAA is highly present in the chickling pea (Lathyrus sativus) of which consumption can cause lathyrism [32, 33]. This substance is an AMPA receptor agonist [34, 35], comparable to glutamate, which can cause motor neuron degeneration [36, 37] and alternative effects on the central nervous system [34, 35]. Another excitotoxic substance is discovered by a high prevalence of ALS on the island of Guam, also known as the Western Pacific amyotrophic lateral sclerosis-parkinsonism dementia, or the amyotrophic lateral sclerosis parkinsonism dementia complex (ALS/PDC). Consumption of cycad seed products (Cycas circinalis) is responsible for the neurodegeneration in ALS/PDC of which β-methylamino-alanine (BMAA) has been identified as a damaging substance [38-40]. BMAA is also a glutamate receptor agonist that is known to cause a motor neuron syndrome [41-43] and damages motor neurons [44], cholinergic neurons in vitro [45, 46] and hippocampal neurons in vivo [47].

THE ACCOMPLICE: AMPA RECEPTORS

Calcium, which causes neuronal death in excitotoxicity, can originate from either the extracellular space or from intracellular stores. As the resting concentration of calcium in the extracellular space is approximately a 3-4 orders of magnitude higher than in the intracellular stores [48] and as more research has been performed on the role of extracellular calcium in ALS, this chapter will focus on the role of extracellular calcium in excitotoxicity.

After the release of glutamate from the pre-synaptic neuron into the synaptic cleft, glutamate binds to NMDA, AMPA, kainate and to the metabotropic receptors. Activation of metabotropic receptors increases intracellular calcium increase by releasing calcium from intracellular stores. Normally, calcium enters through the NMDA receptors, but it is the AMPA receptor that allows extracellular calcium influx into motor neurons, of which high levels will cause neuronal death. Little is known about the role of kainate receptors in excitotoxicity. The AMPA receptor is formed as a tetramer combining, usually pairwise, a combination of its four different subunits (glutamate receptor unit 1-4 (GluR1-4)) [49]. Each subunit can bind glutamate and the channels opens after occupation of at least 2 binding locations [50]. The importance of this receptor in ALS is demonstrated by the ablation of glutamate induced apoptosis in vitro in cortical neurons [25] and motor neurons [51] and in vivo when administering an AMPA receptor antagonist [52].

The AMPA receptor plays an imperative role in excitotoxicity by its calcium permeability that is determined by the incorporation of the GluR2 subunit in the receptor complex. In most conditions, the AMPA receptor complex contains at least one GluR2 subunit and this prevents the influx of extracellular calcium into the neuron [53]. In contrast, receptors lacking the GluR2 subunit are highly calcium permeable [53]. A general decrease of GluR2 is found in the ALS model mice, portraying an increased vulnerability of these mice to excitotoxic insults [54, 55]. The role of GluR2 in ALS is further investigated by genetically ablating GluR2 in ALS mice, which decreases survival in vivo and decreases cell survival in vitro [56]. The opposite has been shown by up-regulating GluR2 expression in motor neurons of ALS mice, as hereby survival is increased [57]. In addition, pharmacological inhibition of the AMPA receptor prolonged survival in ALS model mice [52, 55, 58]. Although the role of AMPA receptors is established, there is no genetic evidence that polymorphisms in the GluR2 gene increase susceptibility to ALS [59].

In view of the crucial role of AMPA receptor composition (as the absence or presence of the GluR2 subunit determines the calcium permeability of the AMPA receptors), it is highly relevant to understand the regulation of this subunit. Interestingly, the surrounding astrocytes influence the expression level of the GluR2 subunit in motor neurons, as soluble factor(s) released from astrocytes affect GluR2 gene expression and neuronal vulnerability to excitotoxic insults, both in vitro and in vivo [60]. Intriguingly, the presence of mutant SOD1 interferes with the production and/or secretion of this factor(s) [60]. Although not all of these influencing factors are known, secreted vascular endothelial growth factor (VEGF), brain-derived neurotrophic factor (BDNF) and glial cell-derived neurotrophic factor (GDNF) are shown to up-regulate GluR2expression [61, 62].

The GluR2 subunit's special characteristic of blocking calcium influx through the AMPA receptor is due to RNA editing at the Q/R site. This editing in the GluR2 pre-mRNA results in the introduction of a positively charged arginine at the Q/R site of the GluR2 peptide instead of the genetically encoded neutral glutamine [63]. Under normal conditions, GluR2 pre-mRNA editing is virtually complete. However, under pathological conditions the editing process could become less efficient resulting in more calcium permeable AMPA receptors. Indeed, evidence exists that the editing of the pre-mRNA of GluR2 is defective in the spinal motor neurons of individuals affected by sporadic ALS [64]. In addition, a decrease of GluR2 gene expression and reduced GluR2 RNA editing was also detected in the ventral spinal cord of ALS patients [65]. Furthermore, the enzyme responsible for the RNA editing, adenosine deaminase acting on RNA 2 (ADAR2), was detected in all motor neurons of controls, but only in 50% of the motor neurons in post mortem tissue from sporadic ALS patients [66]. Reduced editing at the Q/R site of GluR2 in mice results in a lethal phenotype accompanied with seizures and neurodegeneration [67, 68]. Transgenic mice carrying a minigene with the GluR2 gene encoding an asparagine (GluR2-N) at the Q/R site, which makes editing impossible, are viable, fertile [69] and are a useful tool to investigate the effect of calcium permeable AMPA receptors, as AMPA receptors incorporating GluR2-N are always permeable to calcium [63]. The combined expression of the GluR2-N transgene and endogenous GluR2 alleles result in a twofold increase in permeability for calcium in these mice [70]. Interestingly, these transgenic mice develop motor neuron degeneration late in life [70] and GluR2-N overexpression induces a progressive decline in function, as well as a degeneration of spinal motor neurons [69]. In accordance to the previously described results, GluR2-N expression in ALS mice exacerbates disease progression and reduces survival confirming the role for edited GluR2 in ALS [69]. A similar approach was taken by Hideyama et al. who conditionally knocked down ADAR2 in motor neurons. These mice also develop a late onset neurodegenerative condition [71].

THE CLEANERS: GLUTAMATE TRANSPORTERS

After glutamate release from the pre-synaptic neuron and binding of this neurotransmitter to ionotropic or metabotropic receptors on the post-synaptic neuron (leading to depolarisation and increase in the concentration of intracellular calcium), glutamate is recycled for further use by the glial and endothelial cells, including astrocytes. As these star-shaped supportive cells are localised perisynaptically in the spinal cord, this chapter shall focus on their role in glutamate re-uptake. Astrocytic glutamate re-uptake occurs by the glutamate transporters: excitatory amino acid transporter 1 (EAAT1) and excitatory amino acid transporter 2 (EAAT2; also known as glutamate aspartate transporter (GLAST1) and glutamate transporter 1 (GLT-1) in rodents, respectively, but in this chapter only EAAT2 will be used for both human and rodent forms). These transporters internalise glutamate, e.g. into the astrocyte, for conversion to glutamine which is secreted and taken up by the neurons. In the neuron, glutamine is converted to glutamate and concentrated in presynaptic vesicles [72].

Decreased levels of glutamate uptake and lower EAAT2 protein are common features in both sporadic and familial ALS and model systems, both in vitro and in vivo [73]. In vitro transfection of primary cultured astrocytes with either mutant SOD1 or wild type human SOD1 down-regulates EAAT2 post transcriptionally [74], although it was not investigated whether this down-regulation of EAAT2 affected neuronal survival in vitro. Decreased glutamate transport was also detected in SH-SY5Y cells after mutant SOD1 transfection [75]. Interestingly, this down-regulation was also found in ALS model rats at pre-symptomatic stages through to end stage [76], at end stage only [77], in ALS model mice at end stage [78] and in post mortem patient spinal cords by staining for EAAT2 [79]. In addition, the loss of EAAT2 and decreased tissue glutamate transport does not coincide with decreased levels of gene expression in patient material [80], indicating that the loss is induced post transcriptionally, also in humans. Moreover, the decreased ability of re-uptake of glutamate in ALS patients has also been confirmed in platelets [81], although other groups were unable to confirm these results [82]. Interestingly, a decrease of EAAT2 protein levels was not only found in the mutant SOD1 mouse model, but was also found in an environmental model of ALS/PDC (wild-type mice fed with washed cycad flour containing BMAA, which causes an ALS-like phenotype [40]) [83]. Although the loss of EAAT2 in ALS is apparent, it remains unclear whether this loss of EAAT2 proceeds or follows the loss of motor neurons.

To assess whether the loss of glutamate transport or the loss of EAAT2 specifically results in motor neuron loss, pharmacological and genetic tools have been employed. To begin, research conducted by pharmacological inhibition of glutamate transport in the rat spinal cord, failed to show any motor neuron loss despite the increased levels of glutamate [84]. This experiment has not (yet) been performed in ALS mice, leaving it to be elucidated if decreased glutamate transport negatively affects motor neuron survival in ALS. In contrast, a similar experiment has been performed to address whether EAAT2 loss specifically would induce motor neuron loss. EAAT2 null mice have been generated that live for approximately 6 weeks before they succumb to epileptic seizures and show increased vulnerability to acute brain injury [85]. The heterozygous mice (containing 1 allele of EAAT2) were used as a tool to assess the effect of approximately 40% knockdown of EAAT2 in the spinal cord in ALS mice [86]. This knockdown results in a non-significant decrease of symptom onset and significant, but moderate, decrease of lifespan in ALS mice [86].

To assess the expected beneficial role of EAAT2 in ALS, transgenic mice overexpressing human EAAT2 in astrocytes only were crossbred with mutant SOD1 mice. Glutamate uptake was increased in these mice and protected primary cortical neurons in culture. Despite these effects, there was no significant effect on symptom onset or lifespan [87]. Possibly, the expression levels were too low to induce an effect or human EAAT2 is not as efficient as murine EAAT2 in mouse, as administration of ceftriaxone (a β-lactam antibiotic) and GPI-1046 (a synthetic, non-immunosuppressive derivative of FK506) increases EAAT2 protein levels and significantly extends lifespan of ALS mice [88, 89]. In addition, EAAT2 is also expressed by other cells types than astrocytes alone [90], which were not targeted with this genetic experimental design.

The beneficial effect of EAAT2 is often used as an explanation of beneficial effects found by cell transfer in ALS model rodents. For instance, the systemic transplantation of c-kit positive cells from bone marrow in mutant SOD1 mice significantly increases the lifespan, which is, at least in part, attributed to increased EAAT2 expression induced by the transferred cells [91]. The same holds true for the prolonged survival of ALS rats when treated with focal transplantation-based astrocyte replacement with wild type glial-restricted precursors (GRPs) [92]. Interestingly, this study also focussed on the precise role of EAAT2 by also transplanting EAAT2 overexpressing GRPs and EAAT2 null GRPs. The ALS mice treated with the EAAT2 overexpressing GRPs showed no additional increase of lifespan compared to wild type GRP treated ALS mice (which is already increased compared to controls). Intriguingly, this positive effect of transplantation of the wild type GRPs is diminished in mice transplanted with EAAT2 null GRPs [92]. In addition, co-culturing of human adipose-derived stem cells with astrocytes induces higher levels of EAAT2 in the astrocytes [93], although this treatment has not (yet) been shown to affect motor neuron survival in vitro or in vivo.

THE VICTIM: MOTOR NEURONS

Within ALS, the motor neurons specifically degenerate, both in patients and in ALS models based on an ubiquitous overexpression of mutant SOD1 [94]. A number of different reasons for this have been proposed varying from vulnerability due to the very long axons, to the large cell soma and to vulnerability to excitotoxic insults. It is the latter which is of interest in this chapter.

As discussed previously in this chapter, motor neurons are excited by glutamate from the pre-synaptic neuron that binds to glutamate receptors on the post synaptic motor neuron, which are, among others, the AMPA receptors. Interestingly, the AMPA receptors found on motor neurons are mainly calcium permeable in vitro [51, 95, 96], which may explain the selective vulnerability of motor neurons to excitotoxic cell death. In addition, extracellular calcium entry via these calcium permeable AMPA receptors is responsible for selective motor neuron death, as motor neuron death is inhibited by selective blockers of calcium permeable AMPA receptors [95]. Also electrophysiological experiments showed that AMPA receptors of motor neurons had a lower rectification index and a higher relative calcium permeability ratio than other neurons [97]. Not only in vitro, but also in vivo it has been demonstrated that motor neurons express calcium permeable AMPA receptors [98]. Interestingly, the increased vulnerability of motor neurons in comparison to other cell types in vivo has been shown by infusing the spinal cord of wild type rats with AMPA receptor agonists [99, 100]. This experiment induced specific neurodegeneration of motor neurons and paralysis, which was blocked by co-administration of a selective blocker of calcium permeable AMPA receptors [99, 100]. Moreover, also the above described combination of subunits that is responsible for the calcium permeability of AMPA receptors (AMPA receptors lacking the GluR2 subunit) is specific for motor neurons. Wild type murine spinal cords contain significantly lower levels of GluR2 mRNA in motor neurons compared to other neurons [97]. In addition, laser capture microscopy and quantitative PCR demonstrated that the expression level of the GluR2 subunit was lower in (human) spinal motor neurons compared to other neurons [101, 102]. In conclusion, motor neurons express calcium permeable AMPA receptors, which could (partially) explain their pronounced and selective vulnerability to excitotoxic insults.

An additional explanation for selective motor neuron vulnerability is the capability this cell type has to deal with the increased amount of intracellular calcium. Studies into the calcium homeostasis in motor neurons have shown a diminished calcium buffering capacity distinguishing ALS-vulnerable from resistant motor neuron types. To begin, ALS-vulnerable spinal and brain stem motor neurons in mice display a low endogenous calcium buffering capacity as demonstrated by patch clamp and microfluorometirc calcium measurements [103, 104]. In addition, ALS-resistant oculomotor neurons contain a larger calcium buffering capacity than ALS-vulnerable motor neurons, as measured by similar microfluorometirc calcium measurements [105]. Others have shown that this difference in calcium buffering capacity is directly due to the differential expression levels of the calcium binding proteins calbindin-D28k and parvalbumin [106]. The beneficial effect of calcium buffering by calcium binding proteins is shown by experiments of acute neurodegeneration in a mouse overexpressing the calcium binding protein parvalbumin [107]. According to expectations, parvalbumin overexpressing cells are protected against neurodegeneration induced by axotomy in vivo [107].

CONCLUSION

This chapter summarises the current basic knowledge in the field of excitotoxicity and how this has been implemented and studied in ALS patients and ALS model organisms. This began at the detected heightened levels of glutamate in (patient) spinal cords. In addition, the dysregulation is shown for AMPA receptor formation rendering these channels calcium permeable by GluR2 subunit exclusion by inefficient pre-RNA editing. Furthermore, the re-uptake of glutamate to protect the motor neurons in ALS is decreased. These findings may also explain the selective motor neuron death in ALS on basis of motor neuron calcium permeable AMPA receptors and the cell's limited capacity of calcium buffering. Future directions of research may include pharmacologically targeting the mechanism of excitotoxicity as this mechanism plays an important role in ALS.

REFERENCES

[1] Logroscino, G., et al., Incidence of amyotrophic lateral sclerosis in Europe. *J. Neurol. Neurosurg Psychiatry*, **81**(4): p. 385-90.

[2] Kotchoubey, B., et al., Cognitive processing in completely paralyzed patients with amyotrophic lateral sclerosis. *Eur. J. Neurol.*, 2003. 10(5): p. 551-8.

[3] Bensimon, G., L. Lacomblez, and V. Meininger, A controlled trial of riluzole in amyotrophic lateral sclerosis. ALS/Riluzole Study Group. *N. Engl. J. Med.*, 1994. 330(9): p. 585-591.

[4] Gurney, M.E., et al., Motor neuron degeneration in mice that express a human Cu,Zn superoxide dismutase mutation. *Science*, 1994. 264(5166): p. 1772-1775.

[5] Reaume, A.G., et al., Motor neurons in Cu/Zn superoxide dismutase-deficient mice develop normally but exhibit enhanced cell death after axonal injury. *Nat. Genet*, 1996. 13(1): p. 43-47.

[6] Shefner, J.M., et al., Mice lacking cytosolic copper/zinc superoxide dismutase display a distinctive motor axonopathy. *Neurology*, 1999. 53(6): p. 1239-46.

[7] Bruijn, L.I., T.M. Miller, and D.W. Cleveland, Unraveling the mechanisms involved in motor neuron degeneration in ALS. *Annu. Rev. Neurosci.*, 2004. 27: p. 723-49.

[8] Van Deerlin, V.M., et al., TARDBP mutations in amyotrophic lateral sclerosis with TDP-43 neuropathology: a genetic and histopathological analysis. *Lancet Neurol*, 2008.

[9] Rutherford, N.J., et al., Novel mutations in TARDBP (TDP-43) in patients with familial amyotrophic lateral sclerosis. *PLoS Genet*, 2008. 4(9): p. e1000193.

[10] Del Bo, R., et al., TARDBP (TDP-43) sequence analysis in patients with familial and sporadic ALS: identification of two novel mutations. *Eur. J. Neurol.*, 2009. 16(6): p. 727-32.

[11] Kwiatkowski, T.J., Jr., et al., Mutations in the FUS/TLS gene on chromosome 16 cause familial amyotrophic lateral sclerosis. *Science*, 2009. 323(5918): p. 1205-8.

[12] Vance, C., et al., Mutations in FUS, an RNA processing protein, cause familial amyotrophic lateral sclerosis type 6. *Science*, 2009. 323(5918): p. 1208-11.

[13] Maruyama, H., et al., Mutations of optineurin in amyotrophic lateral sclerosis. *Nature*. 465(7295): p. 223-6.

[14] Johnson, J.O., et al., Exome sequencing reveals VCP mutations as a cause of familial ALS. *Neuron*. 68(5): p. 857-64.

[15] Boillée, S., C. Vande Velde, and D.W. Cleveland, ALS: a disease of motor neurons and their nonneuronal neighbors. *Neuron*, 2006. 52(1): p. 39-59.

[16] Yamanaka, K., et al., Astrocytes as determinants of disease progression in inherited amyotrophic lateral sclerosis. *Nat. Neurosci.*, 2008. 11(3): p. 251-253.

[17] Boillée, S., et al., Onset and progression in inherited ALS determined by motor neurons and microglia. *Science*, 2006. 312(5778): p. 1389-92.

[18] Lobsiger, C.S., et al., Schwann cells expressing dismutase active mutant SOD1 unexpectedly slow disease progression in ALS mice. *Proc. Natl. Acad. Sci. USA*, 2009. 106(11): p. 4465-70.

[19] Jaarsma, D., et al., Neuron-specific expression of mutant superoxide dismutase is sufficient to induce amyotrophic lateral sclerosis in transgenic mice. *J. Neurosci.*, 2008. 28(9): p. 2075-88.

[20] Siniscalchi, A., et al., Neuroprotective effects of riluzole: an electrophysiological and histological analysis in an in vitro model of ischemia. *Synapse*, 1999. 32(3): p. 147-52.

[21] Liu, A.Y., et al., Neuroprotective drug riluzole amplifies the heat shock factor 1 (HSF1)- and glutamate transporter 1 (GLT1)-dependent cytoprotective mechanisms for neuronal survival. *J. Biol. Chem.* 286(4): p. 2785-94.

[22] Lacomblez, L., et al., Dose-ranging study of riluzole in amyotrophic lateral sclerosis. Amyotrophic Lateral Sclerosis/Riluzole Study Group II. *Lancet*, 1996. 347(9013): p. 1425-1431.

[23] Fiszman, M.L., et al., In vitro neurotoxic properties and excitatory aminoacids concentration in the cerebrospinal fluid of amyotrophic lateral sclerosis patients. Relationship with the degree of certainty of disease diagnoses. *Acta Neurol. Scand.* 121(2): p. 120-6.

[24] Spreux-Varoquaux, O., et al., Glutamate levels in cerebrospinal fluid in amyotrophic lateral sclerosis: a reappraisal using a new HPLC method with coulometric detection in a large cohort of patients. *J. Neurol. Sci.*, 2002. 193(2): p. 73-8.

[25] Cid, C., et al., Low concentrations of glutamate induce apoptosis in cultured neurons: implications for amyotrophic lateral sclerosis. *J. Neurol. Sci.*, 2003. 206(1): p. 91-5.

[26] Wootz, H., et al., Reduced VGLUT2 expression increases motor neuron viability in Sod1(G93A) mice. *Neurobiol. Dis.* 37(1): p. 58-66.

[27] Debonnel, G., L. Beauchesne, and C. de Montigny, Domoic acid, the alleged "mussel toxin," might produce its neurotoxic effect through kainate receptor activation: an electrophysiological study in the dorsal hippocampus. *Can. J. Physiol. Pharmacol,* 1989. 67(1): p. 29-33.

[28] Teitelbaum, J.S., et al., Neurologic sequelae of domoic acid intoxication due to the ingestion of contaminated mussels. *N. Engl. J. Med.*, 1990. 322(25): p. 1781-7.

[29] Scholin, C.A., et al., Mortality of sea lions along the central California coast linked to a toxic diatom bloom. *Nature*, 2000. 403(6765): p. 80-4.

[30] Muha, N. and J.S. Ramsdell, Domoic acid induced seizures progress to a chronic state of epilepsy in rats. *Toxicon.* 57(1): p. 168-71.

[31] Gill, D.A., et al., Neonatal exposure to low-dose domoic acid lowers seizure threshold in adult rats. *Neuroscience.* 169(4): p. 1789-99.

[32] Streifler, M. and D.F. Cohn, Chronic central nervous system toxicity of the chickling pea (Lathyrus sativus). *Clin. Toxicol.*, 1981. 18(12): p. 1513-7.

[33] Spencer, P.S., et al., Lathyrism: evidence for role of the neuroexcitatory aminoacid BOAA. *Lancet*, 1986. 2(8515): p. 1066-7.

[34] Willis, C.L., et al., Neuroprotective effect of free radical scavengers on beta-N-oxalylamino-L-alanine (BOAA)-induced neuronal damage in rat hippocampus. *Neurosci. Lett.,* 1994. 182(2): p. 159-62.

[35] Kunig, G., et al., Excitotoxins L-beta-oxalyl-amino-alanine (L-BOAA) and 3,4,6-trihydroxyphenylalanine (6-OH-DOPA) inhibit [3H] alpha-amino-3- hydroxy-5-methyl-4-isoxazole-propionic acid (AMPA) binding in human hippocampus. *Neurosci. Lett*, 1994. 169(1-2): p. 219-22.

[36] Chase, R.A., et al., Comparative toxicities of alpha- and beta-N-oxalyl-L-alpha, beta-diaminopropionic acids to rat spinal cord. *Neurosci. Lett.*, 1985. 55(1): p. 89-94.

[37] Weiss, J.H., J.Y. Koh, and D.W. Choi, Neurotoxicity of beta-N-methylamino-L-alanine (BMAA) and beta-N-oxalylamino-L-alanine (BOAA) on cultured cortical neurons. *Brain Res.*, 1989. 497(1): p. 64-71.

[38] Steele, J.C. and T. Guzman, Observations about amyotrophic lateral sclerosis and the parkinsonism-dementia complex of Guam with regard to epidemiology and etiology. *Can. J. Neurol. Sci.*, 1987. 14(3 Suppl): p. 358-62.

[39] Hudson, A.J., Amyotrophic lateral sclerosis/parkinsonism/dementia: clinico-pathological correlations relevant to Guamanian ALS/PD. *Can. J. Neurol. Sci.*, 1991. 18(3 Suppl): p. 387-9.

[40] Wilson, J.M., et al., Behavioral and neurological correlates of ALS-parkinsonism dementia complex in adult mice fed washed cycad flour. *Neuromolecular Med.*, 2002. 1(3): p. 207-21.

[41] Murch, S.J., et al., Occurrence of beta-methylamino-l-alanine (BMAA) in ALS/PDC patients from Guam. *Acta Neurol. Scand*, 2004. 110(4): p. 267-9.

[42] Chang, Y.C., S.J. Chiu, and K.P. Kao, beta-N-methylamino-L-alanine (L-BMAA) decreases brain glutamate receptor number and induces behavioral changes in rats. *Chin J. Physiol.*, 1993. 36(2): p. 79-84.

[43] Purdie, E.L., et al., Effects of the cyanobacterial neurotoxin beta-N-methylamino-L-alanine on the early-life stage development of zebrafish (Danio rerio). *Aquat Toxicol*, 2009. 95(4): p. 279-84.

[44] Rao, S.D., et al., BMAA selectively injures motor neurons via AMPA/kainate receptor activation. *Exp. Neurol.*, 2006. 201(1): p. 244-52.

[45] Liu, X.Q., et al., Selective death of cholinergic neurons induced by beta-methylamino-L-alanine. *Neuroreport.* 21(1): p. 55-8.

[46] Brownson, D.M., T.J. Mabry, and S.W. Leslie, The cycad neurotoxic amino acid, beta-N-methylamino-L-alanine (BMAA), elevates intracellular calcium levels in dissociated rat brain cells. *J. Ethnopharmacol.*, 2002. 82(2-3): p. 159-67.

[47] Buenz, E.J. and C.L. Howe, Beta-methylamino-alanine (BMAA) injures hippocampal neurons in vivo. *Neurotoxicology*, 2007. 28(3): p. 702-4.

[48] Foskett, J.K., et al., Inositol trisphosphate receptor Ca^{2+} release channels. *Physiol. Rev.*, 2007. 87(2): p. 593-658.

[49] Shi, S.H., et al., Rapid spine delivery and redistribution of AMPA receptors after synaptic NMDA receptor activation. *Science,* 1999. 284(5421): p. 1811-6.

[50] Mayer, M.L., Glutamate receptor ion channels. *Curr. Opin. Neurobiol.*, 2005. 15(3): p. 282-8.

[51] Carriedo, S.G., H.Z. Yin, and J.H. Weiss, Motor neurons are selectively vulnerable to AMPA/kainate receptor- mediated injury in vitro. *J. Neurosci.*, 1996. 16(13): p. 4069-4079.

[52] Van Damme, P., et al., The AMPA receptor antagonist NBQX prolongs survival in a transgenic mouse model of amyotrophic lateral sclerosis. *Neurosci. Lett.*, 2003. 343(2): p. 81-84.

[53] Seeburg, P.H., et al., Genetic manipulation of key determinants of ion flow in glutamate receptor channels in the mouse. *Brain Res.*, 2001. 907(1-2): p. 233-43.

[54] Zhao, P., et al., Altered presymptomatic AMPA and cannabinoid receptor trafficking in motor neurons of ALS model mice: implications for excitotoxicity. *Eur. J. Neurosci.*, 2008. 27(3): p. 572-9.

[55]   Tortarolo, M., et al., Glutamate AMPA receptors change in motor neurons of SOD1(G93A) transgenic mice and their inhibition by a noncompetitive antagonist ameliorates the progression of amytrophic lateral sclerosis-like disease. *J. Neurosci. Res.*, 2006. 83(1): p. 134-46.

[56]   Van Damme, P., et al., GluR2 deficiency accelerates motor neuron degeneration in a mouse model of amyotrophic lateral sclerosis. *J. Neuropathol. Exp. Neurol.*, 2005. 64: p. 605-612.

[57]   Tateno, M., et al., GluR2 overexpression in motor neurons renders AMPA receptors impermeable to calcium and delays disease onset in an ALS transgenic mouse model. *Soc. for Neurosci. Abstr.*, 2002. 789.21.

[58]   Canton, T., et al., RPR 119990, a novel a-amino-3-hydroxy-5-methyl-4-isoxazolepropionic acid antagonist: synthesis, pharmacological properties, and activity in an animal model of amyotrophic lateral sclerosis. *J. Pharmacol. Exp. Ther.*, 2001. 299(1): p. 314-322.

[59]   Bogaert, E., et al., Polymorphisms in the GluR2 gene are not associated with amyotrophic lateral sclerosis. *Neurobiol Aging.* 2010.doi:10.1016/j.neurobiolaging. 2010.03.007

[60]   Van Damme, P., et al., Astrocytes regulate GluR2 expression in motor neurons and their vulnerability to excitotoxicity. *Proc. Natl. Acad. Sci. USA*, 2007. 104(37): p. 14825-30.

[61]   Bogaert, E., et al., VEGF protects motor neurons against excitotoxicity by upregulation of GluR2 *Neurobiol Aging*, 2010. 31(12):p. 2185-91.

[62]   Brene, S., et al., Regulation of GluR2 promoter activity by neurotrophic factors via a neuron-restrictive silencer element. *Eur. J. Neurosci.*, 2000. 12(5): p. 1525-1533.

[63]   Burnashev, N., et al., Divalent ion permeability of AMPA receptor channels is dominated by the edited form of a single subunit. *Neuron*, 1992. 8(1): p. 189-198.

[64]   Kawahara, Y., et al., Glutamate receptors: RNA editing and death of motor neurons. *Nature*, 2004. 427(6977): p. 801.

[65]   Takuma, H., et al., Reduction of GluR2 RNA editing, a molecular change that increases calcium influx through AMPA receptors, selective in the spinal ventral gray of patients with amyotrophic lateral sclerosis. *Ann. Neurol.*, 1999. 46(6): p. 806-815.

[66]   Aizawa, H., et al., TDP-43 pathology in sporadic ALS occurs in motor neurons lacking the RNA editing enzyme ADAR2. *Acta Neuropathol.* 120(1): p. 75-84.

[67]   Brusa, R., et al., Early-onset epilepsy and postnatal lethality associated with an editing-deficient GluR-B allele in mice. *Science*, 1995. 270(5242): p. 1677-80.

[68]   Higuchi, M., et al., Point mutation in an AMPA receptor gene rescues lethality in mice deficient in the RNA-editing enzyme ADAR2. *Nature*, 2000. 406(6791): p. 78-81.

[69]   Kuner, R., et al., Late-onset motoneuron disease caused by a functionally modified AMPA receptor subunit. *Proc. Natl. Acad. Sci. USA*, 2005. 102(16): p. 5826-31.

[70]   Feldmeyer, D., et al., Neurological dysfunctions in mice expressing different levels of the Q/R site-unedited AMPAR subunit GluR-B. *Nat. Neurosci*, 1999. 2(1): p. 57-64.

[71]   Hideyama, T., et al., Induced loss of ADAR2 engenders slow death of motor neurons from Q/R site-unedited GluR2. *J. Neurosci.* 30(36): p. 11917-25.

[72]   Laake, J.H., et al., Glutamine from glial cells is essential for the maintenance of the nerve terminal pool of glutamate: immunogold evidence from hippocampal slice cultures. *J. Neurochem.*, 1995. 65(2): p. 871-81.

[73] Staats, K.A. and L. Van Den Bosch, Astrocytes in amyotrophic lateral sclerosis: direct effects on motor neuron survival. *J. Biol. Phys.*, 2009. 35(4): p. 337-46.

[74] Tortarolo, M., et al., Expression of SOD1 G93A or wild-type SOD1 in primary cultures of astrocytes down-regulates the glutamate transporter GLT-1: lack of involvement of oxidative stress. *J. Neurochem.*, 2004. 88(2): p. 481-93.

[75] Sala, G., et al., Impairment of glutamate transport and increased vulnerability to oxidative stress in neuroblastoma SH-SY5Y cells expressing a Cu,Zn superoxide dismutase typical of familial amyotrophic lateral sclerosis. *Neurochem. Int.,* 2005. 46(3): p. 227-34.

[76] Howland, D.S., et al., Focal loss of the glutamate transporter EAAT2 in a transgenic rat model of SOD1 mutant-mediated amyotrophic lateral sclerosis (ALS). *Proc. Natl. Acad. Sci. USA*, 2002. 99(3): p. 1604-1609.

[77] Warita, H., et al., Tardive decrease of astrocytic glutamate transporter protein in transgenic mice with ALS-linked mutant SOD1. *Neurol. Res.*, 2002. 24(6): p. 577-81.

[78] Bendotti, C., et al., Transgenic SOD1 G93A mice develop reduced GLT-1 in spinal cord without alterations in cerebrospinal fluid glutamate levels. *J. Neurochem.*, 2001. 79(4): p. 737-746.

[79] Sasaki, S., et al., EAAT1 and EAAT2 immunoreactivity in transgenic mice with a G93A mutant SOD1 gene. *Neuroreport*, 2001. 12(7): p. 1359-1362.

[80] Bristol, L.A. and J.D. Rothstein, Glutamate transporter gene expression in amyotrophic lateral sclerosis motor cortex. *Ann. Neurol.*, 1996. 39(5): p. 676-679.

[81] Ferrarese, C., et al., Decreased platelet glutamate uptake in patients with amyotrophic lateral sclerosis. *Neurology,* 2001. 56(2): p. 270-2.

[82] Bos, I.W., et al., Increased glutamine synthetase but normal EAAT2 expression in platelets of ALS patients. *Neurochem. Int*, 2006. 48(4): p. 306-11.

[83] Wilson, J.M., et al., Decrease in glial glutamate transporter variants and excitatory amino acid receptor down-regulation in a murine model of ALS-PDC. *Neuromolecular Med.*, 2003. 3(2): p. 105-18.

[84] Tovar, Y.R.L.B., et al., Chronic elevation of extracellular glutamate due to transport blockade is innocuous for spinal motoneurons in vivo. *Neurochem. Int.,* 2009. 54(3-4): p. 186-91.

[85] Tanaka, K., et al., Epilepsy and exacerbation of brain injury in mice lacking the glutamate transporter GLT-1. *Science,* 1997. 276(5319): p. 1699-702.

[86] Pardo, A.C., et al., Loss of the astrocyte glutamate transporter GLT1 modifies disease in SOD1(G93A) mice. *Exp. Neurol.*, 2006. 201(1): p. 120-30.

[87] Guo, H., et al., Increased expression of the glial glutamate transporter EAAT2 modulates excitotoxicity and delays the onset but not the outcome of ALS in mice. *Hum. Mol. Genet.*, 2003. 12(19): p. 2519-2532.

[88] Ganel, R., et al., Selective up-regulation of the glial Na+-dependent glutamate transporter GLT1 by a neuroimmunophilin ligand results in neuroprotection. *Neurobiol. Dis.*, 2006. 21(3): p. 556-67.

[89] Rothstein, J.D., et al., Beta-lactam antibiotics offer neuroprotection by increasing glutamate transporter expression. *Nature*, 2005. 433(7021): p. 73-7.

[90] Anderson, C.M. and R.A. Swanson, Astrocyte glutamate transport: review of properties, regulation, and physiological functions. *Glia,* 2000. 32(1): p. 1-14.

[91] Corti, S., et al., Systemic transplantation of c-kit+ cells exerts a therapeutic effect in a model of amyotrophic lateral sclerosis. *Hum. Mol. Genet.* 19(19): p. 3782-96.

[92] Lepore, A.C., et al., Focal transplantation-based astrocyte replacement is neuroprotective in a model of motor neuron disease. *Nat. Neurosci.*, 2008. 11(11): p. 1294-301.

[93] Gu, R., et al., Human adipose-derived stem cells enhance the glutamate uptake function of GLT1 in SOD1(G93A)-bearing astrocytes. *Biochem. Biophys Res. Commun.* 393(3): p. 481-6.

[94] Pasinelli, P. and R.H. Brown, Molecular biology of amyotrophic lateral sclerosis: insights from genetics. *Nat. Rev. Neurosci,* 2006. 7(9): p. 710-23.

[95] Van Den Bosch, L., et al., Ca^{2+}-permeable AMPA receptors and selective vulnerability of motor neurons. *J. Neurol. Sci.*, 2000. 180(1-2): p. 29-34.

[96] Van Den Bosch, L., et al., An alpha-mercaptoacrylic acid derivative (PD150606) inhibits selective motor neuron death via inhibition of kainate-induced Ca^{2+} influx and not via calpain inhibition. *Neuropharmacology,* 2002. 42(5): p. 706-713.

[97] Van Damme, P., et al., GluR2-dependent properties of AMPA receptors determine the selective vulnerability of motor neurons to excitotoxicity. *J. Neurophysiol.*, 2002. 88(3): p. 1279-1287.

[98] Greig, A., et al., Characterization of the AMPA-activated receptors present on motoneurons. *J. Neurochem.*, 2000. 74(1): p. 179-191.

[99] Corona, J.C. and R. Tapia, Ca^{2+}-permeable AMPA receptors and intracellular Ca^{2+} determine motoneuron vulnerability in rat spinal cord in vivo. *Neuropharmacology,* 2007. 52(5): p. 1219-28.

[100] Sun, H., et al., Slow and selective death of spinal motor neurons in vivo by intrathecal infusion of kainic acid: implications for AMPA receptor-mediated excitotoxicity in ALS. *J. Neurochem.*, 2006. 98(3): p. 782-91.

[101] Heath, P.R., et al., Quantitative assessment of AMPA receptor mRNA in human spinal motor neurons isolated by laser capture microdissection. *NeuroReport*, 2002. 13(14): p. 1753-1757.

[102] Kawahara, Y., et al., Human spinal motoneurons express low relative abundance of GluR2 mRNA: an implication for excitotoxicity in ALS. *J. Neurochem.*, 2003. 85(3): p. 680-689.

[103] Palecek, J., M.B. Lips, and B.U. Keller, Calcium dynamics and buffering in motoneurones of the mouse spinal cord. *J. Physiol.*, 1999. 520 Pt 2: p. 485-502.

[104] Lips, M.B. and B.U. Keller, Endogenous calcium buffering in motoneurones of the nucleus hypoglossus from mouse. *J. Physiol.*, 1998. 511(Pt 1): p. 105-117.

[105] von Lewinski, F. and B.U. Keller, Ca^{2+}, mitochondria and selective motoneuron vulnerability: implications for ALS. *Trends Neurosci.*, 2005. 28(9): p. 494-500.

[106] Obal, I., J.I. Engelhardt, and L. Siklos, Axotomy induces contrasting changes in calcium and calcium-binding proteins in oculomotor and hypoglossal nuclei of Balb/c mice. *J. Comp. Neurol.*, 2006. 499(1): p. 17-32.

[107] Paizs, M., et al., Hypoglossal motor neurons display a reduced calcium increase after axotomy in mice with upregulated parvalbumin. *J. Comp. Neurol.* 518(11): p. 1946-61.

In: Motor Neuron Diseases
Editors: Bradley J. Turner and Julie B. Atkin

ISBN 978-1-61470-101-9
© 2012 Nova Science Publishers, Inc.

Chapter VII

STEM CELL APPLICATION IN AMYOTROPHIC LATERAL SCLEROSIS: GROWTH FACTOR DELIVERY AND CELL THERAPY

Ksenija Bernau[1], Michael G. Meyer[2], and Masatoshi Suzuki[2,3]

[1]Deparment of Biomedical Engineering
[2]Department of Comparative Biosciences,
[3]The Stem Cell and Regenerative Medicine Center
University of Wisconsin-Madison, Madison, WI, U. S.

ABSTRACT

Amyotrophic lateral sclerosis (ALS) is a neurodegenerative disease where motor neurons within the brain and spinal cord are lost, leading to paralysis and death. Recent studies suggest the involvement of neuronal-glial interactions in ALS pathogenesis where motor neuron degeneration may be due in part to dysfunction of the surrounding astrocyte populations. Stem cells may be able to help in the battle against ALS in many different ways: cell therapy, disease modeling, drug delivery, and drug screening. But how close are we to using these cells to treat ALS? While the obvious use for stem cells would be to make new neurons to replace those that are lost in ALS, a more practical and immediate approach may be to use stem cells to protect the patients' own motor neurons that are undergoing degeneration. Transplantation of different types of stem cells into the spinal cord of either rat or mouse models of ALS have previously resulted in some motor neuron protection and functional improvement. We also demonstrated that transplantation of human stem cells releasing glial cell line-derived neurotrophic factor (GDNF) directly into the spinal cord or skeletal muscle results in robust cellular migration into degenerating regions, efficient delivery of GDNF, and remarkable preservation of host

* Correspondence: Masatoshi Suzuki, 2015 Linden Drive, Madison, WI 53706, USA. Tel: (608) 262-4264. Fax: (608) 263-3936. E-mail: msuzuki@svm.vetmed.wisc.edu

motor neurons. Taken together, *ex vivo* cell therapy targeting both the skeletal muscles (*i.e.* nerve terminals of motor neurons) and spinal cord (*i.e.* cell body) could provide the optimum combination for future human clinical studies.

INTRODUCTION

Amyotrophic lateral sclerosis (ALS) is a fatal, progressive neurodegenerative disease characterized by motor neuron cell death in the brain and spinal cord accompanied by rapid loss of muscle control and eventual complete paralysis [1]. ALS is an ideal candidate for novel gene and cell therapy approaches as it is an incurable and terminal disease. Trophic factors promote motor neuron survival and are excellent candidates for gene therapy in both familial and sporadic forms of ALS. In the last decade, our group has investigated the efficacy of *ex vivo* cell therapy targeting spinal cord and/or skeletal muscles to ameliorate motor neuron death in ALS. Here we summarize recent approaches in which growth factors and stem cells are being used to protect, generate, or regenerate specific sets of motor neurons in rodent models of ALS. We also discuss the prospects and problems of translating these laboratory findings into clinically useful therapies.

Amyotrophic Lateral Sclerosis (ALS)

The clinical features of ALS are rapid loss of muscle control and eventual paralysis due to the death of large motor neurons in the motor cortex, brainstem, and spinal cord [1, 2]. The onset of disease is usually between 40 and 60 years of age. The annual incidence rate for ALS in developed countries ranges from 0.4 to 2.4 per 100,000 individuals [3] and there are approximately 5,000 new cases of ALS in the USA each year. Currently, the only available treatment, riluzole (Rilutek, a glutamate release inhibitor), extends survival only by a matter of months. Motor neuron loss probably involves multiple pathways including formation of protein aggregates, axonal transport defects, oxidative damage, mitochondrial defects, glutamate toxicity, and alterations in calcium homeostasis [4, 5] [for review see [1]].

The vast majority of ALS cases are of a sporadic nature, while ~10% are familial (FALS) [6]. While the cause of sporadic ALS remains unclear,15-20% of FALS patients have point mutations in cytosolic Cu^{2+}/Zn^{2+} superoxide dismutase 1 (SOD1), suggesting that an abnormal function of this enzyme may play a pivotal role in the pathogenesis and progression of disease in these patients [7-10]. There is good reason to suspect that mutant SOD1 acts through a toxic gain of function rather than loss of dismutase activity, since SOD1 knockout mice do not exhibit motor neuron degeneration [11].

In contrast, both mouse and rat models over-expressing mutant forms of the human SOD1 gene have been developed which show a similar disease phenotype and progression to that seen in humans [12-14]. Clearly there are caveats that limit extrapolation of data from rodents directly to patients with regard to predicting outcomes in clinical trials [15], as the FALS cases linked to the mutations in SOD1 represent such a small population of ALS patients. However, success in slowing motor neuron death in rodent models is still the best predictor of success in ALS patients currently available.

Growth Factors and Gene Therapy in ALS

Trophic/growth factors promote motor neuron survival and are excellent candidates for gene therapy in both familial and sporadic forms of ALS. Growth factors are naturally occurring proteins which are essential for neuronal survival and differentiation during development. They are also required for the maintenance of normal function in the adult nervous system. Several growth factors such as glial cell line-derived growth factor (GDNF), insulin-like growth factor I (IGF-I), ciliary neurotrophic factor (CNTF), brain-derived growth factor (BDNF), and vascular endothelial growth factor (VEGF) have been evaluated in experimental models of ALS [for review see [2, 16]]. In nearly all cases these factors have been shown to have positive effects on both function and motor neuron survival when delivered to rodents carrying the SOD1 mutation [17-20]. However, human trials in ALS using these growth factors have all been negative using classical approaches of protein delivery [21-24]. Administration of these proteins *in vivo* has been possibly hindered by (i) inability of some to cross the blood-brain barrier or surface of the ventricles, (ii) unwanted side effects in non-targeted sites, and (iii) a relatively short half-life. These types of problems are significantly increased when dealing with the human nervous system which has far greater mass than the rodent and thus requires far more penetration of the growth factor to reach deep structures within the brain and spinal cord from the blood, ventricular system, or pial surface. These may be overcome in part by implanting catheters directly into the region of the brain requiring the growth factor [25, 26]. However, to deliver growth factors to the spinal cord using this approach is far more complex. The implanted catheter may interrupt descending and/or ascending white matter tracts, and the natural movement of the spinal cord in patients increases the chances of shearing forces causing further tissue damage.

Gene therapy approaches using viral vectors have the potential to circumvent these protein delivery issues. Motor neuron death in ALS is a complex process accompanied by muscular atrophy. Targeting location of vector delivery (spinal cord vs. muscle) seems to be crucial for these approaches. Vectors based on lentivirus, adenovirus, and adeno-associated virus (AAV) have a natural tropism for infecting neurons when injected into the living brain or spinal cord and can be readily engineered to encode therapeutic proteins. There is extensive literature on the use of AAV to deliver growth factors and enzymes to specific brain regions, cumulating in a series of clinical trials in Parkinson's disease [27]. Interestingly, most of the studies on ALS have focused on injecting viruses encoding the growth factors described above into the muscle of mice and rats expressing mutant SOD1 [17-19, 28-31]. While there have been some results in the SOD1^{G93A} mouse with IGF1 and GDNF, there is also mounting evidence that sick motor neurons may detach from the muscle early in disease progression [32] or have defects in transport mechanisms even if still attached [33, 34] Furthermore, retrograde transport may be more severely affected in larger species such as rats, monkeys, and humans when compared to very small mice where the distance is relatively short. This problem appears to have slowed translation of muscle growth factor delivery from these animal studies to patient clinical trials. Direct injection of viral constructs to the spinal cord would be a solution to avoid the need for retrograde transport of the protein from the muscle [35]. Surprisingly, there is only one published study delivering a growth factor (GDNF) directly to the motor neurons within the spinal cord of the SOD1^{G93A} mouse using viruses (35). However, there were only modest effects of GDNF on survival of facial motor neurons and no effect on lumbar motor neuron survival or function, even though high levels of GDNF were expressed directly around dying motor neurons [35]. In support of this study, another report used promoter-driven transgenic mice to overexpress GDNF locally in either the muscle or spinal cord of these SOD1^{G93A}animals and showed that muscle expression of GDNF was able to slow disease progression and onset, but expression in the spinal cord had no effect [36]. One caveat to both of these studies is that the expression of GDNF is achieved in older cells that are already compromised and undergoing degeneration due to the mutant SOD1 expression. The effects of added viral infection or protein production on degenerating neurons is poorly understood, but may potentially add further stress to an already sick cell and not be optimal for protein delivery.

Cellular Therapies – How Can We Use Stem Cells?

Much attention has been placed on stem cell therapy as a promising new treatment for ALS. There are at least two major strategies for using stem cells to treat ALS. The first, and most obvious, is to replace motor neurons which would result in the eventual recovery of neuromuscular function. There is some evidence that adult stem cells derived from bone marrow or umbilical cord may be able to produce "neural like" cells which may be useful for diseases such as ALS [37, 38]. However, the differentiation, survival, and integration of these cells into functional motor neurons or glia, either in the dish or after transplantation into the adult central nervous system, have yet to be proven.

Progressive advances in tissue culture now allow the production of human neural stem cells from either embryonic stem (ES) cells or fetal brain tissue [39]. In contrast to adult cells, there are many papers showing that these can produce functional motor neurons and glia both in the dish and following transplantation [40-43]. Several studies have shown that it is possible to generate motor neurons *in vitro* from mouse ES cells. These cells initiate a motor neuron-specific transcriptional pattern [44] and acquire immunohistochemical and electrophysiological features of mature neurons *in vitro* [45]. Furthermore, mouse ES cell-derived motor neurons transplanted into embryonic chick spinal cord extend a few axons into the periphery and form neuromuscular junctions [44]. In very exciting new studies, this work has been extended to show that these motor neurons can be encouraged to put out a few axons towards the muscle which then make functional connections that lead to an improvement in limb function [46]. This required a combination of approaches including addition of drugs which increased fiber outgrowth from the spinal cord, and cells releasing GDNF along the sciatic nerves to further encourage growth towards the muscle. Human ES cells can also generate motor neurons which have similar properties to those from the mouse [47, 48]. However, the major mechanistic limitation of neural replacement is that this strategy would first have to recapitulate the synaptic inputs from upper motor neurons and interneurons, and then extend axons to an appropriate target muscle which would require months to years in humans. Furthermore, the other challenge in translating this idea to the clinic for patients may be obtaining good survival of the transplanted motor neurons in a diseased spinal cord environment, which has proven difficult in the past. Finally, the human body is orders of magnitude larger than the mouse and rat models currently used. Will it be possible to guide a motor axon all the way from the spinal cord to distant muscles that may be over one meter away? Although potentially of great interest for future cell replacement therapies, application of ES cell-derived motor neurons for functional replacement in patients may take some time.

The focus is now on how to get more axons from the motor neurons to grow out through the ventral horns and make contact with the muscle in a time frame that would be useful to ALS patients.

Whereas neuronal replacement in ALS patients seems a distant goal, using stem cells to prevent sick motor neurons from dying may be a more realistic clinical approach. Therefore, a more practical strategy of stem cell application in ALS might be to deliver a stem cell population that migrates to sites of motor neurodegeneration. This would provide a protective environment to maintain motor neuron survival and function. Several direct strategies to modulate the host environment have already been used in the SOD1^{G93A} rodent model: (1) human neural stem cells grafted into the spinal cord [49], (2) hNT neurons derived from the human teratocarcinoma cell line grafted into the spinal cord [50], (3) mouse Sertoli cells grafted into the parenchyma of the spinal cord [51], (4) human umbilical cord blood cells transfused into the systemic circulation [52], or (5) human [52] or mouse [53] bone marrow transplants. In each of these studies there was some effect on motor neuron survival and lifespan of the animals, which in many cases was associated with growth factor release from the transplanted cells [for a review of these studies see [54]]. However, it is important to note that while Sertoli cells and mesenchymal stem cells may also be beneficial through release of certain growth factors, they are, by nature, unlikely to integrate as well into the nervous system or differentiate completely into glial cells when compared to neural stem cells that naturally do this very efficiently. Furthermore, the use of autologous cell transplantation in ALS, while reducing immune rejection issues, raises the potential problem that the patients' own cells may carry and be affected by whatever genetic traits originally contributed to the disease process. Interestingly, based on extensive literature on primary neuronal transplants for Parkinson's disease, it is likely that immune suppression will only be required for short periods of time even for non-autologous tissues transplanted to the brain [55].

The other approach is to replace nearby glial cells and protect existing motor neurons from ongoing degeneration, either with or without genetic modification to express enzymes, transporters, or specific neuroprotective trophic/growth factors. This idea has gained much momentum recently due to inroads regarding the contribution of different cellular subtypes to disease initiation and progression. In the central nervous system, glial cells play key roles to modulate many neuronal functions including glutamate uptake, synaptic plasticity, trophic factor support, and even neural transmission [56]. Astrocytes and microglia surrounding motor neurons have now also been shown to play a crucial role in motor neuron health and survival in ALS [57, 58]. The initial onset of motor neuron damage may trigger secondary abnormal responses in astrocytes and microglia carrying the SOD1 mutation, leading to further propagation of the disease [59]. Most of the studies to date have attempted to modify the environment surrounding motor neurons by altering levels of mutant SOD in non-neural support cells. Reducing the number of glia expressing the mutation can have a significant impact on motor neuron survival and disease progression [60, 61]. Studies with chimeric mice showed that increasing the proportion of healthy, wild-type non-neuronal cells in proximity to mutant SOD1-expressing motor neurons reduces mortality of those motor neurons and extends survival in these animals [60]. It was also found that a reduction in mutant SOD1 selectively from astrocytes or microglia using a CRE-lox system in mice modulates disease progression [62, 63]. Meanwhile, a recent study showed that spinal cord transplantation of rodent glial restricted precursors (GRP) led to extensive differentiation of grafts into mature astrocytes, extended survival and disease duration, and slowed declines in forelimb motor and respiratory physiological functions [64]. Therefore, focal delivery of astrocytes into the spinal cord ultimately presents a new therapeutic strategy to prevent motor neuron loss in ALS.

Combined Growth Factor and Stem Cell Therapy for ALS

Replacing support cells within the spinal cord of ALS mice and rats may improve motor neuron survival, in part, through trophic factor release. It seems logical to try enhancing this effect further using the cells genetically modified to secrete neuroprotective trophic/growth factors that are difficult to deliver in any other way.

In the last decade, our group has investigated the efficacy of *ex vivo* cell therapy targeting spinal cord or skeletal muscles to ameliorate motor neuron death in ALS. We prepared genetically modified human neural progenitor cells (hNPC) to release GDNF, and transplanted them into the lumbar spinal cord in SOD1^{G93A} rats [65]. hNPC are isolated from fetal brain cortical tissue [66-69] and can be maintained for over 50 weeks in the presence of mitogens [70] while retaining the ability to produce astrocytes. These cells could thus serve as "mini pumps," being a source of glial replacement and trophic factor delivery following transplantation into specific regions of the rodent and primate brain [71]. Following transplantation into the spinal cord of SOD1^{G93A} rats, there was robust cellular migration into degenerating areas, efficient delivery of GDNF, and remarkable preservation of motor neurons at early and end stages of the disease within chimeric regions. The progenitors retaining immature markers, and those not secreting GDNF had no effect on motor neuron survival. Interestingly, this robust motor neuron survival was not accompanied by continued innervation of muscle end plates and therefore resulted in no improvement in ipsilateral hindlimb use. To maintain these neuromuscular connections, we subsequently engineered human mesenchymal stem cells (hMSC) derived from bone marrow to secrete GDNF and transplanted them into three muscle groups in SOD1^{G93A} rats [70]. These cells survived within muscle, released GDNF, and significantly increased the number of neuromuscular connections and motor neuron survival in the spinal cord at mid-stages of disease. Furthermore, intramuscular transplantation of these cells delayed disease progression and increased the overall lifespan of animals.

Together, our studies have provided an initial outline for the future development of a combined growth factor and stem cell therapy (Figure 1). The potential to maintain dying motor neurons by delivering GDNF using neural progenitor cells represents a novel and powerful treatment strategy for ALS. While this approach represents a unique way to prevent motor neuron loss, our data also suggest that additional strategies may be required as well for maintenance of neuromuscular connections and full functional recovery. However, simply maintaining motor neurons in patients would be the first step of a therapeutic advance for this devastating and incurable disease, whereas future strategies would focus on the maintenance of the neuromuscular junction [72].

Possible Clinical Trial Designs

While a number of centers in and outside the United States advertise stem cell therapies for ALS, very few of these have been subject to serious pre-clinical and post-operative follow up. A clinical trial was carried out in Italy with autologous mesenchymal stem cells transplanted into the thoracic region of 9 ALS patients [73]. While there were no adverse effects or significant improvements in these patients, the location of the transplants was below the main cervical regions of the spinal cord controlling arm movement and breathing. Furthermore, as discussed above, the use of bone marrow derived cells may be less than optimal for maximal integration and full differentiation into functional cells within the spinal cord. However, this study does provide "proof of concept" that large volumes (1ml) can be infused into the spinal cord without the formation of cysts or other pathology based on MRI data. More recently, the first U.S. ALS phase I clinical trial began early last year, injecting hNPC in ALS patients' spinal cords (Emory ALS Center, 2010). Although these trials are still in early stages, stem cells have demonstrated to be a promising method for treatment of ALS and potentially other neurodegenerative diseases.

So what's to come in the future? The holy grail of stem cell therapy for ALS is to replace dead motor neurons with new ones. This will only happen in the clinic when we learn more about how to differentiate human embryonic stem cells into pure populations of motor neurons, find out how to make them survive in the degenerating environment of the ALS spinal cord, and then force them to form a new long range connection to the muscle.

A lofty goal, but one that is worth striving towards given the early encouraging studies in the mouse [44].

A more realistic alternative is astrocyte replacement combined perhaps with growth factor delivery. As most patients with ALS will only be diagnosed after starting to exhibit symptoms, it is of particular interest that glial cells seem to modulate disease progression rather than onset [60] – again making the approach practical in clinical terms. Interestingly, it is now becoming clear that astrocytes carrying the SOD1 mutation may also release factors that are toxic to motor neurons, at least *in vitro* [74].

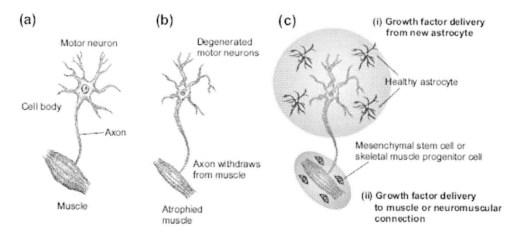

Figure 1.Combined stem cell and growth factor therapy in ALS. (a) In the intact nervous system, motor neurons are innervated to target muscle. (b) In familial ALS with SOD1 mutation, both motor neurons and astrocytes may be affected leading to a complex cascade of degeneration. It is currently not known whether the motor neurons or astrocytes are the primary target in sporadic ALS. (c) Stem cell generated astrocytes, growth factors, or a combination of both may be able to re-establish physiological interactions with dying motor neurons, thus delaying the degeneration process. However, it is also possible that further growth factor delivery to the muscle will be required to maintain full innervation of the muscle and prevent paralysis.

Thus, replacement of glial cells via stem cell transplants will need to have effects on many levels, including perhaps diluting out toxic effects of host astrocytes while releasing factors that protect motor neurons from ongoing degeneration.

We would contend that using stem cells that produce astroglia, either alone or modified to release factors such as GDNF, IGF1 or VEGF, represents a combined approach that may be worthy of future testing in clinical trials. This approach does not require host cell infection with viruses, provides new astroglial cells to detoxify the local environment, and represents a one-time transplant into a focal region of the spinal cord. Obviously, one caveat is that this is a segmental approach which is difficult to deliver to the entire spinal cord. Furthermore, the upper motor neurons in the brain will not be targeted, although there is always the possibility of retrograde transport of the growth factor produced in the spinal cord or additional transplants to the motor cortex. However, providing "proof of concept" that motor neurons within a small region of the spinal cord can be maintained or rejuvenated in humans would be a major step forward. In addition, monitoring a very specific set of muscles associated with the transplant region may provide the first clear evidence that this protection, if evident, has any functional relevance. Given that motor neurons in the SOD1 mutant models of ALS can survive without being connected to the muscle, it is clear that other interesting approaches to protect endplates may be required. As muscle is an accessible tissue, it is not difficult to think of delivery strategies to achieve this. Given the seriousness of ALS and the lack of current treatment options, perhaps growth factor delivery using stem cells to both the spinal cord (to protect the motor neuron) and muscle (to protect the connection) would be the ultimate protective strategy. Furthermore, if this were shown to be safe in patients, it would also pave the way towards transplanting motor neurons derived from human ES or induced-pluripotent stem cell (iPS) cells in future studies as a replacement, rather than protection, strategy. In fact, providing new astroglial support cells that secrete growth factors along with the human motor neuron transplant may be crucial for keeping the cells alive long enough to begin projecting to the muscle.

CONCLUSION

Given the lack of current treatment options for ALS, the development of novel strategies is of high priority. Current preclinical studies collectively suggest that gene and/or cellular therapies are promising approaches. Particularly, stem cell transplants aimed toward protecting, rather than replacing, motor neurons is very feasible for treating humans with ALS in the near future. Our recent results suggest that approaches to protect axons within muscle endplates may also be required. As muscle is an accessible tissue, the development of successful cell and growth factor delivery strategies here seem to be more straightforward than for the spinal cord. Perhaps the most powerful future approach would be to target both spinal cord (*i.e.* cell body) and muscle (*i.e.* nerve terminals of motor neurons). However, there are still numerous hurdles which need to be overcome in a rigorous and careful manner to avoid early setbacks. After these putative stem-cell-based therapies pass safety testing, optimal cell dose, source, delivery route, and immunosuppressive regimen must be carefully considered. Clearly, the challenges are great, but the rewards are even greater in the continual fight against this devastating disease.

ACKNOWLEDGMENTS

This work was supported by grants from the ALS Association, NIH/NINDS (PO1NS057778 and R21NS06104), the University of Wisconsin Foundation, and the Les Turner ALS foundation.

REFERENCES

[1]   Cleveland, D. W. and Rothstein, J. D. (2001) *Nat. Rev. Neurosci.* 2, 806-819.

[2]   Boillee, S., Vande, V. C., and Cleveland, D. W. (2006) *Neuron* 52, 39-59.

[3]   Mayeux, V., Corcia, P., Besson, G., Jafari-Schluep, H. F., Briolotti, V., and Camu, W. (2003) *Ann. Neurol.* 53, 815-818.

[4]   Julien, J. P. (2001) *Cell* 104, 581-591.

[5]   Rowland, L. P. and Shneider, N. A. (2001) *N. Engl. J. Med.* 344, 1688-1700.

[6]   Brown, R. H., Jr. (1995) *Cell* 80, 687-692.

[7]   Andersen, P. M., Sims, K. B., Xin, W. W., Kiely, R., O'Neill, G., Ravits, J., Pioro, E., Harati, Y., Brower, R. D., Levine, J. S. *et al.* (2003) *Amyotroph. Lateral. Scler. Other Motor Neuron Disord.* 4, 62-73.

[8]   Rosen, D. R. (1993) *Nature* 364, 362.

[9]   Shaw, C. E., Enayat, Z. E., Powell, J. F., Anderson, V. E., Radunovic, A., al Sarraj, S., and Leigh, P. N. (1997) *Neurology* 49, 1612-1616.

[10] Orrell, R. W. (2000) *Neuromuscul. Disord.* 10, 63-68.

[11] Reaume, A. G., Elliott, J. L., Hoffman, E. K., Kowall, N. W., Ferrante, R. J., Siwek, D. F., Wilcox, H. M., Flood, D. G., Beal, M. F., Brown, R. H., Jr. *et al.* (1996) *Nat. Genet.* 13, 43-47.

[12] Gurney, M. E. (1994) *N. Engl. J. Med.* 331, 1721-1722.

[13] Nagai, M., Aoki, M., Miyoshi, I., Kato, M., Pasinelli, P., Kasai, N., Brown, R. H., Jr., and Itoyama, Y. (2001) *J. Neurosci.* 21, 9246-9254.

[14] Howland, D. S., Liu, J., She, Y., Goad, B., Maragakis, N. J., Kim, B., Erickson, J., Kulik, J., DeVito, L., Psaltis, G. *et al.* (2002) *Proc. Natl. Acad. Sci. U. S. A* 99, 1604-1609.

[15] Rothstein, J. D. (2004) *Amyotroph. Lateral. Scler. Other Motor Neuron Disord.* 5 Suppl 1, 22-25.

[16] Hedlund, E., Hefferan, M. P., Marsala, M., and Isacson, O. (2007) *Eur. J. Neurosci.* 26, 1721-1737.

[17] Kaspar, B. K., Llado, J., Sherkat, N., Rothstein, J. D., and Gage, F. H. (2003) *Science* 301, 839-842.

[18] Acsadi, G., Anguelov, R. A., Yang, H., Toth, G., Thomas, R., Jani, A., Wang, Y., Ianakova, E., Mohammad, S., Lewis, R. A. *et al.* (2002) *Hum. Gene Ther.* 13, 1047-1059.

[19] Azzouz, M., Ralph, G. S., Storkebaum, E., Walmsley, L. E., Mitrophanous, K. A., Kingsman, S. M., Carmeliet, P., and Mazarakis, N. D. (2004) *Nature* 429, 413-417.

[20] Pun, S., Santos, A. F., Saxena, S., Xu, L., and Caroni, P. (2006) *Nat. Neurosci.* 9, 408-419.

[21] Borasio, G. D., Robberecht, W., Leigh, P. N., Emile, J., Guiloff, R. J., Jerusalem, F., Silani, V., Vos, P. E., Wokke, J. H., and Dobbins, T. (1998) *Neurology* 51, 583-586.

[22] Lai, E. C., Felice, K. J., Festoff, B. W., Gawel, M. J., Gelinas, D. F., Kratz, R., Murphy, M. F., Natter, H. M., Norris, F. H., and Rudnicki, S. A. (1997) *Neurology* 49, 1621-1630.

[23] (1999) *Neurology* 52, 1427-1433.

[24] (1996) *Neurology* 46, 1244-1249.

[25] Gill, S. S., Patel, N. K., Hotton, G. R., O'Sullivan, K., McCarter, R., Bunnage, M., Brooks, D. J., Svendsen, C. N., and Heywood, P. (2003) *Nat. Med.* 9, 589-595.

[26] Slevin, J. T., Gerhardt, G. A., Smith, C. D., Gash, D. M., Kryscio, R., and Young, B. (2005) *J. Neurosurg.* 102, 216-222.

[27] Svendsen, C. (2007) *Lancet Neurol.* 6, 754-756.

[28] Cisterni, C., Henderson, C. E., Aebischer, P., Pettmann, B., and Deglon, N. (2000) *J. Neurochem.* 74, 1820-1828.

[29] Hottinger, A. F., Azzouz, M., Deglon, N., Aebischer, P., and Zurn, A. D. (2000) *J. Neurosci.* 20, 5587-5593.

[30] Haase, G., Kennel, P., Pettmann, B., Vigne, E., Akli, S., Revah, F., Schmalbruch, H., and Kahn, A. (1997) *Nat. Med.* 3, 429-436.

[31] Wang, L. J., Lu, Y. Y., Muramatsu, S., Ikeguchi, K., Fujimoto, K., Okada, T., Mizukami, H., Matsushita, T., Hanazono, Y., Kume, A. *et al.* (2002) *J. Neurosci.* 22, 6920-6928.

[32] Fischer, L. R., Culver, D. G., Tennant, P., Davis, A. A., Wang, M., Castellano-Sanchez, A., Khan, J., Polak, M. A., and Glass, J. D. (2004) *Exp. Neurol.* 185, 232-240.

[33] Williamson, T. L. and Cleveland, D. W. (1999) *Nat. Neurosci.* 2, 50-56.

[34] De Vos, K. J., Chapman, A. L., Tennant, M. E., Manser, C., Tudor, E. L., Lau, K. F., Brownlees, J., Ackerley, S., Shaw, P. J., McLoughlin, D. M. *et al.* (2007) *Hum. Mol. Genet.* 16, 2720-2728.

[35] Guillot, S., Azzouz, M., Deglon, N., Zurn, A., and Aebischer, P. (2004) *Neurobiol. Dis.* 16, 139-149.

[36] Li, W., Brakefield, D., Pan, Y., Hunter, D., Myckatyn, T. M., and Parsadanian, A. (2006) *Exp. Neurol.*

[37] McGuckin, C. P., Forraz, N., Allouard, Q., and Pettengell, R. (2004) *Exp. Cell Res.* 295, 350-359.

[38] Croft, A. P. and Przyborski, S. A. (2006) *Stem Cells* 24, 1841-1851.

[39] Tai, Y. T. and Svendsen, C. N. (2004) *Curr. Opin. Pharmacol.* 4, 98-104.

[40] Shihabuddin, L. S., Horner, P. J., Ray, J., and Gage, F. H. (2000) *J. Neurosci.* 20, 8727-8735.

[41] Karimi-Abdolrezaee, S., Eftekharpour, E., Wang, J., Morshead, C. M., and Fehlings, M. G. (2006) *J. Neurosci.* 26, 3377-3389.

[42] Vroemen, M., Aigner, L., Winkler, J., and Weidner, N. (2003) *Eur. J. Neurosci.* 18, 743-751.

[43] Cao, Q. L., Zhang, Y. P., Howard, R. M., Walters, W. M., Tsoulfas, P., and Whittemore, S. R. (2001) *Exp. Neurol.* 167, 48-58.

[44] Wichterle, H., Lieberam, I., Porter, J. A., and Jessell, T. M. (2002) *Cell* 110, 385-397.

[45] Miles, G. B., Yohn, D. C., Wichterle, H., Jessell, T. M., Rafuse, V. F., and Brownstone, R. M. (2004) *J. Neurosci.* 24, 7848-7858.

[46] Deshpande, D. M., Kim, Y. S., Martinez, T., Carmen, J., Dike, S., Shats, I., Rubin, L. L., Drummond, J., Krishnan, C., Hoke, A. *et al.* (2006) *Ann. Neurol.* 60, 32-44.

[47] Li, X. J., Du, Z. W., Zarnowska, E. D., Pankratz, M., Hansen, L. O., Pearce, R. A., and Zhang, S. C. (2005) *Nat. Biotechnol.* 23, 215-221.

[48] Lee, H., Al Shamy, G., Elkabetz, Y., Schoefield, C. M., Harrsion, N. L., Panagiotakos, G., Socci, N. D., Tabar, V., and Studer, L. (2007) *Stem Cells.*

[49] Yan, J., Xu, L., Welsh, A. M., Chen, D., Hazel, T., Johe, K., and Koliatsos, V. E. (2006) *Stem Cells* 24, 1976-1985.

[50] Garbuzova-Davis, S., Willing, A. E., Milliken, M., Saporta, S., Zigova, T., Cahill, D. W., and Sanberg, P. R. (2002) *Exp. Neurol.* 174, 169-180.

[51] Hemendinger, R., Wang, J., Malik, S., Persinski, R., Copeland, J., Emerich, D., Gores, P., Halberstadt, C., and Rosenfeld, J. (2005) *Exp. Neurol.* 196, 235-243.

[52] Habisch, H. J., Janowski, M., Binder, D., Kuzma-Kozakiewicz, M., Widmann, A., Habich, A., Schwalenstocker, B., Hermann, A., Brenner, R., Lukomska, B. *et al.* (2007) *J. Neural Transm.*

[53] Corti, S., Locatelli, F., Donadoni, C., Guglieri, M., Papadimitriou, D., Strazzer, S., Del Bo, R., and Comi, G. P. (2004) *Brain* 127, 2518-2532.

[54] Hedlund, E., Hefferan, M. P., Marsala, M., and Isacson, O. (2007) *Eur. J. Neurosci.* 26, 1721-1737.

[55] Piccini, P., Pavese, N., Hagell, P., Reimer, J., Bjorklund, A., Oertel, W. H., Quinn, N. P., Brooks, D. J., and Lindvall, O. (2005) *Brain* 128, 2977-2986.

[56] Kirchhoff, F., Dringen, R., and Giaume, C. (2001) *Eur. Arch. Psychiatry Clin. Neurosci.* 251, 159-169.

[57] Hall, E. D., Oostveen, J. A., and Gurney, M. E. (1998) *Glia* 23, 249-256.

[58] Barbeito, L. H., Pehar, M., Cassina, P., Vargas, M. R., Peluffo, H., Viera, L., Estevez, A. G., and Beckman, J. S. (2004) *Brain Res. Brain Res. Rev.* 47, 263-274.

[59] Rao, S. D. and Weiss, J. H. (2004) *Trends Neurosci.* 27, 17-23.

[60] Clement, A. M., Nguyen, M. D., Roberts, E. A., Garcia, M. L., Boillee, S., Rule, M., McMahon, A. P., Doucette, W., Siwek, D., Ferrante, R. J. *et al.* (2003) *Science* 302, 113-117.

[61] Beers, D. R., Henkel, J. S., Xiao, Q., Zhao, W., Wang, J., Yen, A. A., Siklos, L., McKercher, S. R., and Appel, S. H. (2006) *Proc. Natl. Acad. Sci. U. S. A* 103, 16021-16026.

[62] Boillee, S., Yamanaka, K., Lobsiger, C. S., Copeland, N. G., Jenkins, N. A., Kassiotis, G., Kollias, G., and Cleveland, D. W. (2006) *Science* 312, 1389-1392.

[63] Yamanaka, K., Chun, S. J., Boillee, S., Fujimori-Tonou, N., Yamashita, H., Gutmann, D. H., Takahashi, R., Misawa, H., and Cleveland, D. W. (2008) *Nat. Neurosci.* 11, 251-253.

[64] Lepore, A. C., Rauck, B., Dejea, C., Pardo, A. C., Rao, M. S., Rothstein, J. D., and Maragakis, N. J. (2008) *Nat. Neurosci.* 11, 1294-1301.

[65] Suzuki, M., McHugh, J., Tork, C., Shelley, B., Klein, S. M., Aebischer, P., and Svendsen, C. N. (2007) *PLoS. ONE.* 2, e689.

[66] Svendsen, C. N., Clarke, D. J., Rosser, A. E., and Dunnett, S. B. (1996) *Exp. Neurol.* 137, 376-388.

[67]   Keyoung, H. M., Roy, N. S., Benraiss, A., Louissaint, A., Jr., Suzuki, A., Hashimoto, M., Rashbaum, W. K., Okano, H., and Goldman, S. A. (2001) *Nat. Biotechnol.* 19, 843-850.

[68]   Tamaki, S., Eckert, K., He, D., Sutton, R., Doshe, M., Jain, G., Tushinski, R., Reitsma, M., Harris, B., Tsukamoto, A. *et al.* (2002) *J. Neurosci. Res.* 69, 976-986.

[69]   Suslov, O. N., Kukekov, V. G., Ignatova, T. N., and Steindler, D. A. (2002) *Proc. Natl. Acad. Sci. U. S. A* 99, 14506-14511.

[70]   Wright, L. S., Li, J., Caldwell, M. A., Wallace, K., Johnson, J. A., and Svendsen, C. N. (2003) *J. Neurochem.* 86, 179-195.

[71]   Behrstock, S., Ebert, A., McHugh, J., Vosberg, S., Moore, J., Schneider, B., Capowski, E., Hei, D., Kordower, J., Aebischer, P. *et al.* (2006) *Gene Ther.* 13, 379-388.

[72]   Suzuki, M. and Svendsen, C. N. (2008) *Trends Neurosci.* 31, 192-198.

[73]   Mazzini, L., Mareschi, K., Ferrero, I., Vassallo, E., Oliveri, G., Nasuelli, N., Oggioni, G. D., Testa, L., and Fagioli, F. (2007) *J. Neurol. Sci.*

[74]   Nagai, M., Re, D. B., Nagata, T., Chalazonitis, A., Jessell, T. M., Wichterle, H., and Przedborski, S. (2007) *Nat. Neurosci.* 10, 615-622.

In: Motor Neuron Diseases
Editors: Bradley J. Turner and Julie B. Atkin

ISBN 978-1-61470-101-9
© 2012 Nova Science Publishers, Inc.

Chapter VIII

THERAPEUTIC INTERVENTION IN SPINAL AND BULBAR MUSCULAR ATROPHY (SBMA)

Haruhiko Banno[1,2], Masahisa Katsuno[1,*],
Keisuke Suzuki[1], Fumiaki Tanaka[1], and Gen Sobue[1,*]

[1]Department of Neurology, Nagoya University Graduate School of Medicine /
65 Tsurumai-cho, Showa-ku, Nagoya 466-8550, Japan
[2]Institute for Advanced Research, Nagoya University / Furo-cho, Chikusa-ku,
Nagoya 464-8601, Japan

ABSTRACT

Spinal and bulbar muscular atrophy (SBMA), also known as Kennedy's disease, is an adult-onset, X-linked motor neuron disease characterized by muscle atrophy, weakness, contraction fasciculations and bulbar involvement. SBMA is caused by the expansion of a CAG triplet repeat, encoding a polyglutamine tract within the first exon of the androgen receptor (AR) gene. The histopathological finding in SBMA is the loss of lower motor neurons in the anterior horn of the spinal cord as well as in the brainstem motor nuclei. There is no well-established disease-modifying therapy for SBMA. Animal studies have revealed that the pathogenesis of SBMA depends on the level of serum testosterone, and that androgen deprivation mitigates neurodegeneration through inhibition of nuclear accumulation and/or stabilization of the pathogenic AR. Heat shock proteins, ubiquitin-proteasome system and transcriptional regulation are also potential targets of therapy development for SBMA. Among these therapeutic approaches, androgen deprivation has been translated into clinic. Surgical castration is shown to reverse motor dysfunction in mouse models of SBMA. The luteinizing hormone-releasing hormone analogue, leuprorelin, prevents nuclear translocation of aberrant AR proteins, resulting in a significant improvement of disease phenotype in a mouse model of SBMA. These results of animal studies were verified in a phase 2 clinical trial of leuprorelin, in which the patients treated with this drug exhibited decreased mutant AR

---

* Author to whom correspondence should be addressed; E-Mails: ka2no@med.nagoya-u.ac.jp (M.K.); sobueg@
med.nagoya-u.ac.jp (G.S.); Tel. +81-52-744-2385; Fax: +81-52-744-2384.

accumulation in scrotal skin biopsy and significantly better swallowing parameters than those receiving placebo. An autopsy of one patient who received leuprorelin suggested that androgen deprivation inhibits the nuclear accumulation of mutant AR in the motor neurons of the spinal cord and brainstem. Phase 3 clinical trial showed the possibility that leuprorelin treatment is associated with improved swallowing function particularly in patients with a disease duration less than 10 years. These observations suggest that pharmacological inhibition of the toxic accumulation of mutant AR is a potential therapy for SBMA.

Keywords: Spinal and bulbar muscular atrophy (SBMA); polyglutamine; androgen receptor (AR); leuprorelin acetate.

INTRODUCTION

Spinal and bulbar muscular atrophy (SBMA) is also referred to as Kennedy disease (KD), named after William R. Kennedy, whose study on 11 patients from 2 families described the clinical and pathological features of this disorder in 1968 [1]. Alternative names for this disease include bulbospinal neuronopathy and bulbospinal muscular atrophy. SBMA is the first of the neurodegenerative diseases, for which the molecular basis was discovered to be the expansion of a trinucleotide CAG repeat in the causative gene.

SBMA chiefly affects adult males. The prevalence of this disease is estimated to be 1-2 per 100,000, whereas a considerable number of patients may have been misdiagnosed as other neuromuscular diseases including amyotrophic lateral sclerosis [2, 3]. Patients of various ethnic backgrounds have been reported throughout the world. Major symptoms of SBMA are weakness, atrophy and fasciculations of bulbar, facial and limb muscles [1]. The onset of weakness is usually between 30 and 60 years, but is often preceded by non-specific symptoms such as postural tremor and muscle cramps. Typically, affected individuals require a wheel chair 15-20 years after the onset of weakness [4, 5, 6]. Patients with SBMA occasionally demonstrate signs of androgen insensitivity such as gynecomastia, testicular atrophy, impaired erection and decreased fertility, some of which are detected before the onset of motor impairment. Female carriers are usually asymptomatic, but some express subclinical phenotypes including high amplitude motor unit potentials on electromyography. The progression of SBMA is usually slow, but life-threatening respiratory tract infection often occurs in the advanced stages of the disease, resulting in early death in some patients. The cardinal cause of death is aspiration pneumonia [4].

The molecular basis of SBMA is the expansion of a trinucleotide CAG repeat, which encodes the polyglutamine tract in the first exon of the androgen receptor (AR) gene [7]. The CAG repeat within AR ranges in size from 11 to 35 in normal subjects, but from 40 to 62 in SBMA patients [2, 7, 8]. The number of CAGs is correlated with disease severity and inversely correlated with the age of onset, as observed in other polyglutamine-related neurodegenerative diseases, including Huntington's disease (HD) and several forms of spinocerebellar ataxia (SCA) [9, 10, 11]. In a nerve conduction study of SBMA, the CAG repeat size and the age at onset were significantly different among the patients with motor- and sensory-dominant phenotypes, indicating that a longer CAG repeat is more closely linked to the motor-dominant phenotype and a shorter CAG repeat is more closely linked to the sensory-dominant phenotype [12].

AR, the causative protein of SBMA, is a 110-kDa nuclear receptor which belongs to the steroid/thyroid hormone receptor family [13]. AR mediates the effects of androgens, testosterone and dihydrotestosterone, through binding to an androgen response element in the target gene to regulate its expression. AR is essential for major androgen effects including normal male sexual differentiation and pubertal sexual development, although AR-independent non-genomic function of androgen has been reported. AR is expressed not only in primary and secondary sexual organs, but also in non-reproductive organs including the kidney, skeletal muscle, adrenal gland, skin, and nervous system, suggesting its far-reaching influence on a variety of mammalian tissues. In the central nervous system, the expression level of AR is relatively high in spinal and brainstem motor neurons, the same cells which are vulnerable in SBMA.

Molecular Mechanisms of SBMA

The fundamental histopathological finding in SBMA is the loss of lower motor neurons in the anterior horn of the spinal cord as well as in the brainstem motor nuclei except for the third, fourth and sixth cranial nerves [14]. The number of nerve fibers is reduced in the ventral spinal nerve root, reflecting motor neuronopathy. Sensory neurons in the dorsal root ganglia are less severely affected, and large myelinated fibers demonstrate a distally accentuated sensory axonopathy in the peripheral nervous system. Muscle histopathology includes both neurogenic and myogenic findings: there are groups of atrophic fibers with a number of small angular fibers, fiber type grouping and clamps of pyknotic nuclei as well as variability in fiber size, hypertrophic fibers, scattered basophilic regenerating fibers and central nuclei.

In general, the abnormal polyglutamine protein forms inclusion bodies in affected neurons, which is a unifying histopathological hallmark of polyglutamine diseases [15]. These neuronal inclusion bodies are often detected in the nucleus, although they may be formed within the cytoplasm or neurites. The deposition of inclusion bodies is not only found in the postmortem neural tissues from patients, but has also been reported in animal models of polyglutamine diseases. The abnormal polyglutamine proteins in the inclusion bodies are often truncated, indicating that proteolytic cleavage appears to enhance the toxicity of the causative gene products [16]. The abnormal polyglutamine proteins are also expressed outside the nervous system, leading to non-neuronal pathology, such as diabetes mellitus, in some polyglutamine diseases [17, 18].

In SBMA, nuclear inclusions (NIs) containing the pathogenic AR are found in the residual motor neurons in the brainstem and spinal cord as well as in non-neuronal tissues including the prostate, testes, and skin [19]. These inclusions are detectable using antibodies recognizing a small portion of the N-terminus of the AR protein, but not by those against the C-terminus of the protein. This observation implies that the C-terminus of the AR is truncated or masked upon formation of NI. A full-length AR protein with an expanded polyglutamine tract is cleaved by caspase-3, releasing a polyglutamine-containing toxic fragment, and the susceptibility to cleavage is polyglutamine repeat length-dependent [20]. Thus, proteolytic cleavage is likely to enhance the toxicity of the pathogenic AR protein. Electron microscopic immunohistochemistry shows dense aggregates of AR-positive granular material without limiting membrane, both in the neural and non-neural inclusions, in contrast to the other polyglutamine diseases where NIs take the form of filamentous structures.

Although NIs are a disease-specific histopathological finding, their role in pathogenesis has been heavily debated. Several studies have suggested that NIs may indicate a cellular response coping with the toxicity of abnormal polyglutamine protein [21]. Instead, the diffuse nuclear accumulation of the mutant protein has been considered essential for inducing neurodegeneration in polyglutamine diseases including SBMA (Figure 1). Recent data suggests that the toxic species of protein in polyglutamine diseases may be soluble mutant conformers which can exist as oligomers or monomers containing beta-sheet conformation [22, 23, 24]. Although it is difficult to determine the toxic protein species in human histopathology, diffuse accumulation of the causative gene products has been construed as an important finding. An immunohistochemical study on autopsied SBMA patients using an anti-polyglutamine antibody demonstrated that diffuse nuclear accumulation of the pathogenic AR is more frequently observed than NIs in the anterior horn of the spinal cord [25]. Intriguingly, the frequency of diffuse nuclear accumulation of the pathogenic AR in spinal motor neurons strongly correlates with the length of the CAG repeat in the AR gene. No such correlation has been found between NI occurrence and the CAG repeat length. A similar observation has been reported in DRPLA [26]. Taken together, it appears that the pathogenic AR containing an elongated polyglutamine tract principally accumulates within the nuclei of motor neurons in a diffusible form, leading to neuronal dysfunction and eventual cell death in SBMA. In support of this hypothesis, neuronal dysfunction is halted by genetic modulation preventing nuclear import of the pathogenic polyglutamine-containing protein in cellular and animal models of polyglutamine diseases [11].

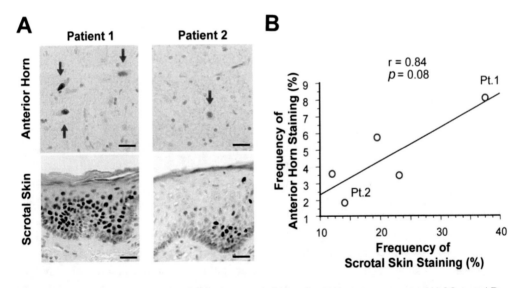

Figure 1. Mutant AR nuclear accumulation in scrotal skin and spinal motor neurons. (A) Mutant AR accumulation was remarkable in both spinal motor neurons and scrotal skin of Patient 1, but less remarkable in both motor neurons and skin in Patient 2. Scale bar = 30 μm. (B) The extent of mutant AR accumulation in scrotal skin epithelial cells showed a tendency to correlate with that in anterior horn cells.

Since the human AR is widely expressed in various organs, nuclear accumulation of the pathogenic AR protein is detected not only in the central nervous system, but also in non-neuronal tissues such as scrotal skin. The degree of pathogenic AR accumulation in scrotal skin epithelial cells tends to be correlated with that in the spinal motor neurons in autopsy specimens, and it is well correlated with CAG repeat length and inversely correlated with the motor functional scale [27]. These findings indicate that scrotal skin biopsy with anti-polyglutamine immunostaining is a good biomarker with which to monitor SBMA pathogenic processes (Figure 1).

A number of studies have indicated that transcriptional dysregulation underlies the molecular mechanism of neuronal dysfunction in polyglutamine diseases. Transcriptional co-activators such as cAMP-response element binding protein-binding protein (CBP) have been shown to be sequestrated into the NIs through protein-protein interaction in mouse models and patients with SBMA [28]. It has also documented that the histone acetyltransferase activity of CBP is inhibited in animal models of polyglutamine diseases, and that the level of histone acetylation is decreased in a mouse model of SBMA [29]. Taken together, polyglutamine-mediated transcriptional dysregulation appears to play an important role in the pathogenesis of SBMA. Mitochondrial impairment and oxidative stress have also been stipulated as a causative molecular event in polyglutamine diseases. Depolarization of the mitochondrial membrane and an elevated level of reactive oxygen species have been observed in a cellular model of SBMA [30]. Moreover, the pathogenic AR protein represses the transcription of the subunits of peroxisome proliferator-activated receptor gamma co-activator-1 (PGC-1), a transcriptional co-activator that regulates the expression of various nuclear-encoded mitochondrial proteins [30]. Similar findings have been reported in cellular and animal models of polyglutamine diseases, suggesting that mitochondrial dysfunction is a unifying molecular mechanism whereby abnormal polyglutamine proteins induce neuronal damage. Obstruction of axonal transport has also gained attention as a cause of neuronal dysfunction in SBMA. The pathogenic AR has been shown to impair axonal transport through a pathway that involves activation of cJun N-terminal kinase (JNK) activity [31]. In a mouse model of SBMA, the nuclear accumulation of the abnormal AR protein induces transcriptional dysregulation of dynactin 1, an axonal motor protein that regulates axonal trafficking [32]. A recent study, however, demonstrated no disruption of axonal transport in another mouse model of SBMA, suggesting the need for further investigation of the relationship between axonal trafficking and the pathogenic AR [33].

Therapeutic Strategies for SBMA

For any given polyglutamine disease including SBMA, more than one mechanism likely contributes to neuronal dysfunction and eventual cell death. They include: (i) misfolding of the disease protein resulting in altered function; (ii) deleterious protein interactions engaged in by the mutant protein; (iii) formation of toxic oligomeric complexes; (iv) transcriptional dysregulation; (v) mitochondrial dysfunction resulting in impaired bioenergetics and oxidative stress; (vi) impaired axonal transport; (vii) aberrant neuronal signaling including excitotoxicity; (viii) cellular protein homeostasis impairment; and (ix) RNA toxicity [34]. Although each of these molecular mechanisms could be subject to therapeutic interventions, upstream events are more plausible targets than secondary cellular changes.

There is no well-established disease-modifying therapy for SBMA. Potential therapeutics, however, have emerged from basic research using animal models. Among these therapeutic approaches, androgen deprivation has been translated into clinic [35]. Several animal studies demonstrated that neurological symptoms and histopathological findings are profound in male SBMA mice, and that the accumulation of the pathogenic AR proteins is dependent on the circulating level of testosterone [36, 37]. In support of this view, surgical castration is shown to reverse motor dysfunction in mouse models of SBMA [36, 38]. Similar results were obtained in a pre-clinical study of leuprorelin. Leuprorelin is a potent luteinizing hormone-releasing hormone (LHRH) analog suppressing the releases of gonadotrophins, luteinising hormone and follicle-stimulating hormone. This drug has been used for a variety of sex hormone-dependent diseases including prostate cancer, endometriosis, and pre-puberty. Within about 2 to 4 weeks of leuprorelin administration, human serum testosterone level decreases to the extent achieved by surgical castration. Leuprorelin successfully inhibits nuclear accumulation of the pathogenic AR, resulting in marked amelioration of neuromuscular phenotypes seen in the male SBMA mice. Leuprorelin initially increases the serum testosterone level by agonizing the LHRH receptor, but subsequently reduces it to undetectable levels. Androgen blockade effects were also confirmed by reduced weights of the prostate and seminal vesicle. The leuprorelin-treated SBMA mice show longer lifespan, larger body size, and better motor performance compared with vehicle-treated mice. Leuprorelin appears to improve neuronal dysfunction by preventing ligand-dependent nuclear translocation of the pathogenic AR in the same way as castration [39].

Activation of the cellular defense machinery is another promising therapeutic approach for SBMA. Over-expression of heat shock proteins (HSPs), stress-inducible molecular chaperones, inhibits toxic accumulation of abnormal AR protein and suppresses neurodegeneration in a mouse model of SBMA [40]. Similar beneficial effects have also been achieved by the pharmacological induction of HSPs [41]. On the other hand, inhibition of Hsp90 has been demonstrated to arrest neurodegeneration by activating the ubiquitin-proteasome system in SBMA. Treatment with 17-allylamino geldanamycin (17-AAG), a potent Hsp90 inhibitor, dissociated p23 from the Hsp90-AR complex, and thus facilitated proteasomal degradation of the pathogenic AR in cellular and mouse models of SBMA [42, 43]. Similar effects were observed in the SBMA mice being treated with an oral Hsp 90 inhibitor, 17-(dimethylaminoethylamino)-17-demethoxygeldanamycin (17-DMAG) [44].

Transcriptional dysregulation is another target for therapeutic intervention. Because suppression of histone deacetylase (HDAC) activities results in an augmentation of histone acetylation and a subsequent restoration of gene transcription, HDAC inhibitors have been considered to be of therapeutic benefit in polyglutamine diseases [45]. Butyrate was the first HDAC inhibitor to be discovered, and the related compound, phenylbutyrate, has been successfully employed in experimental cancer therapy. Oral administration of sodium butyrate ameliorates the symptomatic and histopathological phenotypes of a mouse model of SBMA through upregulation of histone acetylation in nervous tissues [22].

Clinical Trials of Leuprorelin Acetate

The results of animal studies were verified in a phase 2 clinical trial of leuprorelin, in which the patients treated with this drug exhibited decreased mutant AR accumulation in scrotal skin biopsy, significantly higher functional scores and better swallowing parameters than those receiving placebo (Figure 2).

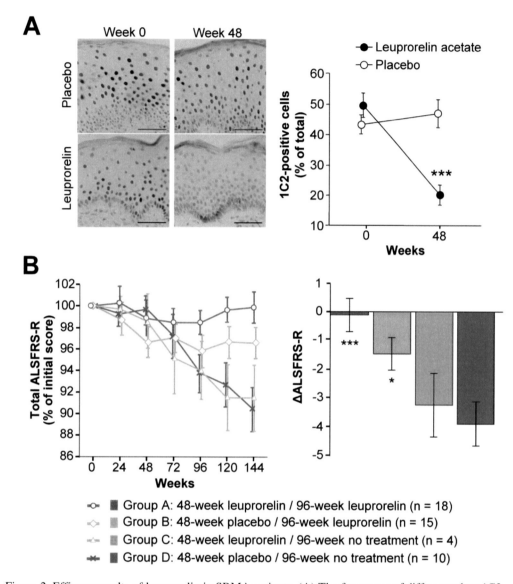

Figure 2. Efficacy results of leuprorelin in SBMA patients. (A) The frequency of diffuse nuclear 1C2 staining (indicative of mutant AR) in the scrotal epithelial cells was significantly decreased after the 48-week administration of leuprorelin acetate. (B) Changes in the ALSFRS-R scores showed treatment duration-dependent improvements in the leuprorelin-treated groups. Scale bars = 50 μm. Data is expressed as means ± SEM. *p < 0.05; **p < 0.005; ***p < 0.001 with respect to Group D [36].

Autopsy of one patient who received leuprorelin suggested that androgen deprivation inhibits the nuclear accumulation and/or stabilization of mutant AR in the motor neurons of the spinal cord and brainstem (Figure 3). These observations suggest that administration of leuprorelin suppresses the deterioration of neuromuscular impairment in SBMA by inhibiting the toxic accumulation of mutant AR [46].

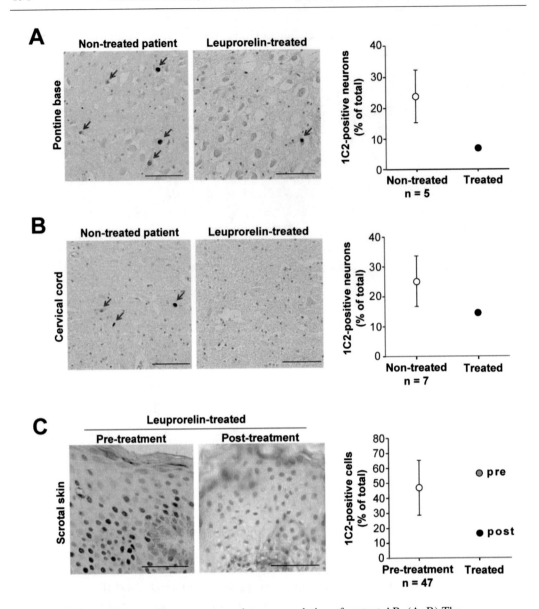

Figure 3. Effects of leuprorelin acetate on nuclear accumulation of mutant AR. (A, B) The accumulation of mutant AR in neurons was remarkable both in the pontine base and in the spinal anterior horn of all the control, non-treated autopsied patients, but the number of 1C2-positive neurons was relatively small in the leuprorelin-treated patient. Scale bars=100 μm. (C) Mutant AR accumulation in biopsied scrotal skin epithelial cells was markedly reduced by leuprorelin. Scale bars=50 μm. Data is expressed as means±SD [36].

These promising results of the phase 2 clinical trial, together with the well-known tolerability of LH-RH agonists, led us to undertake a, randomized, placebo-controlled clinical trial of leuprorelin in SBMA. The primary endpoint was pharyngeal barium residue, which indicates incomplete bolus clearance, measured at week 48 by videofluorography. 204 patients were randomly assigned and 199 started treatment; 100 with leuprorelin and 99 with placebo. At week 48, the pharyngeal barium residue had changed by −5.1% (SD 21.0) in the leuprorelin group and by 0.2% (18.2) in the placebo group (difference between groups −5.3%

(p=0.063). In a pre-defined subgroup analysis, leuprorelin treatment was associated with a greater reduction in barium residue than was placebo in patients with a disease duration less than 10 years difference between groups (–9.8%, p=0·009) (Figure 4) [47].

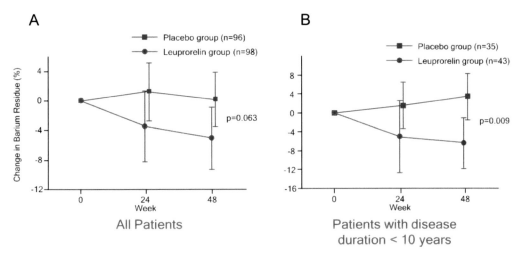

Figure 4. Effects of leuprorelin acetate on mean change in pharyngeal barium residue after initial swallowing. (A) In all patients. (B) Patients with disease duration <10 years. Bars=95% CI.

These results suggest that the disease duration of the patients might have influenced the efficacy. A disease-modifying treatment that prevents the accumulation of abnormal proteins might be more powerful before downstream molecular events have irreversibly damaged neurons: for example, anti-amyloid β vaccines might be effective in patients with pre-symptomatic or early-stage Alzheimer's disease. The results of the subgroup analysis in patients with a disease duration of less than 10 years were not conclusive, and thus the effect of disease duration on outcome measures should be further investigated in clinical trials.

Recently, the results of a randomized, placebo-controlled trial of the 5-α-reductase inhibitor dutasteride were also presented. This clinical trial showed that dutasteride was safe but did not have a significant effect on the progression of muscle weakness, measured by quantitative muscle assessment. Although the difference was not significant, the placebo group showed a decrease of 4.5% (–0.30 kg/kg) in this primary outcome measure, and the dutasteride group showed an increase in strength of 1.3% (0.14 kg/kg). Moreover, the results showed a tendency that dutasteride slows the deterioration of swallowing function as assessed by videofluorography [48]. Although these studies provided no conclusive results, their findings do not exclude the possibility that androgen-depleting therapies slow the progression of SBMA. Given the strong evidence shown in studies in animals, this hypothesis needs to be further verified in clinical trials with a rigorous and efficient design [49].

CONCLUSION

Given that SBMA is a slowly progressive disease, extremely long-term clinical trials are likely necessary to verify clinical benefits of disease-modifying therapies by targeting clinical endpoints such as the occurrence of aspiration pneumonia or becoming wheelchair-bound.

Suitable surrogate endpoints, which reflect the pathogenesis and severity of SBMA, are thus substantial to assess the therapeutic efficacy in drug trials. To this end, appropriate biomarkers should be identified and validated in translational researches. We might need to combine several parameters to appropriately use biomarkers in the development of therapeutics [50]. Quantitative analysis of natural history, including genetic, biological, and clinical data, is also necessary for long term evaluation of therapeutic agents for SBMA.

In view of the limited availability of participants and funds, clinical trials of neurodegenerative diseases such as SBMA should be carefully designed in terms of endpoints, sample size, duration, and inclusion and exclusion criteria. Although not a big leap, the recent clinical trials of androgen-modulating therapies for SBMA provide substantial information to guide the design of future clinical trials and pre-clinical animal studies.

ACKNOWLEDGMENTS

Figure 1 is reproduced from Banno *et al.* [27]. Figures 2 and 3 are reproduced from Banno *et al.* [46]. Figure 4 is reproduced from Katsuno *et al.* [47]. This work was supported by grants from the Ministry of Education, Culture, Sports, Science and Technology, Japan, grants from the Ministry of Health, Labor and Welfare, Japan.

REFERENCES

[1]   Kennedy, WR; Alter, M; Sung, JH. Progressive proximal spinal and bulbar muscular atrophy of late onset. A sex-linked recessive trait. Neurology 1968, 18, 671-680.

[2]   Fischbeck, KH. Kennedy disease. *J. Inherit. Metab. Dis.* 1997, 20, 152-158.

[3]   Guidetti, D; Sabadini, R; Ferlini, A; Torrente, I. Epidemiological survey of X-linked bulbar and spinal muscular atrophy, or Kennedy disease, in the province of Reggio Emilia, Italy. *Eur. J. Epidemiol.* 2001, 17, 587-591.

[4]   Atsuta, N; Watanabe, H; Ito, M; Banno, H; Suzuki, K; Katsuno, M; Tanaka, F; Tamakoshi, A; Sobue, G. Natural history of spinal and bulbar muscular atrophy (SBMA): A study of 223 Japanese patients. *Brain* 2006, 129, 1446-1455.

[5]   Katsuno, M; Adachi, H; Waza, M; Banno, H; Suzuki, K; Tanaka, F; Doyu, M; Sobue G. Pathogenesis, animal models and therapeutics in spinal and bulbar muscular atrophy (SBMA). *Exp. Neurol.* 2006, 200, 8-18.

[6]   Sinnreich, M; Sorenson, EJ; Klein, CJ. Neurologic course, endocrine dysfunction and triplet repeat size in spinal bulbar muscular atrophy. *Can. J. Neurol. Sci.*, 2004, 31, 378-382.

[7]   La Spada, AR; Wilson, EM; Lubahn, DB; Harding, AE; Fischbeck, KH. Androgen receptor gene mutations in X-linked spinal and bulbar muscular atrophy. *Nature* 1991, 352, 77-79.

[8]   Tanaka, F; Doyu, M; Ito, Y; Matsumoto, M; Mitsuma, T; Abe, K; Aoki, M; Itoyama, Y; Fischbeck, KH; Sobue, G. Founder effect in spinal and bulbar muscular atrophy (SBMA). *Hum. Mol. Genet.* 1996, 5, 1253-1257.

[9]   Doyu, M; Sobue, G; Mukai, E; Kachi, T; Yasuda, T; Mitsuma, T; Takahashi, A. Severity of X-linked recessive bulbospinal neuronopathy correlates with size of the tandem CAG repeat in androgen receptor gene. *Ann. Neurol.* 1992, 32, 707-710.

[10] La Spada, AR; Roling, DB; Harding, AE; Warner, CL; Spiegel, R; Hausmanowa-Petrusewicz, I; Yee, WC; Fischbeck, KH. Meiotic stability and genotype-phenotype correlation of the trinucleotide repeat in X-linked spinal and bulbar muscular atrophy. *Nat. Genet.* 1992; 2, 301-304.

[11] Gatchel, JR; Zoghbi, HY. Diseases of unstable repeat expansion: Mechanisms and common principles. *Nat. Rev. Genet.* 2005, 6, 743-755.

[12] Suzuki, K; Katsuno, M; Banno, H; Takeuchi, Y; Atsuta, N; Ito, M; Watanabe, H; Yamashita, F; Hori, N; Nakamura, T; Hirayama, M; Tanaka, F; Sobue, G. CAG repeat size correlates to electrophysiological motor and sensory phenotypes in SBMA. *Brain* 2008, 131, 229-239.

[13] Poletti, A. The polyglutamine tract of androgen receptor: from functions to dysfunctions in motor neurons. *Front. Neuroendocrinol.* 2004, 25, 1-26.

[14] Sobue, G; Hashizume, Y; Mukai, E; Hirayama, M; Mitsuma, T; Takahashi, A. X-linked recessive bulbospinal neuronopathy - A clinicopathological study. *Brain* 1989, 112, 209-232.

[15] Bates, G. Huntingtin aggregation and toxicity in Huntington's disease. *Lancet* 2003, 361, 1642-1644.

[16] Martindale, D; Hackam, A; Wieczorek, A; Ellerby, L; Wellington, C; McCutcheon, K; Singaraja, R; Kazemi-Esfarjani, P; Devon, R; Kim, SU; Bredesen, DE; Tufaro, F; Hayden, MR. Length of huntingtin and its polyglutamine tract influences localization and frequency of intracellular aggregates. *Nat. Genet.* 1998, 18, 150-154.

[17] Podolsky, S; Sax, DS; Leopold, NA. Increased frequency of diabetes mellitus in patients with Huntington's chorea. *Lancet* 1972, 1, 1356-1358.

[18] Sinnreich, M; Klein, CJ. Bulbospinal muscular atrophy - Kennedy's disease. *Arch. Neurol.* 2004, 61, 1324-1326.

[19] Li, M; Miwa, S; Kobayashi, Y; Merry, D.E; Yamamoto, M; Tanaka, F; Doyu, M; Hashizume, Y; Fischbeck, KH; Sobue, G. Nuclear inclusions of the androgen receptor protein in spinal and bulb muscular atrophy. *Ann. Neurol.* 1998, 44, 249-254.

[20] Kobayashi, Y; Miwa, S; Merry, DE; Kume, A; Mei, L; Doyu, M; Sobue, G. Caspase-3 cleaves the expanded androgen receptor protein of spinal and bulbar muscular atrophy in a polyglutamine repeat length-dependent manner. *Biochem. Biophys. Res. Commun.* 1998, 252, 145-150.

[21] Arrasate, M; Mitra, S; Schweitzer, ES; Segal, MR; Finkbeiner, S. Inclusion body formation reduces levels of mutant huntingtin and the risk of neuronal death. *Nature* 2004, 431, 805-810.

[22] Truant, R; Atwal, RS; Desmond, C; Munsie, L; Tran, T. Huntington's disease: Revisiting the aggregation hypothesis in polyglutamine neurodegenerative diseases. *FEBS J.* 2008, 275, 4252-4262.

[23] Nagai, Y; Inui, T; Popiel, HA; Fujikake, N; Hasegawa, K; Urade, Y; Goto, Y; Naiki, H; Toda, T. A toxic monomeric conformer of the polyglutamine protein. Nat. Struct. Mol. Biol. 2007, 14, 332-340.

[24] Takahashi, T; Kikuchi, S; Katada, S; Nagai, Y; Nishizawa, M; Onodera, O. Soluble polyglutamine oligomers formed prior to inclusion body formation are cytotoxic. *Hum. Mol. Genet.* 2008, 17, 345-356.

[25] Adachi, H; Katsuno, M; Minamiyama, M; Waza, M; Sang, C; Nakagomi, Y; Kobayashi, Y; Tanaka, F; Doyu, M; Inukai, A; Yoshida, M; Hashizume, Y; Sobue, G. Widespread nuclear and cytoplasmic accumulation of mutant androgen receptor in SBMA patients. *Brain* 2005, 128, 659-670.

[26] Yamada, M; Sato, T; Tsuji, S; Takahashi, H. Oligodendrocytic polyglutamine pathology in dentatorubral-pallidoluysian atrophy. *Ann. Neurol.* 2002, 52, 670-674.

[27] Banno, H; Adachi, H; Katsuno, M; Suzuki, K; Atsuta, N; Watanabe, H; Tanaka, F; Doyu, M; Sobue, G. Mutant androgen receptor accumulation in spinal and bulbar muscular atrophy scrotal skin: A pathogenic marker. *Ann. Neurol.* 2006, 59, 520-526.

[28] McCampbell, A; Taylor, JP; Taye, AA; Robitschek, J; Li, M; Walcott, J; Merry, D; Chai, Y; Paulson, H; Sobue, G; Fischbeck, KH. CREB-binding protein sequestration by expanded polyglutamine. *Hum. Mol. Genet.* 2002, 9, 2197-2202.

[29] Minamiyama, M; Katsuno, M; Adachi, H; Waza, M; Sang, C; Kobayashi, Y; Tanaka, F; Doyu, M; Inukai, A; Sobue, G. Sodium butyrate ameliorates phenotypic expression in a transgenic mouse model of spinal and bulbar muscular atrophy. *Hum. Mol. Genet.* 2004, 13, 1183-1192.

[30] Ranganathan, S; Harmison, GG; Meyertholen, K; Pennuto, M; Burnett, BG; Fischbeck, KH. Mitochondrial abnormalities in spinal and bulbar muscular atrophy. *Hum. Mol. Genet.* 2009, 18, 27-42.

[31] Morfini, G; Pigino, G; Szebenyi, G; You, Y; Pollema, S; Brady, ST. JNK mediates pathogenic effects of polyglutamine-expanded androgen receptor on fast axonal transport. *Nat. Neurosci.* 2006, 9, 907-916.

[32] Katsuno, M; Adachi, H; Minamiyama, M; Waza, M; Tokui, K; Banno, H; Suzuki, K; Onoda, Y; Tanaka, F; Doyu, M; Sobue, G. Reversible disruption of dynactin 1-mediated retrograde axonal transport in polyglutamine-induced motor neuron degeneration. *J. Neurosci.* 2006, 26, 12106-12117.

[33] Malik, B; Nirmalananthan, N; Bilsland, LG; La Spada, AR; Hanna, MG; Schiavo, G; Gallo, JM; Greensmith, L. Absence of disturbed axonal transport in spinal and bulbar muscular atrophy. *Hum Mol Genet.* 2011, 20, 1776-1786.

[34] Williams, AJ; Paulson, HL. Polyglutamine neurodegeneration: Protein misfolding revisited. *Trends Neurosci.* 2008, 31, 521-528.

[35] Katsuno, M; Banno, H; Suzuki, K; Takeuchi, Y; Kawashima, M; Tanaka, F; Adachi, H; Sobue, G. Molecular genetics and biomarkers of polyglutamine diseases. *Curr. Mol. Med.* 2008, 8, 221-234.

[36] Katsuno, M; Adachi, H; Kume, A; Li, M; Nakagomi, Y; Niwa, H; Sang, C; Kobayashi, Y; Doyu, M; Sobue, G. Testosterone reduction prevents phenotypic expression in a transgenic mouse model of spinal and bulbar muscular atrophy. *Neuron* 2002, 35, 843-854.

[37] Takeyama, K; Ito, S; Yamamoto, A; Tanimoto, H; Furutani, T; Kanuka, H; Miura, M; Tabata, T; Kato, S. Androgen-dependent neurodegeneration by polyglutamine-expanded human androgen receptor in Drosophila. *Neuron* 2002, 35, 855-864.

[38] Chevalier-Larsen, ES; O'Brien, CJ; Wang, HY; Jenkins, SC; Holder, L; Lieberman, AP; Merry, DE. Castration restores function and neurofilament alterations of aged

symptomatic males in a transgenic mouse model of spinal and bulbar muscular atrophy. *J. Neurosci.* 2004, 24, 4778-4786.

[39]   Katsuno, M; Adachi, H; Doyu, M; Minamiyama, M; Sang, C; Kobayashi, Y; Inukai, A; Sobue, G. Leuprorelin rescues polyglutamine-dependent phenotypes in a transgenic mouse model of spinal and bulbar muscular atrophy. *Nat. Med.* 2003, 9, 768-773.

[40]   Adachi, H; Katsuno, M; Minamiyama, M; Sang, C; Pagoulatos, G; Angelidis, C; Kusakabe, M; Yoshiki, A; Kobayashi, Y; Doyu, M; Sobue, G. Heat shock protein 70 chaperone overexpression ameliorates phenotypes of the spinal and bulbar muscular atrophy transgenic mouse model by reducing nuclear-localized mutant androgen receptor protein. *J. Neurosci.* 2003, 23, 2203-2211.

[41]   Katsuno, M; Sang, C; Adachi, H; Minamiyama, M; Waza, M; Tanaka, F; Doyu, M; Sobue, G. Pharmacological induction of heat-shock proteins alleviates polyglutamine-mediated motor neuron disease. *Proc. Natl. Acad. Sci. USA* 2005, 102, 16801-16806.

[42]   Waza, M; Adachi, H; Katsuno, M; Minamiyama, M; Sang, C; Tanaka, F; Inukai, A; Doyu, M; Sobue, G. 17-AAG, an Hsp90 inhibitor, ameliorates polyglutamine-mediated motor neuron degeneration. *Nat. Med.* 2005, 11, 1088-1095.

[43]   Thomas, M; Harrell, JM; Morishima, Y; Peng, HM; Pratt, WB; Lieberman, AP. Pharmacologic and genetic inhibition of hsp90-dependent trafficking reduces aggregation and promotes degradation of the expanded glutamine androgen receptor without stress protein induction. *Hum. Mol. Genet.* 2006, 15, 1876-1883.

[44]   Tokui, K; Adachi, H; Waza, M; Katsuno, M; Minamiyama, M; Doi, H; Tanaka, K; Hamazaki, J; Murata, S; Tanaka, F; Sobue, G. 17-DMAG ameliorates polyglutamine-mediated motor neuron degeneration through well-preserved proteasome function in a SBMA model mouse. *Hum. Mol. Genet.* 2009, 18, 898-910.

[45]   Steffan, JS; Bodai, L; Pallos, J; Poelman, M; McCampbell, A; Apostol, BL; Kazantsev, A; Schmidt, E; Zhu, YZ; Greenwald, M; Kurokawa, R; Housman, DE; Jackson, GR; Marsh, JL; Thompson, LM. Histone deacetylase inhibitors arrest polyglutamine-dependent neurodegeneration in Drosophila. Nature 2001, 413(6857): 739-743.

[46]   Banno, H; Katsuno, M; Suzuki, K; Takeuchi, Y; Kawashima, M; Suga, N; Takamori, M; Ito, M; Nakamura, T; Matsuo, K; Yamada, S; Oki, Y; Adachi, H; Minamiyama, M; Waza, M; Atsuta, N; Watanabe, H; Fujimoto, Y; Nakashima, T; Tanaka, F; Doyu, M; Sobue, G. Phase 2 trial of leuprorelin in patients with spinal and bulbar muscular atrophy. *Ann. Neurol.* 2009, 65, 140-150.

[47]   Katsuno, M; Banno, H; Suzuki, K; Takeuchi, Y; Kawashima, M; Yabe, I; Sasaki, H; Aoki, M; Morita, M; Nakano, I; Kanai, K; Ito, S; Ishikawa, K; Mizusawa, H; Yamamoto, T; Tsuji, S; Hasegawa, K; Shimohata, T; Nishizawa, M; Miyajima, H; Kanda, F; Watanabe, Y; Nakashima, K; Tsujino, A; Yamashita, T; Uchino, M; Fujimoto, Y; Tanaka, F; Sobue, G. Japan SBMA Interventional Trial for TAP-144-SR (JASMITT) study group. Efficacy and safety of leuprorelin in patients with spinal and bulbar muscular atrophy (JASMITT study): a multi-center, randomized, double-blind, placebo-controlled trial. *Lancet Neurol.* 2010, 9, 875-884.

[48]   Fernández-Rhodes, LE; Kokkinis, AD; White, MJ; Watts, CA; Auh, S; Jeffries, NO; Shrader, JA; Lehky, TJ; Li, L; Ryder, JE; Levy, EW; Solomon, BI; Harris-Love, MO; La Pean, A; Schindler, AB; Chen, C; Di Prospero, NA; Fischbeck, KH. Efficacy and safety of dutasteride in patients with spinal and bulbar muscular atrophy: a randomized placebo-controlled trial. *Lancet Neurol.* 2011, 10, 140-147.

[49] Banno, H; Katsuno, M; Suzuki, K; Sobue, G. Dutasteride for spinal and bulbar muscular atrophy. *Lancet Neurol.* 2011, 10, 113-115.

[50] Borovecki, F; Lovrecic, L; Zhou, J; Jeong, H; Then, F; Rosas, HD; Hersch, SM; Hogarth, P; Bouzou, B; Jensen, RV; Krainc, D. Genome-wide expression profiling of human blood reveals biomarkers for Huntington's disease. *Proc. Natl. Acad. Sci. USA* 2005, 102, 11023-11028.

In: Motor Neuron Diseases
Editors: Bradley J. Turner and Julie B. Atkin

ISBN 978-1-61470-101-9
© 2012 Nova Science Publishers, Inc.

Chapter IX

EXPERT COMMENTARY: MOTOR NEURON DISEASE: ASSISTIVE TECHNOLOGY

Louisa Ng[*1,2] *and Fary Khan*[1,2]

[1]Neurological Rehabilitation Physician, Royal Melbourne Hospital,
Parkville, Melbourne VIC 3052, Australia
[2]Department of Rehabilitation Medicine, University of Melbourne, Australia

INTRODUCTION

Motor Neuron Disease (MND) is an adult-onset neurodegenerative disease, which leads to progressive weakness of limb, bulbar and respiratory muscles resulting in death often within three to five years, generally from respiratory failure. The burden of disease of MND upon patients and their caregivers (often family members) is substantial, often beginning long before the actual diagnosis is made, and increasing with worsening disability and the need for medical equipment and assisted care [1]. The course of MND is relentless and in the absence of a cure, management relies mostly on symptomatic, rehabilitative and palliative care. Assistive technology can have a dramatic effect on restoring and maintaining independence, a sense of control and quality of life and is an integral component of the rehabilitative process in the care of persons with MND (pwMND).

The use of assistive technology in MND can be broadly divided into 1) technology that assists with mobility; 2) communication, including computer access, and 3) environmental control units (ECU), with significant overlap and integration amongst the three categories. In a recent study [2] of 44 pwMND currently receiving multidisciplinary care, limited understanding and availability of assistive technology to facilitate function and decrease reliance on caregivers was identified as an area for improvement. There is a general lack of awareness especially around available environmental control technology even amongst health

* Ph: +61 3 83872000, fax: +61 3 83872222, email: louisa.ng@mh.org.au

professionals [3]. It must however also be stressed that, in general, it is essential for patients, families and therapists to work closely together when prescribing and using assistive technology to ensure the correct, safe and optimal use of such aids and equipment; and to anticipate future needs especially with the expense of such technology. Close collaboration with specialised providers of assistive technology that can also supply back-up technical support is also crucial.

ASSISTIVE TECHNOLOGY FOR MOBILITY

Difficulties in bed mobility can result in significant complications including the development of pressure areas and pain. It also increases caregiver burden and stress [4] especially if caregivers have to wake overnight to turn the patient or to assist with any body posture changes. Electrically controlled beds facilitate management of dependent oedema, transferring in/out of bed and can ameliorate pain, which may or may not be related to spasticity [5]. Controls should be appropriate for the patient's disability (mounted close to a functional limb) or an ECU could be used [6].

Powered wheelchairs are essential for independent mobility as lower limb weakness progresses. Persons with MND often wish they had received their powered chairs sooner and generally feel satisfied that their chair is good value for money despite the high costs (range USD$20,000-35,000) [7]. They are suitable for indoor and/or outdoor use although features may vary depending on the terrain. These chairs can be controlled in a variety of ways and further integrated with systems to enable communication and ECUs [8]. Additional features such as recline, tilt-in-space and custom seating serve to optimise independence and social interaction whilst preventing contractures, compression nerve palsies, skin breakdown and aspiration [4] and facilitate swallowing and breathing.

ASSISTIVE TECHNOLOGY FOR COMMUNICATION
AND COMPUTER ACCESS

As intelligibility in MND worsens, Augmentative and Alternative Communication (AAC) is required. AACs can improve quality of life by optimising function and assisting with decision making [9]. AACs range from no or low technology (gestures, communication boards with letters) to high-tech electronic communication devices or computers that allow the user to have voice output, send e-mail and surf the web [9]. For example, speech-generating devices such as LightWRITERs are commonly used. These devices can be used as long as there is voluntary motor movement (including eye gaze). The specific access method depends on the abilities of the patient – for example, pointing with a body part or pointer, adapted mice or joysticks or switches and scanning technology can be used. For those who have no voluntary motor control for communication, a recent case study using a brain-computer interface system has been reported and appears promising [10]. The emotional aspect of using an alternative form of communication however can result in significant patient resistance and acceptance as the ability to speak and use language is what distinguishes us from all other species [9,11]. Hence, acceptance of an AAC may take weeks to months.

A source of significant frustration for those with speech difficulties is use of the telephone. Technology is available and varies from country to country. In the United States, "Speech to Speech" technology can be used, where trained communication assistants are used by the patient to complete phone calls. They are trained to use superior equipment to hear the caller and place the call, then repeat verbatim what the caller says so the call is completed successfully [12].

Computer technology is fast advancing and options include different types of keyboards, mouse alternatives, switches, interfaces, mounting systems, integrated communication/computer access packages, software and systems. For those who have some proximal arm control, track balls, type writing sticks and forearm supports may be useful. In pwMND who have more severe upper limb weakness, head tracking systems, on-screen keyboards and voice recognition software may be required. Text-entry software such as Dasher (which is free) can be used whenever a full-size keyboard cannot be used such as on a palmtop computer or with a joystick, touchscreen, trackball, headpointer, or eyetracker [12]. There are also many mouse alternatives available -- eyegaze system, foot control mouse, head tracking mouse, joysticks and switch-adapted mouse.

ENVIRONMENTAL CONTROL UNITS

Environmental control systems offer sophisticated electronics to enable people with a range of impairments and severe disability to use a wide variety of electrical devices. Aids may include unobtrusive control units (eg. remote control for TV), home security (door intercoms, door release and alarms), adapted telephones (such as hands-free control) and lighting and heating/cooling systems [13]. These environmental control units may be used to facilitate function and decrease reliance on carers, improve family dynamics and improve patients' self-esteem [13].

"Smart homes" refer to any technology that automates a home-based activity but are used by many to describe interactive systems that allow an occupant to control home activities from a central access point (eg. computer, personal digital assistant or remote-control device) [14]. They are becoming increasingly common and affordable (range from USD$200 to $100,000) and in relation to people with disability, can be divided into five classes: 1) incorporation of intelligent objects such as doors or window shade via remote control or motion-activation 2) use of wired or wireless networks for information exchange such as computer-controlled thermostat or lighting 3) "connected homes" that use of electronic networks that reach beyond the home such as management of appliances remotely or internet grocery shopping or a falls monitoring system that triggers external alerts 4) "learning homes" that link to computers which analyse patterns of activity and mange appliances accordingly and 5) "attentive homes" that control technology in anticipation of human needs [15]. The later two classes are still in development phases; however, there is a growing body of evidence supporting the first three classes of smart homes. A randomized controlled trial (n=104) found that provision of individualized assistive technology and home modifications (eg. ramps, bath rails, medical alert bracelets and security lighting) in frail elderly patients resulted in less decrease in functional independence, reduced medical care costs and reduced hospitalizations [16]. As for class 3 homes, a randomized trial of spinal cord injury patients showed that telehealth interventions improved one-year health outcomes [17]; similarly telerehabilitation interventions in stroke, brain in jury and multiple sclerosis found improvements in arm/hand function [18]. In an MND population, as disability becomes severe and travelling difficult and a proportion of patients stop coming to clinic; telehealth could supplement the provision of care.

Some pwMND themselves or have family members that have engineering or technological backgrounds and create their own ECU. For example, a pwMND reports that with little functional use of upper or lower limbs, and with voice commands, line-of-sight or through the head array on his electric wheelchair, he is able to control the computer pointer without a mouse. He has integrated software systems, which allows him to control many electronic devices from his bed or wheelchair with microphones and other input devices. For example, he is able to control lights, heating, television (on/off, volume, record programs), internet radio, speak to visitors at his door using audio/video cameras, lock or unlock his front door, call for help regardless of where he is in the house through intercoms, access the emergency helpline, use word processors with speech recognition and mouse pointer control, access the internet (e-mail and browse internet), speak to family and caregivers using audio/video cameras through internet access and adjust his electric bed [19].

There are many possible ways to increase independence and quality of life in those who have disability. Assistive technology should be considered in pwMND. Patients and therapists should push the boundaries and be creative. Especially as newer generations become more technologically savvy, the potential is unlimited and inventors, researchers, manufacturers, vendors, clinicians and consumers need to work together to realise that potential.

REFERENCES

[1]   Klein LM, Forshew DA. The economic impact of ALS. *Neurology.* 1996 Oct;47(4 Suppl 2):S126-9.

[2]   Ng L, Talman P, Khan F. Motor Neurone Disease: Disability profile and service needs in an Australian cohort. *Int. J. Rehabil Res.* 2011;in press.

[3]   Martins B, Fitzsimons C. Towards a more comprehensive AT service for people with neurological disabilities in Ireland. In: Craddock GM, editor. *Assistive technology - shaping the future.* Amsterdam: IOS press; 2003.

[4]   Francis K, Bach JR, DeLisa JA. Evaluation and rehabilitation of patients with adult motor neuron disease. *Arch. Phys. Med. Rehabil.* 1999 Aug;80(8):951-63.

[5]   Frank A. Motor neurone disease: practical update ignores rehabilitative approaches - particularly assistive technology. *Clinical Medicine.* 2010;10(6):640-1.

[6]   Paul SN, Frank AO, Hanspal RS, Groves R. Exploring environmental control unit use in the age group 10-20 years. *Int. J. Ther Rehabil.* 2006;13:511-6.

[7]   Ward AL, Sanjak M, Duffy K, Bravver E, Williams N, Nichols M, et al. Power wheelchair prescription, utilization, satisfaction, and cost for patients with amyotrophic lateral sclerosis: preliminary data for evidence-based guidelines. *Arch. Phys. Med. Rehabil.* 2010 Feb;91(2):268-72.

[8]   Williams E. Electronic assistive technology: a working party report of the British Society of Rehabilitation Medicine. London: British Society of Rehabilitation Medicine2000.

[9]   Brownlee A, Palovcak M. The role of augmentative communication devices in the medical management of ALS. *NeuroRehabilitatio*n. 2007;22(6):445-50.

[10] Sellers EW, Vaughan TM, Wolpaw JR. A brain-computer interface for long-term independent home use. *Amyotroph. Lateral Scler.* 2010 Oct;11(5):449-55.

[11] Pinker S, Jackendoff R. The faculty of language: what's special about it? *Cognition.* 2005 Mar;95(2):201-36.

[12] [cited 2011 January]; Available from: http://www.fctd.info/resources?on= disabilityandtag=Neurological+Disorders.

[13] Wellings DJ, Unsworth J. Fortnightly review. Environmental control systems for people with a disability: an update. *BMJ.* 1997 Aug 16;315(7105):409-12.

[14] Gentry T. Smart homes for people with neurological disability: state of the art. *NeuroRehabilitation.* 2009;25(3):209-17.

[15] Aldrich F. Smart homes past, present and future. In: Harper R, editor. *Inside the Smart Home.* London: Springer; 2003. p. 17-39.

[16] Mann WC, Ottenbacher KJ, Fraas L, Tomita M, Granger CV. Effectiveness of assistive technology and environmental interventions in maintaining independence and reducing home care costs for the frail elderly. A randomized controlled trial. *Arch. Fam. Med.* 1999 May-Jun;8(3):210-7.

[17] Phillips VL, Temkin A, Vesmarovich S, Burns R, Idleman L. Using telehealth interventions to prevent pressure ulcers in newly injured spinal cord injury patients post-discharge. Results from a pilot study. *Int. J. Technol. Assess Health Care.* 1999 Fall;15(4):749-55.

[18] Huijgen BC, Vollenbroek-Hutten MM, Zampolini M, Opisso E, Bernabeu M, Van Nieuwenhoven J, et al. Feasibility of a home-based telerehabilitation system compared to usual care: arm/hand function in patients with stroke, traumatic brain injury and multiple sclerosis. *J. Telemed. Telecare.* 2008;14(5):249-56.

[19] New Assistive Technology For All Is Possible Holland Landing2010 [cited 2011 19th January]; Available from: http://www.alsforums.com/forum/general-discussion-about-als-mnd/11963-new-assistive-technology-all-possible.html.

In: Motor Neuron Diseases
Editors: Bradley J. Turner and Julie B. Atkin

ISBN 978-1-61470-101-9
© 2012 Nova Science Publishers, Inc.

Chapter X

COMPARATIVE STUDY ON APPLICATION OF INVASIVE AND NON-INVASIVE VENTILATION TO ALS PATIENTS IN JAPAN, THE USA AND EUROPE

Rika Yamauchi, Jun Kawamata and Shun Shimohama[*]
Department of Neurology, School of Medicine,
Sapporo Medical University, Japan

ABSTRACT

We reviewed the published documents on application of mechanical ventilation to amyotrophic lateral sclerosis (ALS) patients and analyzed the influential factors of decision making for applying mechanical ventilation by looking into how it is practiced in Japan, the USA, and Europe. In Japan, 29.3% of ALS patients were on invasive ventilation via tracheostomy (TV), 7.2% on non-invasive ventilation (NIV) in 2005. The significant difference in the prevalence of mechanical ventilation was observed among prefectures or hospitals. In the USA, the prevalence rates of TV and NIV were reported to be 3% and 36.2%, respectively, in 2006. NIV is less applied in European nations compared with its usage in Japan and the USA. It is confirmed that the number of patients who choose TV is gradually growing, yet relatively small, in European nations, where an inconsistency in the introduction rate of mechanical ventilation to ALS patients was also observed in accordance with the national, regional and hospital levels. According to the analysis of influential factors in the introduction of mechanical ventilation, it seems that the heavy economic burden is the main factor to decrease the usage rate of mechanical ventilation for ALS patients.

---

* Correspondence: Shun Shimohama, MD, PhD, Department of Neurology, School of Medicine, Sapporo Medical University, shimoha@sapmed.ac.jp

Keywords: amyotrophic lateral sclerosis (ALS), decision making, invasive ventilation via tracheostomy (TV), non-invasive ventilation (NIV), mechanical ventilation

I. INTRODUCTION

Amyotrophic lateral sclerosis (ALS) is a neurodegenerative disease characterized by degeneration of motor neurons in the cerebral cortex, brainstem and spinal cord, and is also known as "Lou Gehrig's disease" in the USA and as "Maladie de Charcot" in France. A combination of upper and lower motor neuron dysfunction produces progressive weakness of voluntary muscles. ALS patients gradually lose their ability to work, walk, speak, and swallow, so they need to be assisted in daily living activities, with equipments, such as wheelchairs and communication aids, life-sustaining therapy, such as percutaneous endoscopic gastrostomy (PEG), and mechanical ventilation. Respiratory failure, mainly due to respiratory muscle dysfunction, is the most common cause of death of ALS patients within five years from the onset of disease. Invasive ventilation via tracheostomy (TV) was the only life-sustaining therapy known to support ALS patients for a long period of time. Recently, some studies have reported that non-invasive ventilation (NIV) improved survival and quality of life of ALS patients almost as much as TV did. ALS does not deprive its patients of their sensation, cognitive faculty and consciousness, so that the patients must decide their own treatment at some stages of the disease. We attempt in this chapter to review the published documents and analyze the influential factors of decision making in applying NIV and TV to ALS patients by looking into how it is practiced in Japan, the USA and Europe.

II. THE EFFICACY OF TV AND NIV ON ALS PATIENTS

TV began to be used, worldwide, for treating the respiratory muscle paralysis by the poliomyelitis in 1950's, and for neuromuscular diseases in 1960's. NIV has carried out for neuromuscular diseases since 1987 in USA. In Japan, initially TV began to be used for neuromuscular diseases in 1970's, and for ALS patients in the latter half of 1980's. NIV began to be used for patients of Duchenne muscular dystrophy (DMD) in 1988. The number of ALS patients with NIV has increased slowly since 1990. As the efficacy of NIV became apparent, some guidelines had already become open to public, which includes "Practice Parameter" updated by the American Academy of Neurology (AAN) in 2009 [1], "Good Practice in the Management of ALS" by the EALSC Working Group in 2007 [2], and "ALS Care Guideline" by the Societas Neurologica Japonica in 2002 [3] for managing respiratory insufficiency of ALS patients at advanced stages.

The content which is common in these guidelines is as follows.

1.   NIV and TV are used to relieve respiratory symptoms, improve quality of life and prolong survival.
2.   There is no verified timing and criteria of introduction of NIV and TV in ALS patients.

3.   Physicians and patients should discuss, in advance, the end of life issues, palliative care, and advance directives, so that they can avoid unplanned TV.
4.   NIV should be applied to relieve respiratory symptoms before TV.
5.   TV may be proposed in a case that NIV is not effective, which is caused by the difficulty to secure the upper airway due to worsen bulbar palsy or increased secretion.

i. The Survival of ALS Patients with Mechanical Ventilation

There are 2 studies that adopted survival as an endpoint, both of which reported prolonged survival of ALS patients with TV. Cazzolli PA *et al.* reported survival rate of 50 patients with TV. They described that 4 of 23 deceased lived for 9-12 years after starting TV, 2 of 27 alive lived after 7-8 years, and 3 were alive after 11-14 years of TV. Most of them were provided with tracheostomy care by family members, as skillfully as trained respiratory care practitioners and registered nurses. TV might extend survival for up to more than 10 years despite significant bulbar impairment when effective respiratory care is given [4]. Lo Coco D *et al.* reported that ALS patients with TV had a high chance of long-term survival; the mean survival time was 37 months [5].

Of ALS patients with NIV, 6 studies used survival as an endpoint and all reported prolonged survival. Bach JR *et al.* showed that 14-17 months prolonged survival in ALS patients who succeeded in use of NIV for 24 hours [6]. Aboussouan LS *et al.* showed that ALS patients who are tolerant of NIV have better survival than those who are intolerant in an observational cohort study [7]. Although NIV has no impact on the rate of decline of lung function, median survivals in ALS patients intolerant and tolerant of NIV were 5 and 20 months, respectively [8]. Kleopa KA *et al.* showed that ALS patients using NIV more than 4hr / day had longer survival and slower decline in vital capacity in a retrospective chart review [9]. Pinto AC *et al.* showed that ALS patients using NIV had longer survival and later appearance of gas exchanges disorders in a prospective, controlled study [10]. Moreover, Bourke SC *et al.* showed that ALS patients using NIV experienced, in a randomized controlled study, a median survival benefit of 205 days with maintained quality of life, but without effect on rate of decline of respiratory function [11].

ii. The Quality of Life in ALS Patients with Mechanical Ventilation

The quality of life in ALS patients with mechanical ventilation was assessed in 6 studies using questionnaires, and all reported positive effect. Kaub-Wittemer D *et al.* described that there was no difference in quality of life between patients using NIV and patients with TV [12]. Gelinas DF *et al.* reported that most patients using either NIV or TV would choose mechanical ventilation again, being satisfied with their decisions [13]. Lyall RA *et al.* [14] and Aboussouan LS *et al.* [8] concluded that NIV improved quality of life of ALS patients despite their increasing disabilities. Bourke SC *et al.* [15] and Jackson CE *et al.* [16] reported that NIV improved the scores in the subscale of vitality and mental health in the Short Form 36 Health Survey (SF-36) that is a self-assessment measure of the quality of life.

III. THE PREVALENCE OF TV AND NIV ON ALS PATIENTS

These evidences given above thus have come to prove the utility of NIV and TV. Although some guidelines recommended mechanical ventilation for management of respiratory insufficiency in ALS patients, the prevalence of NIV and TV has not actually increased.

i. The Prevalence in Japan

In Japan, 7.2% of 4202 ALS patients were on NIV, 29.3% on TV according to the report from the Ministry of Health, Labour and Welfare in 2005. In the report, the significant difference in the prevalence of mechanical ventilation was observed in relation with where it is practiced. Some prefectures, such as Aomori, Yamagata, Kagawa and Oita had a quite high rate, as much as 60%, whereas Yamanashi, Nara and Hiroshima had only 10~15%. In Hokkaido, the prevalence rates of NIV and TV were expected to be 20% and 20%, respectively, in 2010. Many patients on NIV receive medical treatment as outpatients, and nearly half of patients on TV are hospitalized.

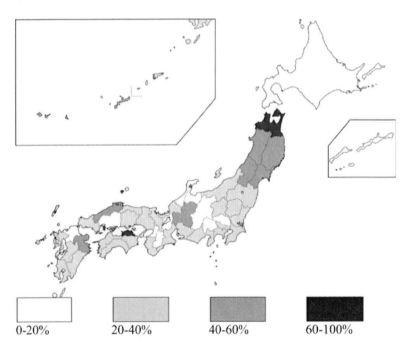

Figure 1. The prevalence of mechanical ventilation by prefecture in Japan.

The prevalence of whole mechanical ventilation is uneven at each prefecture, and there is no tendency according to the district and the population.

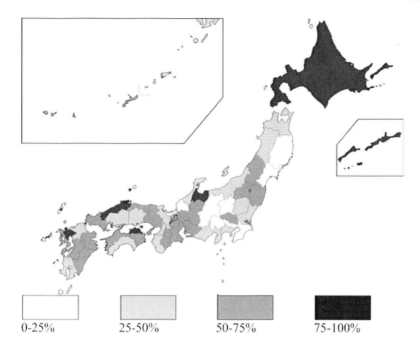

Figure 2. The ratio of hospitalization of the ALS patients with mechanical ventilation by prefectures in Japan.

Among the prefectures where the prevalence of mechanical ventilation is high, some prefectures have high ratios of hospitalization and the other have high ratios of home medical care.

Similarly, the same kind of inconsistency was also observed among hospitals. The investigation on the prevalence of NIV and TV at individual medical institutions has not yet been done throughout Japan. So far, 22 reports from hospitals and visiting nurse stations have been published in Japan, which describe the usage rate of both NIV and/or TV. 9 of these described the usage rate of both NIV and TV all of which was reported between 2003 and 2007. These institutions would be divided into three groups as follows.

1.   Institutions where TV is provided for most ALS patients. The usage rates of NIV and TV were 0%-5% vs. 25%-80%, respectively.
2.   Institutions where TV is more provided for ALS patients than NIV. The usage rates of NIV and TV were 20%-25% vs. 40%-50%, respectively.
3.   Institutions where NIV is more provided for ALS patients than TV. The usage rate of NIV was slightly higher than TV.

The deflection of the usage rate was not seen among districts or prefectures. The following table shows details [17-25].

The majority of institutions seem to have reluctance toward NIV and/or TV. As shown above, even among a few institutions which deal with the management of respiratory insufficiency of patients with neuromuscular disorders such as ALS, there is a wide gap in the usage rate of TV and NIV.

Table 1. The usage rate of NIV and TV in Japan

	Author	Prefecture	Year	Cases	NIV	TV
TV>>NIV	Kimura et al. [17]	Osaka	2003	92	5.4%	29.3%
	Kataoka et al. [18]	Tokyo	2006	12	0.0%	83.3%
	Yoshida et al. [19]	Nagano	2006	136	5.1%	25.0%
	Kondo et al. [20]	Hyogo	2007	59	6.8%	81.4%
TV>NIV	Uehara et al. [21]	Osaka	2003	21	23.8%	47.0%
	Yamamoto et al. [22]	Oita	2003	20	20.0%	65.0%
	Nagahama et al. [23]	Osaka	2004	17	23.5%	41.2%
TV<NIV	Nanba et al. [24]	Okayama	2005	45	33.3%	31.1%
	Kasahara et al. [25]	Tokyo	2005	35	28.6%	25.7%
Total				437	12.4%	39.4%

Some institutions have a lot of ALS patients with TV, other institutions have ALS patients with NIV as many as ALS patients with TV regardless of time, prefectures in Japan.

ii. The Prevalence in the USA

According to ALS CARE database, in the USA, the prevalence rates of NIV and TV were reported to be 15.6% and 2.1%, respectively, in 2004. Though the usage rate of NIV gradually increased to 36.2%, that of TV stayed at 3% from the same database in 2006 [26-28]. The ALS CARE database collected information on 2,500-4,000 ALS patients, of which white prevailed as of 90%. It was estimated that the number of ALS patients in the USA rises up to around 30,000 people. Based on the USA population's distribution in 2009, the total population was 307 million in 2009, white alone was 229.8 million (74.8%), black or African American 38.1 million (12.4%). There was discrepancy between demographic data and ALS CARE database. There was uncertainty as to whether these patients were representative of the ALS patient population at large, and whether the conclusions can be generalized. It could be the tendency in the whole USA, but the selective bias could not be excluded completely.

From those institutions, 9 reports reported the usage rate of both NIV and TV. All was reported between 1997 and 2010, when NIV had begun to infiltrate among developed nations. The number of ALS patients with NIV is reported as about 20-60%. At only two institutions, the number of ALS patients with TV came to around 20%; the number of ALS patients with TV came to a little less than 5% at the other institutions. The following table shows details [6-8, 26, 27, 29-32].

Table 2. The usage rate of NIV and TV in the USA

	Author	State	Year	Cases	NIV	TV
TV=NIV	Sivak ED et al. [29]	NY	2001	27	18.5%	18.5%
	Bach JR et al. [6]	NJ	2002	166	22.3%	23.5%
TV<NIV	Aboussouan LS et al. [7]	OH	1997	66	59.0%	3.0%
	Melo J et al. [30]	All	1999	2537	15.7%	2.8%
	Albert SM et al. [31]	NY	1999	93	19.4%	4.3%
	Aboussouan LS et al. [8]	OH	2000	60	38.3%	5.0%
	Bradley WG et al. [26]	All	2001	2018	28.0%	3.2%
	Cedarbaum JM et al. [32]	All	2001	387	7.0%	2.0%
	Lechtzin N et al. [27]	All	2004	1458	15.6%	2.1%

Most institutions have a few ALS patients with TV regardless of time or place in USA.

iii. The Prevalence in Europe

The NIV is less applied to ALS patients in European nations compared with its usage in the USA and Japan. It is confirmed that there are few patients who choose TV in the continent. In EU survey [33], 1.9 patients (2.6%) selected TV and 7.6 patients (10.3%) selected NIV out of 74 mean patients within a year. From these institutions in UK, Germany, Italy, Portugal, Denmark, 6 reported the usage rate of both NIV and TV. All was reported between 1995 and 2009. It cannot be said that the number of ALS patients with NIV and TV had increased progressively in the period. The numbers of ALS patients with NIV were inconsistent, 5-50%. The ALS patients with TV were around 10% at the only one institution, the ALS patients with TV were 0%-5% at the other institutions. Thus, inconsistency in the introduction rate of NIV and TV was also observed in accordance with the national, prefectural and hospital levels in European nations. The following table shows details [10, 34-39].

Table 3. The usage rate of NIV and TV in Europe

	Author	Nation	Year	Cases	NIV	TV
TV>NIV	Mandrioli J et al. [34]	ITA	2006	123	1.6%	5.7%
TV<NIV	Pinto AC et al. [10]	POR	1995	20	45.0%	5.0%
	Borasio GD et al. [35]	18 nations	2001	74	10.3%	2.6%
	Bourke SC et al. [36]	UK	2002	2280	5.5%	0.4%
	Kuhnlein P et al. [37]	GER	2008	29	93.0%	0.0%
	Nonnenmacher S et al. [38]	GER	2009	65	35.0%	6.0%
	Lorenzen CK et al. [39]	DEN	2009	301	53.5%	11.6%

Most institutions have very few ALS patients with TV regardless of time or nations.

IV. Factors of Difference in Each Nation, Region and Hospital

The prevalence of NIV and TV varies substantially both within and between nations. It is worth analyzing the factors to study the difference of usage rate at each hospital, in the region and the nation. At the national level, the difference in the medical system, the legal system, the state religion and the national traits will be enumerated. At the regional level, the difference in the regional economy, the regional medical service, the trait of the residents will be given as examples. At the institutional level, problems such as the lack of the facilities and trained medical staff that each hospital has, and the difference in physicians' attitudes, experience and training will be enumerated, also.

i. The Difference of the Medical Systems

Firstly, we attempt to consider the difference within the medical systems. Regardless of the use of mechanical ventilator, it became clear in some precedent studies that medical treatment of the ALS patients costs a large amount of expenses [33, 40-43]. Home mechanical ventilation can be expensive. The home health care of 24 hours, which is necessary for ALS patients who choose home mechanical ventilation, costs a lot.

In Japan, the public health insurance system has provided all those living in Japan with tracheostomy and home oxygen therapy since 1985, and with home mechanical ventilation since 1990. Patients pay 0-30% of the medical expense according to age, disability and income. Nitta S *et al.* reported that yearly expenses of 4 ALS patients with TV at home were ¥334,000, ¥350,000, ¥411,000, and ¥872,000, respectively [44]. Uchida T *et al.* reported also that mean monthly medical costs of ALS patients with TV at home was ¥746,219±253,581, at institution was ¥1,049,923±71,147, and the mean monthly out-of pocket expense to families at home was 10%, at institution was 0% [45].

The USA alone, among developed nations, does not have a universal health care system, which will be developed by 2014. The Tax-financed Medicare and Medicaid cover 27.8% of the population. A little over 59% of Americans receive health insurance through employers, leaving a significant number of people without health insurance. As a result, most patients are led to pay all the expense for their own NIV and TV. The average yearly cost of home mechanical ventilation in the USA has been placed at more than $150,000. Some items, such as communication aids, may not be covered. Out-of-pocket expenses borne by families can be amount to $7,200 a month. Moss AH *et al.* also reported that the mean yearly expense of TV was $180,120 ($696-$1,080,000), 91% of patient expenses were covered by insurance, and so the mean yearly out-of pocket expense to families was $10,356 ($0-$240000) [33, 46]. The burden on the patient and their family is large even if some of the expense was covered by insurance. Klein and Forshew also estimated that patients' care with mechanical ventilator cost $16,625 per month, approximately 90% of which was resulted from the intensive nursing care needed by these patients [43]. Most of the expense seems to arise from the part related to the maintenance of the recuperation environment, such as nursing and care, *etc*.

In England, the public health system known as the National Health Service (NHS) has provided free healthcare to all the UK residents since 1948. It has covered NIV from general taxation, but not covered home mechanical ventilation. The ALS patients with TV were forced to spend the whole life in the hospital, which may be the reason that the usage rate of TV does not increase. In France and Germany, the public or private health insurance system has covered all the residents. They provide for NIV, and for some of the home mechanical ventilation, but not entirely. The financial cost of home mechanical ventilation is a less significant factor in nations with national health insurance. There are some reports from European nations on the costs for ALS patients and home mechanical ventilation. In Spain, Lopez-Bastida J *et al.* reported that the annual cost for ALS patients was estimated to be €36,194, and ALS patients have higher mean annual costs compared to other chronic illness such as Parkinson disease (PD), stroke, ataxia and Alzheimer disease (AD) [47]. In the Netherlands, van der Steen I *et al.* reported that the mean monthly expense was €1,336 for ALS patients receiving multidisciplinary care and €1,271 for those receiving general care. It showed that the costs of multi disciplinary ALS care were practically identical to the costs of general care [42]. In Germany, Kaub-Wittemer D *et al.* estimated also the monthly expense of NIV was €230-€1,900, and that of TV was €200-€5,000 [12].

ii. The Advance Directive and the Patient's Autonomy

Next, we attempt to consider the difference within the legal systems. Modern medical ethics are based on "The Hippocratic Oath". Four principles, autonomy, beneficence, nonmaleficence, and justice, are respected throughout the decision making process in the medical treatment. In 1949, "International Code of Medical Ethics" was enacted, which was based on "Declaration of Geneva" in 1948. The new ethics was a revised version of the Hippocratic Oath to make it suitable for the 20th century. "Lisbon declaration" concerning the patients' right was enacted in 1981.

In Japan, the paternalism was the main current in the medical treatment for a long time.The occupation ethics indicator issued by the Japan Medical Association was revised in 2004. Since then, patients' autonomy has been regarded as one of the most important things in the medical treatment.

In the USA, The patients' right movement started in the 1960's in a series of right movement, such as the antidiscrimination movement, the women's liberation movement, and the student movement. "Patient's Bill of Rights" by American Hospital Association was enacted in 1973.

In Europe, the Council of Europe recommended the patients' right several times between the 1970's and the 80's. Movement to enact the law concerning the patients' right had come out after the 1980's.

The advance directives are legally effective in some nations, where people can perform them as they wish. In Japan, the law has not yet come to embrace the concept of advance directives. While several types of advance directive document models were issued by voluntary associations, and the medical workers often follow the documents, they were not authorized legally.

The first law concerning the advance directive was enacted by the state of California, the USA, in 1976. All the 50 states and the District of Columbia now have the law that gives individuals the right to issue advance directive documents and to exercise their will to refuse treatment in certain situations.

In Japan, traditionally, the medical care was offered to patients based on the judgment and the ability of doctor. Patients' own decision making has been given the top priority in the treatment policy since 1980's, just as the USA and European nations. As in the case of ALS, its paternalistic approach, with regards to decisions to start or not to start, or to discontinue the treatment, came to be criticized. Simultaneously, the discussion on how to end one's life gathered a lot of attention in the society. In such public atmosphere, the guideline for patients' own decision making process in the terminal care was issued in 2007 by the Ministry of Health, Labour and Welfare.

1. It is the most important principle to proceed with the terminal care in accordance with decisions made by the patient's oneself. Every decision made by the patient should be based on the appropriate treatment and information provided by medical staff, such as physicians, and the discussion between the patient and the staff.
2. It should be deliberately judged, based on the medical validity, adequacy and the discussions by the medical team which involves multidisciplinary expertise, to start or not to start, modify, and terminate the treatment.
3. It is necessary to provide a patient with the holistic medical treatment, which includes mental and social support for the patient and family, to remove or alleviate, as much as possible, pain and discomfort.
4. This guideline does not concern with the positive euthanasia with the intension to shorten one's life.

In the USA, the prevalence of advance directives is estimated to range from 5%-20% of the population. Moss showed that 79% of ALS patients had completed an advance directive. Only 6% had directives before the ALS diagnosis, while 34% completed directives after diagnosis but before starting mechanical ventilation. 36% completed an advance directive after beginning ventilator support. Only 8% of the patient population did not want to issue an advance directive [46]. Moss AH et al. also found that 58% of physicians favored early discussion of the home ventilation option. 24% felt, however, this issue should not be discussed before respiratory failure occurred. On the other hand, only 75% of ALS patients were aware of the likely development of respiratory failure, fewer than 50% of ALS patients reported that they had discussed this information with their physician. These data suggest that most patients are not well prepared to decide on mechanical ventilation [33].

In EU, the legal significance of autonomy is much less developed than in the USA. Advance directives, however, are believed to be useful at 78% of hospitals. 55% discuss them regularly with their patients, and 30% of patients complete them. The prevalence of advance directives in EU is estimated at less than 5% of the population.

In the scene of the palliative care, most of medical workers feel necessity of the advance directive, there was not the difference of the thought by the international comparison [48]. In EU and Japan, the autonomy of medical therapy is gradually gaining acceptance among ALS patients, their families and treating physicians.

iii. Legal Aspect of Withdrawing and Withholding of TV

Withdrawing of TV means death for ALS patients. In general, it is thought to correspond to passive euthanasia, which is known as accelerating the death of a patient by altering some form of treatment and letting nature take its course. "Active euthanasia" involves causing the death of a patient through a direct action, in response to a request issued by that patient. "Physician-assisted suicide (PAS)" involves supplying information and/or the means of committing suicide to patients, so that the patients can successfully terminate their own lives. PAS is regarded as being in the middle of active and passive euthanasia.

In the USA and European nations where patients' own decision making is given the top priority in shaping the treatment policy, withholding or withdrawing of mechanical ventilation with patient consent (voluntary) is almost unanimously considered to be legal. Although some governments around the world have legalized voluntary euthanasia, generally it remains as a criminal homicide. In the Netherlands and Belgium, where euthanasia has been legalized, it still remains as homicide although it is not prosecuted and not punishable if the doctor meets certain legal exceptions. In 2002, the Netherlands passed a law legalizing euthanasia including physician-assisted suicide. The mandatory conditions of euthanasia in Dutch law consist of four points as follows; (1) The patient has the voluntary intention of euthanasia; (2) The patient has an unbearable pain; (3) The outlook of disease is hopeless; and (4) The treating physician of the patient has consulted the Support and Consultation in Euthanasia in the Netherlands (SCEN) physicians for a second opinion. Maessen M et al. reported that 20% of ALS patients die due to euthanasia or EAS, compared with 5% of cancer patients or 0.5% of cardiac patients [49].

In Japan, euthanasia is illegal, and the application of euthanasia to ALS is not allowed.

The mandatory conditions of euthanasia in Japanese judicial precedents were set nearly half century before; "The Nagoya High Court Decision of 1962" consists of the following six points; (1) The patient's condition is incurable with no hope of recovery, and death should be imminent; (2) The patient suffers from unbearable and severe pain that cannot be relieved; (3) The act of killing is undertaken with the intention of alleviating the patient's pain; (4) The patient himself or herself has made an explicit request of euthanasia; (5) Except for special cases where some other assistances are admitted, in principle the euthanasia must be carried out by a physician; and (6) The euthanasia must be carried out by ethically acceptable methods. These are, however, only a judicial precedent, which cannot be exercised as laws. A constant opinion on the mandatory conditions of euthanasia is still not obtainable today.

The withdrawing of ventilation is not, also, accepted legally. No constant opinions are given on the withholding of ventilation either. The argument on advance directives and palliative care is ongoing even today in the Ministry of Health, Labour and Welfare.

In the USA, while active euthanasia is illegal throughout the USA, Physician-assisted suicide is legal in the three states: Oregon, Washington and Montana. The use of analgesic in order to relieve suffering, even if it hastens death, has been held as legal in several court decisions.

In the UK, euthanasia is illegal. Any person found to be assisting suicide is breaking the law and can be convicted of assisting suicide or attempting to do so.

iv. Attitudes, Beliefs and Opinions of Physicians

It is reported that the doctor who has put on ventilator to a patient tends to put on ventilator to the next patient in Japan, the USA and UK [36, 41, 50]. Bourke SC *et al.* reported also that the majority of UK consultant neurologists did not suggest using NIV to any patients in the preceding 12 months, while only 3 neurologists made as much as 30% of all referrals nationally [36]. Although the guideline recommends NIV and TV, the prevalence of them does not seem to have increased. Neurologists and supporting healthcare professionals can greatly influence patients and their families. Even if physicians do not express their opinions specifically, the attitudes, beliefs, and opinions are conveyed to patients and their families [51]. The indifferent attitude of the neurologists towards application of mechanical ventilation to ALS patients might be one of the reasons that the number of ALS patients with NIV or TV have not increased even after the publication of clinical guidelines on the mechanical ventilation. To our knowledge, there was no research reporting the difficulty in the management of the ALS patient with NIV or TV.

v. The Characteristics of ALS Patients Living with Mechanical Ventilator

Here we report the characteristics of ALS patients living with mechanical ventilator.

In the USA, NIV users were more likely to be male. The evidence suggested that patients receiving NIV were more likely to have a higher income. There was no correlation between age, race, and types of insurance. A higher proportion of patients receiving NIV were using other life-sustaining interventions such as PEG and speech devices [52]. Those who choose TV were younger, more had young children, and had more education and higher incomes than average [41]. The choice of TV was not made from desperation, ignorance, or inability to make wishes clear during a chaotic dying period. Rather, TV choice was consistent with a sustained sense that life was worth living in any way possible, at least for some time and to certain extent [41]. Atkins L *et al.* said that quality of the pre-illness marital relationship is a significant predictor of ongoing marital relationship in both ALS patients and their spouse caregivers. Additionally, social and psychological symptoms rather than disease symptoms are important predictors of marital relationship quality after ALS diagnosis [53]. Murphy PL *et al.* described ALS patients who were more likely to use NIV were more religious and more affected with mobility. Tracheostomy was not correlated with either religiousness or spirituality [54]. Rabkin JG *et al.* also reported that there was no evidence of contribution to the decision on TV for religious and spiritual faith [41].

V. CAREGIVER'S DEPRESSION

The great burden is imposed upon their spouses and their children with the care of the ALS patients. This burden can become one of the causes to hesitate before mechanical ventilation.

In Japan, Miyashita M *et al.* showed that the care burden of caregivers was mainly explained by the intensity of the care and hours spent for giving care per day. The existential and physical burden tended to be higher for the caregivers of ALS compared to those of other neurodegenerative diseases, such as PD and spinocerebellar degeneration (SCD) [55].

In German, Kaub-Wittemer D *et al.* reported that the quality of life evaluated with the Profile of Mood State (POMS) and the Munich Quality of Life Dimensions List (MLDL) in ALS patients did not show any differences between those with NIV and those with TV. The quality of life in their caregivers, on the other hand, showed differences between those with NIV and those with TV. When asked directly, 94% of ALS patients with NIV and 81% of ALS patients with TV would go for the same choice if they went back to the time when they had made a decision to put on the mechanical ventilation, and there was no difference in both groups. However, 94% of the caregivers of ALS patients with NIV and 50% of the caregivers of ALS patients with TV would advise their patients to choose the ventilation again if they returned to that time of the decision, showing that there was difference between two groups. The POMS assessed feeling and emotional states of ALS patients and their caregivers, when applied with mechanical ventilation and summarized the assessment into 4 modes. Not only the patients but also their caregivers felt more fatigue and vigor than depression and anger [12]. In addition, in the UK, Mustfa N *et al.* compared the quality of life of caregivers of patients with NIV with that of caregivers of patients with similar disabilities; the ALS Functional Rating Score (ALSFRS) and the Norris Bulbar Score (NBS), but without ventilation, there was a slight increase of anxiety, but not stress or depression [56]. Contrary to these results, Goldstein LH *et al.* from the UK, Hecht MJ *et al.* from German and Chio A *et al.* from Italy did find an association between greater patients' functional impairment and higher caregivers' depression score [57-59].

VI. THE TOTALLY LOCKED-IN STATE (TLS)

ALS patients progressively lose their ability to control voluntary movements and occasionally enter the totally locked-in state (TLS), in which they cannot move any part of their bodies including the eyes. Majority of ALS patients without TV die of respiratory failure or aspiration pneumonia. Most ALS patients with TV also die of pneumonia, while some ALS patients with TV progress to TLS if the mechanical ventilation could succeed in extending patients' life. It is thought that one of the reasons why many ALS patients do not choose mechanical ventilation is the TLS. Though case reports have occasionally appeared since around 1989, there are no reports on the TLS.

In Japan, Hayashi H *et al.* reported that 47 of 70 ALS patients with TV (67.1%) died within 20 years of the observation, and 27 of those (57.4%) died of pneumonia, 11 of cardiac disease, 2 of chronic renal failure, 2 owing to a ventilator accident, 1 of ischemic colitis, and three of unknown causes. TLS occurred in 8 of 70 ALS patients with TV (11.4%). Of the 33 on TV for more than 5 years, 6 (18.2%) developed TLS, and 11 (33.1%) developed Minimal communication state [60]. To our knowledge, there is no report on the frequency of TLS in the USA and Europe.

Recently, it is reported that cognitive functions and brainstem functions could be preserved in ALS patients in the TLS [61, 62]. Given that, for the patients to use the function to express their thought, there are two kinds of the Brain-Machine Interface (BMI) that utilizes the brain wave. One is invasive type, whose electrodes are buried within the scalp. The other one is non-invasive type, whose electrodes are pasted on the scalp. The devices enable ALS patients to use of a mouse pointer, inputting the letters on the computer screen, and switching on the electric care bed, the light of the room.

VII. DISCUSSION

Decision making on the matters of one's life and death reflects universal value, being, at the same time, extremely personal. Withholding treatment with mechanical ventilation, even if it was requested by the patient who wishes to keep his/her own dignity, might be regarded as a homicide. Even when the mechanical ventilation is available, many patients with ALS do not select life with the mechanical ventilation. If a kind of guilt prevents patients to choose to be supported with mechanical ventilators, it should not be the case. It is ideal if the patients can be assured to be safe and comfortable with the mechanical ventilators. On the other hand, the patients suffering from dyspnea who decide not to receive mechanical ventilation should be treated with utmost palliative therapy. It should be noted that the line between palliative care and euthanasia is a very vague one.

Bach JR warns us that healthcare professionals universally rate a patient's quality of life much lower than the patients rate their own quality of life [63]. Earlier and better communication between physician and patient is needed so that ALS patients can deliberate on mechanical ventilation in advance. In this communication process, information on the patient's expected course, the burdens on the family caregiver, the major expense and the limits to mechanical ventilation need to be disclosed to patients. Neurologist should start to perform and discuss the evaluation with patients and their families, so that patients will be able to make a better choice for their own good. Though physicians must attend each patient and family as individuals, physicians must also endeavor to be objective in evaluating the patient's condition because it can affect patient's outlook.

Though the guidelines are made, the prevalence of NIV has not increased as expected.

The reasons on the patients' side, which impede their willingness for NIV and TV, are the load on the family, the loss of dignity, and depression. The reason on the doctors' side is the lack of experience with NIV. Regarding the present state of the medical care system, the insufficiency of the home care system, such as the house call doctor and the home care service, should be urgently addressed.

It is a well known fact that, just like the prevalence of the mechanical ventilation for the ALS patients, the rate of dialysis for the patients with chronic kidney failure is different from nation to nation as a reflection of the difference in the medical care systems. The dialysis population is 1,230 per 1,000,000 in Japan, but it is 738 in the USA and 229 in the UK [64]. The international comparative cost study has advanced recently because the chronic renal failure has a high morbidity rate. The costs of dialysis per patient a year in Japan was $57,621, while it was $46,000 in the USA and $44,625 in the UK [64]. In Japan, the renal failure requiring hemodialysis is specified as one of "specified diseases", and all of the medical expense that exceeds ¥10,000 within a month is supplied from insurance. In the USA, Medicare covers the patient with chronic renal failure. Although 80% of medical expense is paid by Medicare, 20% of that is covered by the second insurance or is paid individually, which amounts to several thousand dollars per year. It is thought the dialysis is directly leading to the kidney transplant. In the UK, The acceptance of dialysis is severely limited though it is covered with NHS. Although the annual cost is hardly different, the numbers of dialysis population are different among Japan, the USA, and the UK. Small amount of out-of-pocket expenses is needed in Japan and the UK [65]. In addition, the rate of consultation with the specialist in dialysis from general practitioner is low in the present condition in the USA and the UK.

The main reasons that ALS patients with mechanical ventilation did not increase are the large amount of out-of-pocket expenses and the uneasy access to the specialist. It is likely that ALS patients are placed in the similar situation as dialysis patients. Even though some autonomy is given to patients, their treatment is actually very limited in the whole medical care system. Several evidences show that patients' decision making are greatly influenced not by their culture or own value towards life and death, but the medical care system. The economic burdens on the ALS patients force them to give up survival, which causes a lot of difficulties on the medical treatment, and a criticism from ethical point of view. A public policy that will relieve ALS patients of the burden is urgently required.

The report on ALS patients with NIV and TV from Japan is a few. It is perhaps due to its very sensitive nature. A survey at the national level on this matter is essential for shaping a better policy against rare and intractable diseases such as ALS.

VIII. CONCLUSIONS

Each nation has its own medical system and the legislation. Each patient has his/her own lifestyle and values towards life and death, which of course varies from one person to another.

It thus seems difficult to establish standardized systems for decision making in the process of applying mechanical ventilation to ALS patients even at institution or prefectural level, and it is almost impossible to establish the system to function globally that would go beyond the difference in socio-medical, cultural, and religious backgrounds. Such inequality of critical medical service may bear problematic ethical issues. As reviewed in this chapter analysis of influential factors in the introduction of mechanical ventilation would facilitate neurologists and supporting healthcare professionals to avoid paternalistic approach and help ALS patients to make the better decision for their benefit.

ACKNOWLEDGMENTS

This work was supported in part by the grant from the Ministry of Education, Culture, Sports, Science and Technology of Japan and the Smoking Research Foundation. Special thanks to Kimi Kawamata for her help on finalizing, assisting in correcting, and preparing the manuscript.

CONFLICT OF INTEREST STATEMENT

The authors have no conflicts of interest.

REFERENCES

[1]   Miller, RG; Jackson, CE; Kasarskis, EJ; England, JD; Forshew, D; Johnston, W; Kalra, S; Kats, JS; Mitsumoto, H; Rosenfeld, J; Shoesmith, C; Strong, MJ; Woolley, SC. Practice Parameter update: The care of the patient with ALS: Drug, nutritional, and respiratory therapies. *Neurology,* 2009, 73, 1218-1226
[2]   Andersen, PM; Borasio, GD; Dengler, R; Hardiman, O; Kollewe, K; Leigh, PN; Pradat, P-F; Silani ,V; Tomik, B. Good practice in the management of ALS: Clinical guidelines. *Amyotrophic Lateral Sclerosis,* 2007, 8, 195-213
[3]   The Societas Neurologica Japonica. ALS Care Guideline in 2002. *Clinical Neurology,* 2002, 42, 669-719
[4]   Cazzolli, PA; Oppenheimer, EA. Home mechanical ventilation for ALS: nasal compared to tracheostomy-intermittent positive pressure ventilation. *J Neurol Sci,* 1996, 139, S123-128
[5]   Lo Coco, D; Marchese, S; La Bella, V; Piccoli, T; Lo Coco, A. The ALSSFRS predicts survival time in ALS patients on invasive mechanical ventilation. *Chest,* 2007, 132, 64-69
[6]   Bach, JR. Amyotrophic Lateral Sclerosis. *Chest,* 2002, 122, 92-98

[7]   Aboussouan, LS; Khan, SU; Meeker, DP; Stelmach, K; Mitsumoto, H. Effect of noninvasive positive-pressure ventilation on survival in ALS. *Ann Intern Med*, 1997, 127, 450-453

[8]   Aboussouan, LS; Khan, SU; Banerjee, M; Arroliga, AC; Mitsumoto, H. Objective measures of the efficacy of noninvasive positive-pressure ventilation in ALS. *Muscle Nerve,* 2001, 24, 403-409

[9]   Kleopa, KA; Sherman, M; Neal, B; Romano, GJ; Heiman-Patterson, T. Bipap improves survival and rate of pulmonary function decline in patients with ALS. *J Neurol Sci*, 1999, 164, 82-88

[10] Pinto, AC; Evangelista, T; Carvalho, M; Alves, MA; Sales Luis, ML. Respiratory assistance with a non-invasive ventilator in ALS patients: survival rates in a controlled trial. *J Neurol Sci,* 1995, 129, S19-26

[11] Bourke, SC; Tomlinson, M; Williams, TL; Bullock, RE; Shaw, PJ; Gibson, GJ. Effects of non-invasive ventilation on survival and quality of life in patients with ALS: a randomized controlled trial. *Lancet Neurol,* 2006, 5, 140-147

[12] Kaub-Wittemer, D; von Steinbuchel, N; Wasner, M; Laier-Groeneveld, G; Borasio, GD. Quality of life and psychosocial issues in ventilated patients with ALS and their caregivers. *J Pain Symptom Manage,* 2003, 26, 890-896

[13] Gelinas, DF; O'Connor, P; Miller, RG. Quality of life for ventilator-dependent ALS patients and their caregivers. *J Neurol Sci,* 1998, 160, S134-136

[14] Lyall, RA; Donaldson, N; Fleming, T; Wood, C; Newsom-Davis, I; Polkey, MI; Leigh, PN; Moxham, J. A prospective study of quality of life in ALS patients treated with noninvasive ventilation. *Neurology,* 2001, 57, 153-156

[15] Bourke, SC; Bullock, RE; Williams, TL; Shaw, PJ; Gibson, GJ. Noninvasive ventilation in ALS: Indications and effect on quality of life. *Neurology,* 2003, 61, 171-177

[16] Jackson, CE; Rosenfeld, J; Moore, DH; Bryan, WW; Barohn, RJ; Wrench, M; Myers, D; Heberlin, L; King, R; Smith, J; Gelinas, D; Miller, RG. A preliminary evaluation of a prospective study of pulmonary function studies and symptoms of hypoventilation in ALS patients. *J Neurol Sci,* 2001, 191, 75-78

[17] Kimura, F; Shinoda, K; Fujiwara, S; Fujimura, C; Nakajima, H; Furutama, D; Sugino, M; Hanafusa, T. The changes of clinical characteristics in 100 Japanese ALS patients between 1980 and 2000. *Clinical Neurol,* 2003, 43, 385-391

[18] Kataoka, Y; Ooyama, A; Hoshino, K; Kitamura, E; Honma, A; Itoh, T; Yamamoto, T; Okada, Y. A problem of the ALS patients in the end of life. *The Medical Journal of Tokatsu Hospital,* 2005, 2, 14-16

[19] Yoshida, K; Yahikozawa, H; Tabata, K; Ohara, S; Hanyu, N; Ikeda, S. Clinical status and daily-life activity of patients with ALS in Nagano Prefecture. *The Shinshu Medical Journal*, 2007, 55, 181-190

[20] Kondo, K. The management of home mechanical ventilation in the ALS patients. 2007. Available from: *http://www.als.gr.jp/staff/seminar/seminar40/seminar40_05.html*

[21] Uehara, H; Sugino, S; Tsuji, K; Fukuda, K; Nakajima, H; Kimura, F; Hanafusa, T; Tagami, M; Murao, H; Shinoda, K. Studies of non-invasive positive pressure support for respiratory failure in patients with ALS: Appropriate time for introduction and prolonged survival effect. *Neurological Therapeutics*, 2003, 20, 577-581

[22] Yamamoto, M. Intractable disease patients with home mechanical ventilation in Oita Prefectural Hospital. 2003. Available from: http://tenjin.coara.or.jp/~makoty/als/2003NPPV/NPPV_slide01.gif

[23] Nagahama, A. From the experience of the home care of the ALS patients with NIV: The practice of observing and coping. *The Japanese Journal of Home Care Nursing*, 2004, 9, 278-283

[24] Nanba, R. The status and problems for the ALS patients in end of life. *Japanese Journal of National Medical Services*, 2005, 59, 383-388

[25] Kasahara, Y; Michiyama, N; Dekura, Y; Komori, T. A longitudinal study of respiratory dysfunction in patients with ALS. *The Journal of Japanese Physical Therapy Association,* 2005, 32, 66-71

[26] Bradley, WG; Anderson, F; Bromberg, M; Gutmann, L; Harati, Y; Ross, M; Miller, RG. Current management of ALS: Comparison of the ALS CARE Database and the AAN Practice Parameter. *Neurology,* 2001, 57, 500-504

[27] Lechtzin, N; Wiener, CM; Clawson, L; Davidson, MC; Anderson, F; Gowda, N; Diette, GB. Use of noninvasive ventilation in patients with ALS. *Amyotrophic Lateral Sclerosis,* 2004, 5, 9-15

[28] Jackson, CE; Lovitt, S; Gowda, N; Anderson, F; Miller, RG. Factors correlated with NPPV use in ALS. *Amyotrophic Lateral Sclerosis,* 2006, 7, 80-85

[29] Sivak, ED; Shefner, JM; Mitsumoto, H; Taft, JM. The use of non-invasive positive pressure ventilation in ALS patients: A need for improved determination of intervention timing. *Amyotrophic Lateral Sclerosis,* 2001, 2, 139-145

[30] Melo, J; Homma, A; Iturriaga, E; Frierson, L; Amato, A; Anzueto, A; Jackson, C. Pulmonary evaluation and prevalence of non-invasive ventilation in patients with ALS: a multicenter survey and proposal of a pulmonary protocol. *J Neurol Sci,* 1999, 169, 114-117

[31] Albert, SM; Murphy, PL; Del Bene, ML; Rowland, LP. Prospective study of palliative care in ALS: choice, timing, outcomes. *J Neurol Sci*, 1999, 169, 108-113

[32] Cedarbaum, JM; Stambler, N. Disease status and use of ventilatory support by ALS patients. *Amyotrophic Lateral Sclerosis,* 2001, 2, 19-22

[33] Moss, HA; Casey, P; Stocking, CB; Ross, RP; Brooks, BR; Siegler, M. Home ventilation for ALS patients: Outcomes, costs, and patient, family, and physician attitudes. *Neurology,* 1993, 43, 438-43

[34] Mandrioli, J; Faglioni, P; Nichelli, P; Sola, P. Amyotrophic lateral sclerosis: Prognostic indicators of survival. *Amyotrophic Lateral Sclerosis,* 2006, 7, s217-226

[35] Borasio, GD; Shaw, PJ; Hardiman, O; Ludolph, AC; Sales Luis, ML; Silani, V. Standards of palliative care for patients with ALS: results of a European survey. *Amyotrophic Lateral Sclerosis,* 2001, 2, 159 -164

[36] Bourke, SC; Williams, TL; Bullock, RE; Gibson, GJ; Shaw, PJ. Non-invasive ventilation in motor neuron disease: current UK practice. *Amyotrophic Lateral Sclerosis,* 2002, 3, 145-149

[37] Kuhnlein, P; Kubler, A; Raubold, S; Worrell, M; Kurt, A; Gdynia, H-J; Sperfeld, A-D; Ludolph, AC. Palliative care and circumstances of dying in German ALS patients using non-invasive ventilation. *Amyotrophic Lateral Sclerosis,* 2008, 9, 91-98

[38] Nonnenmacher, S; Sorg, S; Lule, D; Hautzinger, M; Ludolph, AC; Kubler, A. Attitudes toward life sustaining treatment in ALS patients. *Amyotrophic Lateral Sclerosis,* 2009, 10, S203

[39] Lorenzen, CK; Schou, L; Dreyer, PS. Survival in ALS patients with non-invasive HMV. *Amyotrophic Lateral Sclerosis,* 2009, 10, S190

[40] Olick, RS; Kimura, R; Kielstein, JT; Hayashi, H; Riedl, M; Siegler, M. Advance care planning and the ALS patients: A cross-cultural perspective on advance directives. *Annual Review of Law and Ethics,* 1996, 4, 529-552

[41] Rabkin, JG; Albert, SM; Tider, T; Del Bene, ML; O'sullivan, I; Rowland, LP; Mitsumoto, H. Predictors and course of elective long-term mechanical ventilation: A prospective study of ALS patients. *Amyotrophic Lateral Sclerosis,* 2006, 7, 86-95

[42] van der Steen, I; van den Berg, J-P; Buskens, E; Lindeman, E; van den Berg, LH. The costs of amyotrophic lateral sclerosis, according to type of care. *Amyotrophic Lateral Sclerosis,* 2009, 10, 27-34

[43] Klein, LM; Forshew, DA. The economic impact of ALS. *Neurology,* 1996, 47, S126-129

[44] Nitta, S; Nitta, S. The expense and necessary home equipment for ALS patients with home mechanical ventilation. *Home Health Care for the People with Intractable Diseases,* 2004, 9, 89-94

[45] Uchida, T; Aizawa, S; Kikuchi, Y; Takao, M; Mihara, B. Analysis of co-payment for medical care in patients with ALS. *Neurological Therapeutics*, 2011, 28, 83-87

[46] Moss, AH; Oppenheimer, EA; Casey, P; Cazzolli, PA; Roos, RP; Stocking, CB; Siegler, M. Patients with ALS receiving long-term mechanical ventilation: Advance care planning and outcomes. *Chest,* 1996, 110, 249-255

[47] Lopez-Bastida, J; Perestelo-Perez, L; Monton-Alvarez, F; Serrano-Aguilar, P; Alfonso-Sanchez, JL. Social economic costs and health-related quality of life in patients with ALS in Spain. *Amyotrophic Lateral Sclerosis*, 2009, 10, 237-243

[48] Voltz, R; Akabayashi, A; Reese, C; Ohi, G; Sass, H-M. End-of-life decisions and advance directives in palliative care: A cross-cultural survey of patients and health-care professionals. *Journal of Pain and Symptom Management,* 1998, 16, 153-162

[49] Maessen, M; Veldink, JH; van den Berg, LH; Schouten, HJ; van der Wal, G; Onwuteaka-Philipsen, BD. Requests for euthanasia: origin of suffering in ALS, heart failure, and cancer patients. *J Neurol,* 2010, 257, 1192-1198

[50] Smyth, A; Riedl, M; Kimura, R; Olick, R; Siegler, M. End of life decisions in ALS: across-cultural perspective. *J Neurol Sci,* 1997, 152, S93-96

[51] Mitsumoto, H; Del Bene, M. Improving the quality of life for people with ALS: The challenge ahead. *Amyotrophic Lateral Sclerosis,* 2000, 1, 329 – 336

[52] Jackson, CE; Lovitt, S; Gowda, N; Anderson, F; Miller, RG. Factors correlated with NPPV use in ALS. *Amyotrophic Lateral Sclerosis,* 2006, 7, 80-85

[53] Atkins, L; Brown, RG; Leigh, PN; Goldstein, LH. Marital relationships in ALS. *Amyotrophic Lateral Sclerosis,* 2010, 11, 344 - 350

[54] Murphy, PL; Albert, SM; Weber, CM; Del Bene, ML; Rowland, LP. Impact of spirituality and religiousness on outcomes in patients with ALS. *Neurology,* 2000, 55, 1581-1584

[55] Miyashita, M; Narita, Y; Sakamoto, A; Kawada, N; Akiyama, M; Kayama, M; Suzukamo, Y; Fukahara, S. Care burden and depression in caregivers caring for patients

with intractable neurological diseases at home in Japan. *J Neurol Sci,* 2009, 276, 148-152

[56] Mustfa, N; Walsh, E; Bryant, V; Lyall, RA; Addington-Hall, J; Goldstein, LH; Donaldson, N; Polkey, MI; Moxham, J; Leigh, PN. The effect of noninvasive ventilation on ALS patients and their caregivers. *Neurology* 2006, 66, 1211-1217

[57] Goldstein, LH; Atkins, L; Landau, S; Brown, R; Leigh, PN. Predictors of psychological distress in carers of people with ALS: a longitudinal study. *Psychol Med,* 2006, 36, 865-875

[58] Hecht, MJ; Graesel, E; Tigges, S; Hillemacher, T; Winterholler, M; Hilz, MJ; Heuss, D; Neundorfer B. Burden of care in amyotrophic lateral sclerosis. *Palliat Med,* 2003, 17, 327-333

[59] Chio, A; Vignola, A; Mastro, E; Dei Giudici, A; Iazzolino, B; Calvo, A; Moglia, C; Montuschi, A. Neurobehavioral symptoms in ALS are negatively related to caregivers' burden and quality of life. *Eur J Neurol,* 2010, 17, 1298-1303

[60] Hayashi, H; Oppenheimer, EA. ALS patients on TPPV: Totally locked-in state, neurologic findings and ethical implications. *Neurology,* 2003, 61, 135-137

[61] Fuchino, Y; Nagao, M; Katura, T; Bando, M; Naito, M; Maki, A; Nakamura, K; Hayashi, H; Koizumi, H; Yoro, T. High cognitive function of an ALS patient in the totally locked-in state. *Neuroscience Letters,* 2008, 435, s85-89

[62] Murguialday, AR; Hill, J; Bensch, M; Martens, S; Halder, S; Nijboer, F; Schoelkopf, B; Birbaumer, N; Gharabaghi, A. Transition from the locked in to the completely locked-in state: A physiological analysis. *Clin Neuro,* 2010, in print

[63] Bach, JR. Ventilator use by muscular dystrophy association patients. *Arch Phys Med Rehabil,* 1992, 72, 179-183

[64] Hidai, H; Hyodo, T. The international comparison of the dialysis medical cost. *Journal of Japanese Society for Dialysis Therapy,* 2001, 34, 91-93

[65] De Vecchi, AF; Dratwa, M; Wiedemann, ME. Healthcare systems end-stage renal disease (ESRD) therapies–an international review: costs and reimbursement/finding of ESRD. *Nephrol Dial Transplant,* 1999, 14, S31-41

In: Motor Neuron Diseases
Editors: Bradley J. Turner and Julie B. Atkin

ISBN 978-1-61470-101-9
© 2012 Nova Science Publishers, Inc.

Chapter XI

MOTOR SPEECH DISORDER IN PATIENTS WITH MOTOR NEURON DISEASE: HOW TO ESTIMATE AND MANAGE THEIR DISTURBED SPEECH SOUNDS CLINICALLY

Hideto Saigusa[*]

Department of Otolaryngology, Nippon Medical School, Tokyo, Japan

INTRODUCTION

Unfortunately, the patients with motor neuron disease (MND) might suffer from not only paralytic movements of the body and the limbs, but also motor speech disorder sooner or later during their clinical history. Once speech sound of the patient with MND is affected, progressive course of dysarthria could not only be avoidable, besides but also might be taken away by severely distorted respiratory function. Thus, clinical estimations of the degree and pathophysiological aspects of affected speech sound should be convenient and timely along with the progression of MND. Also the management for the speech disorder of the patient with MND should be considered and coped along with the progression of MND.

CLINICAL FEATURES OF DYSARTHRIA OF THE PATIENT WITH MND

The clinical features of affected speech sound could be recognized along with the level of motor neurons, i.e., upper motor neurons, lower motor neurons or most often mixed of both upper and lower motor neurons. Sometimes, it could be seen that the symptoms related

[*] Hideto Saigusa, M.D.: Department of Otolaryngology, Nippon Medical School, Tokyo, Japan, 1-1-5 Sendagi, Bunkyo-ku, Tokyo, 113-8603, Japan, e-mail address: s-hideto@nms.ac.jp

speech motor disorder preceded or progressed rather than the other symptoms. It had been reported that the dysarthric features of MND were as a reduced range of articulatory movement and a slowing in the rate of speech synthesis with perceptual impressions as bradylalia and imprecise articulatory sounds. Also, hypernasal emission of the articulatory sounds could be characterized. The pathophysiological features of dysarthria on the patient with MND were previously reported as the result of reduced range and velocity of articulatory muscle movement, causing slowing of the rate of speech synthesis. [1-3] Distorted speech should be largely due to velopharyngeal closure incompetency and partially due to decreased lingual activities during articulation with atrophic changes of the muscles. Limited range of velopharyngeal closure and lingual activities during articulatory movement could result in hypernasality, excessive nasal air emission, vowel distortion, imprecise and weak articulation, and reduced loudness of speech. Slowing rate of speech synthesis could be attributed by fragmentation of sentence with prolonged phonemes, prolonged interval, and inappropriate silence. Reduced muscle strength of respiratory muscles could result reduced utterance length and loudness of speech, short phrasing, reduced stress contrast, and low pitched voice. Those elements of speech disturbance will progress with the progression of MND within an average of two or three years.

To examine how the speech sound is affected in the patient with MND, it could be useful clinically to investigate following three elements along with the progression of MND.

[1] Velopharyngeal function or the pathophysiological aspects of velopharyngeal dysfunction during speech.
[2] Velocity and range of the tongue movement or the pathophysiological aspects of tongue movement disorder during speech.
[3] Respiratory function enough to produce the phonatory sound and muscle strength of the muscles for respirations.

EXAMINATIONS FOR THE VELOPHARYNGAEL FUNCTION AND THE MANAGEMENTS FOR VELOPHARYNGEAL INADEQUACY

Velopharyngeal insufficiency could cause, not only hypernasality of speech sound and weak articulation, but also inadequate respiratory and laryngeal function with excessive air leakage to the nasal cavity during speech. Thus, restoration of velopharyngeal function should be critical for the treatment of dysarthria with velopharyngeal inadequacy. Velopharyngeal function during speech could be examined easily with a mirror held at the nares to detect the nasal airflow, nasopharyngeal fiberscopic examination or x-ray imaging to detect the degree of the closure of the velopharyngeal port during the production of the non-nasal sound. Electromyographic examination for the levator veli palatini muscle is also useful to examine neurogenic change of this muscle.

Also, palpations to estimate the muscle tone for the levator veli palatini muscle (the elevator muscle of the velum) and the palatopharyngeal muscle (the depressor muscle of the velum) [4, 5] should be important (Figure 1.). In some cases, the muscle tone of the palatopharyngeal muscle is increased, i.e., spastic condition, and the muscle tone of the levator veli palatini muscle is not so affected, i.e., extensible condition. For those patients, velopharyngeal closure incompetence could be improved by relaxation approach for the tone of the palatopharyngeal muscle. When the muscle tones of the two muscles is disturbed with atrophic change, it could be considered that the velopharyngeal closure inadequacy of the patient could not be improved with speech therapy or physical medicine, but with the prosthetic or surgical intervention. [3, 6] For the patient with MND, the sensory system of the patient is preserved, causing the prosthetic management for dysarthria difficult in many cases due to discomfort or gag reflex caused by the prosthesis like the palatal lift prosthesis. Additionally, if the lateral pharyngeal wall movement during speech is insufficient to closure the lateral side of the velopharyngeal port, the effect created by the prosthesis is insufficient.

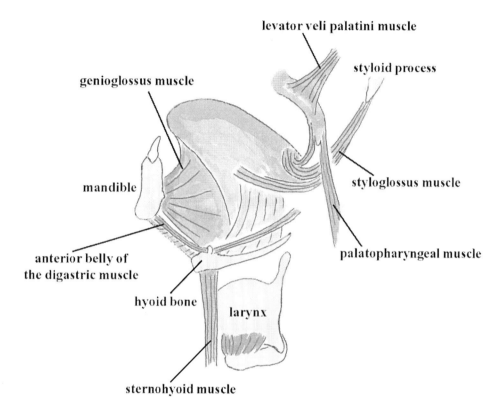

Figure 1. Positioning of the tongue body is controlled by the extrinsic lingual muscles, including the genioglossus and styloglossus muscles. Velopharyngeal closure is adjusted by the levator veli palatini and the palatopharyngeal muscles. And the muscle tones of their muscles could be affected by not only the disturbance of the motor neuron directly, but also the muscle tones of the surrounding muscles including the superior and the inferior hyoid muscles, and the masticatory muscles along with the condition of the posture or the respiratory function secondary.

We have developed and performed the narrowing of lateral palatopharyngeal wall surgery to improve velopharyngeal closure incompetence on the patient with MND at least prolonged survival as functional speech surgery (Figure 2.) [7]. After the surgery, hypernasality of speech sound of the patients were significantly decreased. Intelligibility and quality of the speech sound were improved, and the length of each phrase was elongated postoperatively without any postoperative physical training or speech therapy.

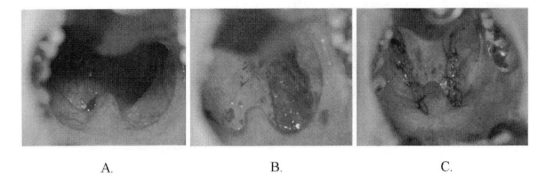

A.   B.   C.

Figure 2. Bilateral narrowing of lateral palapharyngeal wall surgery for improvement of velopharngeal closure inadequacy of the patient with ALS. A: Under general anesthesia with the patient's mouth opened by a mouth gag and the body of the tongue depressed. B: Mucosal incision were made in the posterior palatine arch bilaterally. And next incisions were made in the posterion pharyngeal wall in parallel with mucosal incisions in the posterior palatine arch, and the mucosa of the regions between the two insicions were resected with surgical forceps bilaterally. Then, the pharyngeal constrictor muscle was sectioned along the incision on the pharyngeal wall, and the muscle was separated from the deep fascia bilaterally. C: The stripped flaps of the posterior palatine arch were insterted under the pharyngeal constrictor muscle and sultured with 4-0 Vicryl suture bilaterally.

EXAMINATION OF THE TONGUE MOVEMENT AND THE MANAGEMENT FOR THE DISTURBED TONGUE MOVEMENT DURING SPEECH

To observe and estimate the range and the velocity of the tongue movement during speech, ultrasonic investigation is the most harmless real-time procedure for analyzing articulatory movement for clinicians. In particular, M-mode color Doppler ultrasonic imaging by setting the transducer on the mid-sagittal line of the submental triangle could detect vertical tongue movement and indicate the velocity of the tongue by a color-coded pattern. [8] Upward movement of the tongue was indicated by a blue signal and downward movement was indicated by a red signal. The voice signal was indicated by a green signal by the contact microphone to the anterior neck. The velocity of the tongue could be estimated by color-coded contrast scale on the screen of the ultrasound machine. And the M-mode line could display the locus line of the vertical position of the tongue blade. For articulatory movement associated with the phonation of /ta/, to produce explosive consonant sound /t/, the tongue moves toward the alveolar ridge, and the Doppler signal appears blue. When following the vowel /a/, the tongue moves toward the oral floor, and the Doppler signal is red. Excessive jaw movement, due to "jaw dependency", to conserve the speech sound and some diffused ultrasonic reflections could be canceled out by the comb filter. Figure 3-A is the M-mode color Doppler ultrasonic imaging of a normal subject during repetitive production of monosyllable /ta/ as fast as possible in a single breath. We estimate that the mean velocity of the upward signal (blue signal) was determined to be 19.8 cm/sec. and the mean velocity of the downward signal (red signal) was 23.1cm/sec. And the repetitive rate was 7Hz. On the other hand, Figure 3-B indicated the M-mode color Doppler ultrasonic imaging of a subject with ALS during the production of the same speaking task. The duration of the voice signal, interval between the voice signals were elongated, and the brightness of the up- and downward signals and amplitude of the M-mode line were significantly reduced. The repetitive rate of /ta/ was slow, with a minimum of 2 Hz, whereas the repetition rate was almost consistently preserved. The mean velocity of the upward signal was 4.9 cm/sec., and that of the downward signal was 7.3 cm/sec.

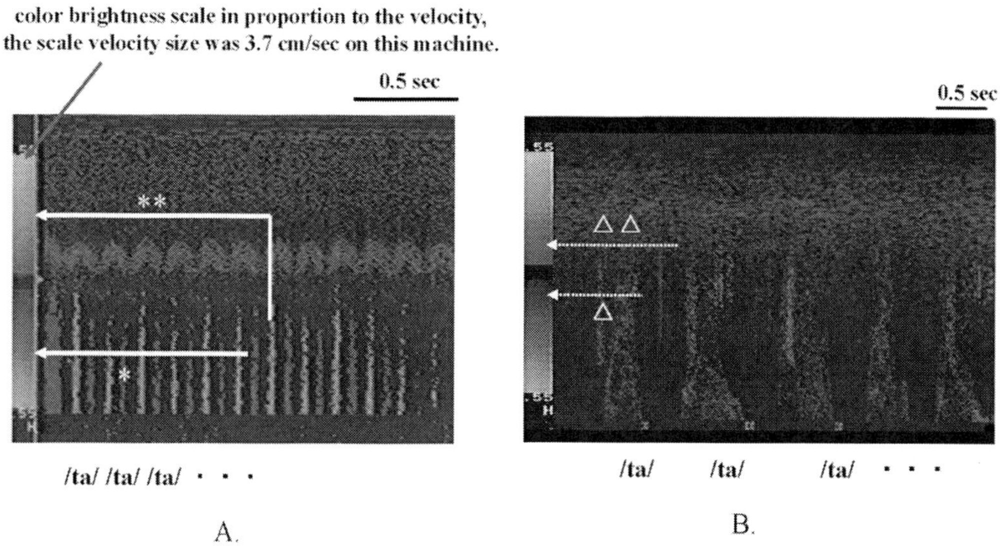

color brightness scale in proportion to the velocity,
the scale velocity size was 3.7 cm/sec on this machine.

/ta/ /ta/ /ta/ · · ·

A.

/ta/   /ta/   /ta/   · · ·

B.

Figure 3. M-mode color Doppler ultrasonic imaging during repetitive production of the monosyllable /ta/as fast as possible in a single breath. A: For a normal subject, mean velocity of the upward (blue) signal (**) was determined to be 19.8 cm/sec., and mean velocity of the downward (red) signal (*) was 23.1 cm/sec. And the repetitive rate was 7Hz. B: For a patient with ALS, mean velocity of the upward (blue) signal (ΔΔ) was determined to be 4.9 cm/sec., and mean velocity of the downward (red) signal (Δ) was 7.3 cm/sec. And the repetive rate was 2Hz. The ampliture of M-mode line was reduced significantly.

Palpations to investigate the muscle tone for the extrinsic lingual muscle including the genioglossus and the styloglossus muscles, and the jaw supporting muscles including the superior hyoid and the masticatory muscles should be useful (Figure 1.). Spastic tones of the genioglossus and the styloglossus muscles could attribute the spastic condition of the tongue positioning during speech. And spastic tones of the jaw supporting muscles could develop to disturb the cooperative movements between the tongue and the mandible during speech. In such cases, relaxation approaches for those muscles could be useful to improve the articulatory movements of not only the tongue, but also the jaw. However, when the tones of those muscles are decreased (flaccid) with atrophic change, it might indicate that the affected speech sound could not be improved already with speech therapy or physical medicine, but with the prosthetic or surgical intervention. However, for the patient with MND, because the sensory system of the patient is preserved, oral prosthetic management might cause discomfort or gag reflex.

Examination of Respiratory Function To Produce The Phonatory Sound and the Management the Affected Muscle Strength of the Muscles for Respirations

We could examine the residual respiratory function of the patient with the spirogram. In the late stage, the patient with MND would complain of shortness or weakness of breath leading to reduced loudness, short phrase of speech, and reduced stress contrast. If the degree of the subglottic pressure is very lower, the phonatory sound leads to the condition of aphonia. In some cases, muscle tones of the trapezius muscle and the inferior hyoid muscles as the supporting muscle of inspiratory function are increased. And spastic tone of the inferior hyoid muscles should cause additional hyper tonicity of the superior hyoid muscles and masticatory muscles as the antagonistic muscles each other. The condition of hyper tonicities of both the superior and the inferior hyoid muscles as extrinsic laryngeal muscles could accomplish to interfere with the tone of the vocal ligament, causing inadequate pitch control and vibration of the vocal fold, and additional hyper tonicity of the masticatory muscles could attribute reduced mobility of the jaw and the tongue. [9] In those cases, it could be useful to encourage the respiratory function and the phonatory sound with relaxation approach for the trapezius muscle and the physical approach to encourage the expiratory function with anteflexion of the neck and the body to squeeze the lung as a traditional oriental respiratory exercise, so called "Tanden Kokyu". Also by pushing the abdominal region or the thorax of the patient during speech to support the subglottal pressure could help the weak phonatory sound. However, when the tones of those muscle are decreased or flaccid with atrophic change, it could be expected the introduction of the artificial ventilator system before long. Atelo-collagen injection to the vocal fold could not improve the weakness of the phonatory sound.

Future For Dysarthria of the Patient with MND

Currently, it has been reported that speech therapy, including behavioral management has very limited value in improving the speech intelligibility of the patients with MND. [3, 10] However, it had not been examined and well documented how to estimate and improve the condition of motor speech disorder along the stage of the progression of MND. Although medical therapies, including artificial ventilator system and enteral alimentation system, for prolonging the life of the patient with MND have been developed, useful therapeutic approach for motor speech disorder of the patient with MND had not been investigated well except augmentative and alternative communication system including, blink response communication system, talking aid, and so on. We should make more our effort to develop useful, concise and useful examination and therapeutic approach, including drug therapy, functional surgery, gene therapy, regenerative medicine, physical approach, and prosthetic approach, for motor speech disorder of the patient with MND.

REFERENCES

[1]   Hirose H (1986): Pathophysiology of motor speech disorders (dysarthria). *Folia Phoniatr Logoped* 38: 61-88.

[2]   Darley FL, Aronson AE, Brown JR (1975): *Motor Speech Disorders*. W.B. Saunders, Philadelphia.

[3]   Duffy JR (2005): *Motor Speech Disorders*. 2nd ed. Elesevier Mosby, St. Louis.

[4]   Bell-Berti F (1976): An electromyographic study of velopharyngeal function in speech. *J Speech Hear Res* 19: 225-240.

[5]   Bell Berti F, Baer T, Harris K, Niimi S (1979). Coarticularory effects of vowel quality on velar function. *Phonetica* 36: 187-193.

[6]   McGuirt WF, Blalock D, Salem W (1980): The otolaryngologist's role in the diagnosis and treatment of amyotrophic lateral sclerosis. *Laryngoscope* 90: 1496-501.

[7]   Saigusa H, Yamaguchi S, Nakamura T, Taro K, Kadosono O, Aino I, Ito H, Saigusa M, Niimi S (2011): Bilateral narrowing of lateral palatopharyngeal wall surgery for improvement of dysarthria on the patient with amyotrophic lateral sclerosis. *Canadian Journal of Speech-Language Pathology and Audiology* (in submitted).

[8]   Saigusa H, Saigusa M, Aino I, Iwasaki C, Li L, Niimi S (2006): M-mode color Doppler ultrasonic imaging of vertical tongue movement during articulatory movement. *J of Voice* 20: 38-45.

[9]   Saigusa H (2010): Comparative anatomy of the larynx and related structures. *J Jp Med Assoc* 139: 803-808.

[10]   Kühnlein P, Gdynia HJ, Sperfeld AD, Pfleghar BI, Ludolph AC, Prosiegel M, Riecker A: (2008): Diagnosis and treatment of bulbar symptoms in amyotrophic lateral sclerosis. *Nature Clin Prac Neurol* 4: 366-374.

INDEX

D

E

F

G

H

I

N

T

triggers, 36, 60, 67, 68, 92, 105, 107, 113, 199
tropism, 173
tumor necrosis factor, 134
tumors, 18, 122

U

ubiquitin-proteasome system, xi, 183, 188
UK, 15, 26, 38, 137, 152, 209, 210, 213, 214, 216, 219
ultrasound, 47, 226
ultrastructure, 95
umbilical cord, 114, 117, 129, 174, 175
underlying mechanisms, viii, 87
United States (USA), viii, xi, 14, 21, 22, 40, 41, 72, 73, 74, 76, 77, 78, 79, 81, 82, 84, 87, 110, 111, 113, 115, 133, 140, 143, 165, 168, 169, 171, 172, 176, 195, 196, 199, 203, 204, 208, 209, 210, 211, 212, 213, 215, 216
urinary tract infection, 33
urine, 65
UV, 107

V

vacuole, 68
validation, 21, 42, 43
variables, 143, 146, 150
variations, ix, 15, 26, 137, 140, 151
vascular endothelial growth factor (VEGF), 161, 173
vector, 126, 173
vehicles, 75
velocity, 18, 224, 226, 227
ventilation, xi, 27, 29, 45, 203, 204, 205, 209, 210, 212, 213, 214, 215, 217, 218, 219, 221
verbal fluency, 34
vesicle, viii, 51, 52, 57, 62, 63, 64, 76, 79, 80, 82, 83, 138, 158

viral gene, 122
viral infection, 63, 174
viral vectors, 173
viruses, 122, 173, 178
vitamin E, 22, 110
vitamins, 22
vomiting, 27
vulnerability, viii, 51, 63, 88, 91, 92, 101, 102, 105, 107, 109, 111, 116, 158, 161, 162, 163, 164, 168, 169, 170

W

Wales, 46
walking, 18, 20, 32, 138
Washington, 140, 151, 213
water, 16, 94
weakness, vii, x, xi, 13, 14, 16, 17, 18, 25, 26, 28, 30, 31, 32, 33, 34, 35, 47, 116, 138, 157, 183, 184, 191, 197, 204, 228
wealth, 57, 100
weight loss, 17, 18, 30, 35
white matter, 121, 173
wild type, 109, 162, 163, 164
wireless networks, 199
Wisconsin, 171, 179
World Health Organization (WHO), 24, 38, 44
wrists, 32

Y

yeast, 76

Z

zinc, 82, 165